PROFESSOR JENNIE BRAND-MILLER'S
LOWGIDIET
Handbook

OTHER TITLES IN **THE LOW GI DIET** SERIES

We have put together this handy guide to help you make the right choice for further reading or for more recipes.

- **GI basics and getting started**
  Low GI Diet Shopper's Guide 2011

- **Cookbooks**
  The Low GI Diet Cookbook
  The Low GI Vegetarian Cookbook
  The Low GI Family Cookbook

- **Diabetes and pre-diabetes**
  The Diabetes and Pre-diabetes Handbook
  The Low GI Diet for Childhood Diabetes

- **Weight loss**
  Low GI Diet 12-week Weight Loss Plan

- **Fertility and PCOS**
  Low GI Diet for Fertility and PCOS

- **Coeliac disease or gluten intolerance**
  The Low GI Guide to Gluten-free Cooking

PROFESSOR JENNIE BRAND-MILLER'S
LOWGIDIET
Handbook

Prof Jennie Brand-Miller • Kaye Foster-Powell • Prof Stephen Colagiuri

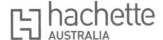

hachette
AUSTRALIA

Although every effort has been made to ensure that the contents of this book are accurate, it must not be treated as a substitute for qualified medical advice. Always consult a qualified medical practitioner. Neither the authors nor the publisher can be held responsible for any loss or claim arising out of the use, or misuse, of the suggestions made or the failure to take medical advice.

The GI values in this book are correct at the time of publication. However, the formulation of commercial foods can change and the GI may change as well. You can rely on foods showing the GI symbol.

 hachette
AUSTRALIA

First published in Australia and New Zealand in 1996 as *The GI Factor*
by Hodder Australia
(an imprint of Hachette Australia Pty Limited)
Level 17, 207 Kent Street, Sydney NSW 2000
www.hachette.com.au

First published as *The GI Factor* in 1996
Revised edition published in 1998
Third edition published as *The New Glucose Revolution* in 2002
Revised and updated fourth edition published as *The Low GI Handbook* in 2008, reprinted in 2010
This revised and updated fifth edition published in 2011

10 9 8 7 6 5 4 3 2

National Library of Australia Cataloguing-in-Publication data

The low GI diet handbook / Prof Jennie-Brand-Miller, Kaye Foster-Powell,
Prof Stephen Colagiuri.
  ISBN: 9780733626449 (pbk.)
  Includes index.
  Dietetics.
  Glycemic index.
  Carbohydrates.
  Food—Carbohydrate content.
  Brand Miller, Jennie, 1952-
613.283

Cover design by Christabella Designs, cover adaptation by Agave Creative
Front cover photograph courtesy Getty Images
Back cover portrait © www.gavinjowitt.com
Interior photograph © 2005 Hachette Australia
Typeset in 12/15pt Bembo by Kirby Jones
Printed in Australia by Griffin Press, Adelaide, an Accredited ISO AS/NZS 4001:2004 Environmental Management Systems printer

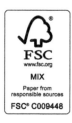

Contents

Preface | The GI story

The concept of the glycemic index was introduced in 1981 by Dr David J. A. Jenkins, now a professor in the Department of Nutritional Sciences at the University of Toronto. Jenkins set out to determine which foods were best for people with diabetes. At the time, the diet most often recommended for people with diabetes was based on a system of carbohydrate exchanges. Each exchange, or portion of food, contained the same amount of carbohydrate. The exchange system assumed that all starchy foods produced the same effect on blood glucose levels – even though some earlier studies had suggested otherwise. Jenkins was one of the first researchers to challenge the use of exchanges and to investigate how individual foods actually affect our blood glucose levels.

Jenkins and his colleagues, including our US co-author Dr Thomas M. S. Wolever, tested a large number of foods that people commonly ate. Their results generated some surprises. First, they found that the starch in foods such as bread, potatoes and many types of rice was digested and absorbed very quickly, not slowly, as had previously been assumed.

Secondly, they found that the sugars in foods such as fruit, chocolate and ice-cream did not produce more rapid or prolonged rises in blood glucose as had always been thought. The truth was that most of the sugars in foods produced quite moderate blood glucose responses, lower than that of many starches.

Because Jenkins's approach was so logical and systematic, yet also contrary to prevailing thinking and recommendations, it attracted an enormous amount of attention from other scientists and medical researchers when the original scientific paper was published in the *American Journal of Clinical Nutrition* in March 1981.

Since that time, nutrition scientists around the world, particularly the authors of this book, have tested the effect of many foods on blood glucose levels, further developing Jenkins's classification of carbohydrates based on what he had termed the glycemic index (GI). Today we know the GI values of about 2000 different items (worldwide) that have been tested in healthy people and people with diabetes. The detailed tables in Part 5 give the GI of many foods you'll find on your supermarket shelves.

What was so revolutionary about the GI?

Before the GI came along, the nature of carbohydrates was described by their chemical structure: *simple* or *complex*. Sugars were simple and starches found in foods like bread and potatoes were complex, only because sugars were small molecules and starches were big ones.

In the early years of nutrition research, scientists had conducted simple experiments on pure solutions of starches and sugars and drawn conclusions about *all foods containing starches and sugars* from the findings. It is important to note, however, that their results did not apply to real foods eaten at realistic meals. For 50 years the findings from these experiments were taught to every medical and biochemistry student as 'fact'. These 'facts', and the assumptions on which they were based, were challenged by the arrival of the GI.

> **Foods with a high GI value contain carbohydrates that cause a dramatic rise in blood glucose levels, while foods with a low GI value contain carbohydrates that have much less of an impact.**

Research on the glycemic index showed that the concept of 'simple' versus 'complex' carbohydrates tells us nothing about how the carbohydrates in food actually affect blood glucose levels in the body. The rise in blood glucose after meals cannot be predicted on the basis of a chemical structure. In other words, the old distinctions that were long made between starchy foods (complex carbohydrates) and sugary foods (simple carbohydrates) have no useful application when it comes to blood glucose levels – and all of the health issues that relate to them.

Summing up, the GI ranks the 'glycemic potency' of the carbohydrates in different foods exactly as they are eaten. Many factors influence whether they will be 'tricklers' or 'gushers'. These findings were revolutionary because they turned assumed knowledge of complex and simple carbohydrates completely upside down.

A growing body of research supports the GI

The GI was a very controversial topic among researchers and health authorities for many years, for a variety of reasons. Initially some criticism was justified. For example, in the early days there was no evidence that the GI values of single foods could influence the resulting blood glucose levels of the entire meals in which they were consumed – or even that low GI foods could bring long-term benefits. There were no studies of the glycemic index's reproducibility, or of the consistency of GI values from one country to another. Many of the early studies used only healthy volunteers rather than those with relevant health conditions. What's more, there was no evidence that the results would improve glucose levels in people with diabetes.

But today, studies from major leading medical institutions and research universities around the world have repeatedly demonstrated that the glycemic index holds up in tests (in scientific terms, it is reproducible) and is a clinically proven tool in its application to weight control, diabetes and coronary health. Studies all around the globe, including the United States, the United Kingdom, France, Italy, Sweden Canada and Australia, have proved the value of the GI. Moreover, diabetes organisations in many countries have endorsed the judicious use of the GI in the dietary management of diabetes.

In 2007, the International Diabetes Federation recommended in their new guidelines for 'Management of Post-meal Glucose' that people with diabetes use the GI to stabilise their blood glucose levels as it 'can provide an additional benefit for diabetes control beyond that of carbohydrate counting'.

Health authorities in the United States have been slower to embrace the GI than many of their counterparts elsewhere in the developed world. This may be the result of a number of factors, including the fact that the earliest research into the GI was conducted outside the United States. In the diabetes realm, the American Diabetes Association (ADA) has for many years endorsed dietary recommendations premised on the idea of carbohydrate counting (which assumes that all starchy foods have the same effect on blood glucose levels).

However, in their 2006 nutrition recommendations for the management of diabetes, the ADA noted, 'The use of the glycemic index/glycemic load may provide a modest additional benefit over that observed when total carbohydrate is considered alone.'

Scientific thinking on the GI has changed to a more positive attitude – as a tool for *everyone*. Several studies have shown that a low GI diet is easier to follow than other diets – meaning you're more likely to stick with it than you would other regimes. In fact, one study from the Royal Children's Hospital Melbourne reported that children and parents found a low GI diet regimen more flexible and family friendly than conventional diets and it 'enhances quality of life in children with [type 1] diabetes'.

The original Low GI Diet bestseller

In 1995, we joined forces to write *The GI Factor*, the first book for the general public about the glycemic index of foods. Research on the glycemic index, or what became known as the GI, clearly showed that different carbohydrate foods had dramatically different effects on blood glucose levels. We believed that it was high time someone brought this story out to the general public. We knew from our own work that understanding the GI of foods made an enormous difference to the diet and lifestyle of people with diabetes. For some it meant, in our experience, a new lease of life.

In the early 1980s Jennie was studying the nutritional composition of Aboriginal bush foods such as acacia seeds and cheeky yam. These foods are unique today because they are uncultivated foods, unlike wheat or potato. Food samples were sent from all over Australia to her laboratory at the University of Sydney for analysis where she took the opportunity to check the metabolic responses they created, that is, how they actually affected blood sugar levels in the body.

The results were telling. Aboriginal bush foods produced only half the blood sugar responses of starchy Western staples like bread and potatoes. So, the question had to be asked: had these traditional foods somehow protected Aborigines from developing diabetes in times past? The answer was yes.

The GI of more than 2000 foods has been tested worldwide, both singly and in combination with mixed meals. Long-term studies on its potential to improve diabetes control have also been carried out. We now know that consuming low GI foods is associated with a lower risk of both type 2 diabetes and coronary heart disease.

Our studies with animal models show that the GI of foods influences the rate at which animals gain body fat and develop abnormalities in insulin secretion. We have also tested the applications of GI for sporting performance and appetite control. It is now obvious, not only to us but to many expert committees and health authorities around the world, that the GI of foods has enormous implications for everybody. It is indeed a 'Glucose Revolution' in that it has changed forever the way we think about carbohydrates.

When this book was first published in 1996, we received a great deal of feedback from readers and health professionals. And still, hardly a day goes by without an email or letter from someone wanting to say thank you and to find out more. The *Low GI Diet Handbook* brings together all the information that we have put together over the years to give readers the most up-to-date and key dietary messages in one package. The *Low GI Diet Handbook* will show you how the GI carbohydrate story fits in with all the other messages about fat, protein, exercise and the many ways you can approach having a healthy diet that suits you and your family's lifestyle, no matter how busy you are. Most importantly the *Low GI Diet Handbook* focuses on individual needs, likes and dislikes and can be adapted to your particular eating habits and food preferences. The *Low GI Diet Handbook* is not about one way of eating a healthy diet – it is about giving you the information to make eating a healthy diet much, much easier.

There's not just one way of eating a healthy diet. What we now know about these different nutritional factors gives us a great deal of flexibility, which is extremely important and helpful in choosing food and food combinations that suit the likes and dislikes of you and your family.

Research conducted by scientists throughout the world has highlighted that the GI has implications for everybody. Research on the GI has changed our understanding of carbohydrates and their effect on our bodies. Included here are some of the latest scientific findings about carbohydrates, blood glucose levels and the GI.

As noted in an interview on Food Ingredients first website: '… while the science of GI can be complex, the consumer application isn't. It's really simple – you swap a high GI food for a low GI food from within food categories – a low GI bread instead of a high GI one, a low GI breakfast cereal for a high GI one. The consumer learnt that there are good fats and bad fats and to swap one for the other. The same applies to carbohydrate.'

Carbohydrates, GI and brain function

Your brain is the hardest working 'muscle' in your body and it never switches off. Of the many nutrients that make up a diet, glucose is the only one that the brain can use. For this, it draws on glucose circulating in the blood. Star-shaped brain cells called astrocytes also store a little glucose in the form of glycogen that acts as a buffer between glucose in the blood and glucose in the fluid nourishing the brain. But after an overnight fast or a long period of mental activity without food, blood glucose levels gradually decline. And they decline more during a period of intense mental effort, such as doing maths versus reading a magazine! When stores of glycogen become limited, your brain benefits greatly from a top-up.

One of the best reasons to include some carbohydrate in every meal is the well-documented effect on mental performance. Studies are showing that intellectual performance, particularly at breakfast time, is improved following the intake of a carbohydrate-rich food. Demanding mental tasks are most improved, while easy tasks are not affected. The improved mental ability following a carbohydrate meal, especially breakfast, has been demonstrated in all types of people – young adults, university students, people with diabetes, the elderly and people with Alzheimer's disease.

Several recent studies suggest that low GI carbohydrates may enhance learning and memory better than high GI carbohydrates. In other words, the type of carbohydrate eaten may be just as important as the quantity, with a low GI breakfast such as traditional oat porridge having a better effect on memory function than a high GI breakfast such as cornflakes. The reason may be related to blood glucose stability and the absence of the 'overshoot' that often accompanies high GI meals. The stress hormone cortisol appears to be involved.

Cortisol's natural function is to prepare the body for fight or flight, with a small amount improving memory, but too much impairs it. Work by Dr Clemens Kirschbaum at the Technical University of Dresden has shown

Did you eat breakfast this morning?

Most of us have been told (countless times) that breakfast is the most important meal of the day. But a lot of us still skip breakfast. Not a good example because alarmingly around 25 per cent of kids are breakfast skippers too. Why? Well, the usual suspects. Too tired. Needed more sleep. Rushed. Not hungry. Don't like breakfast. Dieting. Writing in the *Journal of the American Dietetic Association*, Dr Ruth Striegel-Moore reported that the older a girl gets, the more likely she is to skip breakfast. They found that only 60 per cent of 9-year-old girls regularly ate breakfast, but by age 19 this had plummeted to less than 30 per cent. The diets of the breakfast eaters were consistently higher in calcium and fibre than the skippers and they had a lower body mass index. As it turns out, skipping breakfast is a not such a good idea!

that the consumption of high GI carbohydrates increases the production of cortisol in response to stress. This means there is a trade-off between carbohydrates as brain food and their role as magnifiers of the brain-draining stress response.

Older people with type 2 diabetes have significantly greater risk of performing poorly in cognitive function tests such as recalling word lists. Dr Carol Greenwood at the University of Toronto found that a low GI meal generally results in better verbal memory in the post-meal period, particularly in those who experience the greatest food-induced elevations in blood glucose levels, compared with a high GI meal. She and her colleagues reported their findings of a study involving a group of 20 older adults with type 2 diabetes in the high ranking medical journal *Diabetologia* in 2006. Both the GI of the carbohydrate meal and individual differences in response to the meal contributed to the variation in consequent memory recall. They found that performance following the high GI bread meal was poorer than that following the low GI pasta meal on measures of working memory, executive function and auditory selective attention. Sustained attention showed no sensitivity to the type of carbohydrate food consumed.

In Carbohydrate is brain food in Chapter 3 we discuss what happens when your diet is low in carbohydrate and the brain makes use of ketones, a byproduct of the breakdown of fat.

The GI and dementia

High blood glucose levels are being increasingly linked to dementia, even in its mildest forms. Scientists are already aware that there is a connection between diabetes and cognitive problems. But a four-year study of post-menopausal women found that chronically elevated blood glucose (in technical terms, glycated haemoglobin or HbA1c levels of 7 per cent or higher) was linked with an increased risk of developing mild cognitive impairment.

Dr Kristine Yaffe and her colleagues at the University of California, San Francisco, were interested in the prevalence of mild cognitive impairment in groups of women with and without diabetes. The four-year study looked at 1983 women whose blood glucose levels were tested at the beginning of the study. Over the course of the study, 86 women developed mild cognitive impairment or dementia. For every 1 per cent increase in HbA1c, the women had a greater likelihood of developing mild cognitive impairment or dementia. Women with a HbA1c of 7 per cent or higher were four times more likely to develop mild cognitive impairment or dementia than women who tested at less than 7 per cent. Even when the researchers excluded the women known at the outset to have diabetes, there was still a statistically significant association.

Controlling insulin resistance in middle age may help reduce the risk of dementia in later life. Researchers from the Medical University of South Carolina examined over 7000 healthy adults who were given a series of cognitive tests at the outset and followed up six years later. They reported that those with the highest level of insulinaemia, a condition in which insulin levels in the blood are higher than normal, had significantly greater declines in memory and word tests.

The GI and acne

Most teenagers agonise about their skin, cursing the pimples that appear just before an important social event. Scarring and low self-esteem are sometimes the lifelong products of severe teenage acne. What is not as well known is the fact that many adults also suffer from acne long after they have left adolescence behind. Interestingly, there is an astonishing difference in the incidence of acne in non–Westernised societies. When Dr Staffan Lindeberg from Sweden studied 1200 Papua New Guinea islanders in 1990, he found not a single case of acne, even among the 300 who were aged between 15 and 25 years. The same was true among 115 young Ache hunter-gatherers of Paraguay.

Because acne at any age can be a disfiguring and socially restricting disease, it is understandable that people both young and old are constantly searching for miracle cures. Although diet has been considered in the past as a cause of acne, clinical trials showed no effect in eliminating specific foods, including chocolate, fats, sweets and soft drinks. Dermatologists know that acne results from a combination of three factors:

- overactive sebaceous follicles (oil-producing glands) causing blockages
- increased production of oily sebum, and
- colonisation of the skin follicle with bacteria that generates inflammation.

Consequently, dermatologists and GPs today generally don't make dietary recommendations to their patients with acne. They commonly prescribe hormone-regulating pills, antibiotics and in severe cases Roaccutane™ (a vitamin A analogue). These are effective treatment options but, like all drugs, they have side-effects and they are not for everyone.

A review published in a dermatology journal called *Retinoids* has identified a possible link between diet, high blood insulin levels and acne. Differences in environmental factors rather than genes are thought to explain these findings. When people migrate from a rural to an urban area, or one country to another, increased rates of acne are often noted.

However, Professor Loren Cordain from the University of Colorado suggested that acne may result from the combination of insulin resistance and high insulin levels. His Melbourne colleague Professor Neil Mann has been putting the theory to the test. In the latest of their studies, published in 2006 in the *American Journal of Clinical Nutrition*, they randomly assigned 43 boys to a conventional healthy, low-fat diet or a diet with a lower glycemic load.

A low GI diet will do more for your skin and your waistline than a reduced-fat diet.

To reduce glycemic load, they increased protein intake a little at the expense of carbohydrates, and replaced high GI carbohydrates with low GI ones. After 12 weeks, total lesion counts in the boys on the low glycemic load diet had declined by nearly 25 per cent compared with only 12 per cent in the conventional group. They also reported a little unintended weight loss (around 3 kilograms) and greater improvement in insulin sensitivity in the low GI group.

Further research is needed to say whether it's weight loss or diet composition that makes the difference. But in the meantime, we can be reassured that a low GI diet is going to do more for both your skin and your waistline than the traditional fat-reduced diet.

Low GI for your eyesight's sake

Age-related macular degeneration (AMD) is a devastating disease that affects the central macula of the eye, leaving sufferers with only peripheral vision. The macula is the small yellowish spot in the middle of the retina that provides the greatest visual acuity and colour perception. It's the macula that lets us see fine detail and is critical to central vision helping us to recognise faces, drive a car, read a newspaper, or do close handwork.

Unfortunately, AMD is now one of the most common causes of blindness among older adults in the Western world. As we age, our risk increases: people in their low fifties have only a 2 per cent chance, but it leaps to 30 per cent by age 75. *AMD Alliance International* estimates that 25 to 30 million people are affected worldwide. There's no known cure but there is something you can do.

Just as there are optimum ways of eating for a healthy heart, liver, skin, brain and kidneys, there is one for the eyes. In particular, the red, orange and yellow colours in foods are actually anti-oxidants that belong to a large family of more than 600 carotenoids. Brightly coloured vegetables, dark leafy greens (the yellow colours are hiding there) and egg yolks are rich in these protective compounds. You can eat these vegetables in generous amounts but limit eggs to 5–7 a week because their saturated fat content contributes to other health risks.

Recent studies published in the *American Journal of Clinical Nutrition* suggest that a low GI diet could also be a key part of your AMD prevention plans. Why would that be the case? Well, the retina has among the highest supplies of blood and nutrients, including glucose, and is dependent on adequate glucose delivery from the circulation to maintain its function. Because glucose stores in the retina are negligible and there are no glucose transporters in the cell membrane, it appears that glucose levels in the retina reflect whatever level is found in the blood. High levels spell trouble because excessive uptake produces high reactive charged particles called free radicals that damage all the machinery inside the cell.

Researchers from Tufts and Harvard Universities were the first to notice the link between GI and vision. They had followed 526 women without previous visual problems from the Nurses' Health Study for 10 years. At regular intervals, they assessed the nurses' diets using a food frequency questionnaire. They found that when total carbohydrate intake was constant, consuming a high GI diet was associated with a doubling of the risk of developing AMD.

Similarly, Professor Paul Mitchell, the lead researcher of the Blue Mountains Eye Study in New South Wales, and his colleagues found that a high GI diet, but not a high carbohydrate diet, was linked to an almost 80 per cent higher risk of having age-related macular degeneration within the 10 years of the study. They also found the incidence of cataracts was higher among elderly people who chose a high GI diet.

Although 'observational' data like these cannot establish that the observed association is 'cause-and-effect', they indicate a new direction for further studies.

High GI diets and fatty liver

As the incidence of obesity in adults and children increases, so does a disease of the liver called non-alcoholic fatty liver disease (or NAFL). It is a significant health problem that leaves sufferers feeling tired and unwell. Untreated, the liver cells become inflamed and NAFL turns into non-alcoholic steatohepatitis, or NASH. In time, NASH may develop into cirrhosis of the liver, a life-threatening condition associated with liver failure. The latest figures suggest fatty liver affects 30 per cent of American adults, with Australia and New Zealand probably not far behind, although we don't have detailed statistics.

Although the origins of the disease are still uncertain, it is strongly linked with insulin resistance and relatively common in people with type 2 diabetes. In susceptible people, the cells of the liver have accumulated an excessive amount of fat.

Currently there is no effective treatment other than gradual weight loss, which makes the findings of a new Italian study published in the *American Journal of Clinical Nutrition* timely.

Professor Furio Brighenti and colleagues from the University of Parma in Italy suggest that a low GI diet may help people with NAFL, more so than low carb or high fibre diets, and could be a complementary tool for preventing or treating it. In their study of 247 apparently healthy individuals, the researchers assessed the degree of liver enlargement by ultrasound measurement, as well as their usual diet including the quality and quantity of carbohydrate. They found that the GI of the diet was the best marker for fatty liver – the higher the GI, the greater the prevalence of fatty liver, especially in people with insulin resistance. They found no specific effect of total fibre intake, total carbohydrate intake or glycemic load.

> **Researchers have found that a low GI diet may help people with fatty liver, more so than low carbohydrate or high fibre diets.**

The GI and cancer

There's good evidence from various studies that high blood glucose levels are linked to some types of cancer, too – colon, breast, prostate and ovarian. This is because constant spikes in blood glucose that cause the body to release more insulin also increase a related substance called 'insulin-like growth factor one' (IGF-1). Both these hormones increase cell growth and decrease cell death, and have been shown to increase the risk of developing cancer. Professor Ed Giovannucci at Harvard University was among the first to make the link between insulin levels and cancer growth.

Obesity, particularly abdominal obesity, is a strong predictor of both colorectal cancer and diabetes. Recent reports from the American Cancer Society Cancer Prevention Study and the Iowa Women's Health Study showed an increased risk of colorectal cancer among people with diabetes. Perhaps more importantly, insulin resistance, or factors linked to insulin resistance, have been associated with an increased risk of colorectal cancer.

If insulin resistance and hyperinsulinaemia are risk factors for cancer, and if a high GI or high GL diet increases the risk for insulin resistance, it should follow that such a diet also increases the risk for cancer. Despite the beautiful logic, the scientific findings to date are very mixed.

Some studies support the view that high GI diets increase the risk of cancer. The first study to test the theory found a direct association between dietary glycemic index and colon cancer risk, that is, the higher the GI in the diet, the greater the risk of colorectal cancer. The researchers found that a sedentary lifestyle in conjunction with a high GI diet magnified the risk. Similarly, an Italian study reported that the dietary glycemic index was related to the risk of colorectal cancer among men and breast cancer among women.

As time passes, however, many studies are *not* positive, that is they are finding no relationship between GI or glycemic load and risk of cancer. One reason for the mixed findings could be the lack of validation of the food frequency questionnaires that have been used to assess dietary intake. Some questionnaires are better than others at estimating carbohydrate intake and few of them have been specifically validated to assess the GI. And some studies are smaller and shorter in duration than others.

Dr Alan Barclay from the University of Sydney attempted to make sense of all the conflicting findings by conducting a 'meta-analysis', an analysis that throws all the valid studies together, and 'weighs' better studies more heavily than smaller studies. When all studies were analysed in this way, there were statistically significant relationships between GI and the risk of colorectal cancer, breast cancer, endometrial cancer and all cancers combined. While further studies are necessary, it does no harm to put 'low GI' on your list of cancer prevention strategies.

Sleep and the GI

Tossing and turning at night? You're not alone. Sleep difficulties such as taking a long time to fall asleep, waking up during the night and not falling back easily, and waking too early are increasingly common. According to the Gallup Organisation, nearly 50 per cent of adults do not sleep well on at least five nights per month. Between 10 and 40 per cent say they have intermittent insomnia, and around 15 per cent have long-term sleep difficulties. In Australia, one survey reported that 25 per cent of women had chronic insomnia.

The current treatment options for insomnia are pharmacological (drugs) and cognitive behavioural therapy. Popular remedies used to treat sleep difficulties include prescribed sedatives and tranquillisers, herbal extracts and complementary medicines, massage and relaxation techniques, regular physical activity and avoidance of stimulants such as caffeine before sleeping. Cognitive behavioural therapy of insomina, however, is considered the best practice.

What about food itself? We already know that both the timing of meals and their nutrients can influence your sleep quality. Consuming a meal too close to bedtime, for example, will disturb sleep for reasons that are not entirely clear. Science has shown that nutrients can influence sleep via their effect on levels of the amino acid, tryptophan, a precursor for brain serotonin, a 'feel-good' hormone and sleep–inducing agent.

One factor that promotes the entry of tryptophan into the brain (and therefore serotonin production) is its concentration relative to that of several other amino acids, that is the *tryptophan ratio*. And this is where the GI comes into the picture.

High GI carbohydrates have the ability to increase the *tryptophan ratio* under the direct action of insulin. Thus, a high GI meal might be expected to promote sleep via an increase in brain tryptophan uptake and serotonin production. Paradoxically, the sleep experts believe a meal with a high protein content will reduce serotonin production because it supplies relatively more of the other amino acids, thereby reducing the ratio.

A study led by doctors Chin Moi Chow and Helen O'Connor at the School of Exercise and Sport Science at the University of Sydney tested the theory that a high GI meal might aid sleep. In the setting of a sleep laboratory, 4 hours before bedtime, 12 healthy men aged between 18 and 35 years were given a meal containing 90 per cent of its energy as carbohydrate in the form of either a low GI rice or high GI rice. The researchers found that sleep onset was only 9 minutes after the high GI meal, considerably shorter than the 17 minutes taken to fall asleep after the low GI meal. They also showed that the high GI meal was more effective if it was consumed 4 hours before bedtime rather than 1 hour before. No effects on other sleep variables were observed.

While any natural, safe therapy that improves sleep is good news, much larger, long-term studies are required before we recommend that people with sleep problems start experimenting with high GI meals. Scientists are also exploring the idea that sleepiness and alertness on the job might be affected by the GI of the lunchtime meal. Stay tuned!

Part 1

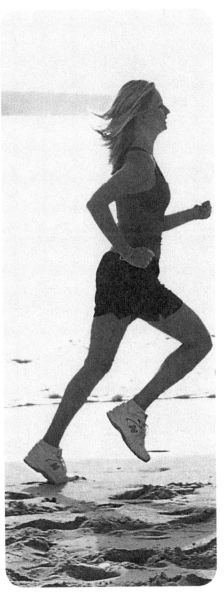

The GI factor

- Understanding the glycemic index
- What's wrong with today's diet?
- Carbohydrate — what it is, why we need it, how we digest it

What are the benefits of a low GI diet?

Knowing the GI values of individual foods is your key to the enormous health benefits of a low GI diet.

Low GI eating has science on its side. It's not a diet. There are no strict rules or regimens to follow. It's essentially about making simple adjustments to your usual eating habits – such as swapping one type of bread or breakfast cereal for another.

You'll find that you can live with it for life.

Low GI eating:

❏ Reduces your insulin levels and helps you burn fat
❏ Lowers your cholesterol levels
❏ Helps control your appetite
❏ Halves your risk of heart disease and diabetes
❏ Is suitable for your whole family
❏ Means you are eating foods closer to the way nature intended
❏ Doesn't defy commonsense!

Not only that. You will feel better and have more energy – and you don't have to deprive or discipline yourself. A low GI diet is easy and has particular benefits for people who are overweight, have diabetes, hypertension, elevated blood fats, heart disease or the metabolic syndrome (Syndrome X).

Understanding the GI of foods helps you choose the right amount of carbohydrate and the right sort of carbohydrate for your longterm health and wellbeing.

Chapter 1

Understanding the glycemic index

Carbohydrate foods are not created equal. In fact, they can behave quite differently in our bodies. The glycemic index, or GI, is a measure of carbohydrate 'potency'. It is a ranking that describes how much the carbohydrates (sugars and starches) in individual foods affect blood glucose levels. It is a physiologically based measure, too – a comparison of carbohydrates based on feeding real foods to real people.

Foods containing carbohydrates that break down quickly during digestion, like those in white bread, have the highest GI values. The blood glucose response is fast and high – in other words, the glucose in the bloodstream increases rapidly. We call them 'fast action carbs', or 'gushers'.

Foods that contain carbohydrates that break down slowly, releasing glucose gradually into the bloodstream like those in legumes, pasta and barley, have low GI values. They can keep you feeling full for longer, help you achieve and maintain a healthy weight and provide you and your brain with more consistent energy throughout the day. They can also have a major effect on the way the body functions and whether or not you develop health problems.

For most people, under most circumstances, foods with low GI values have advantages over those with high GI values. But there are exceptions: some athletes can benefit from high GI foods during and after competition and high GI foods are also useful in the treatment of hypoglycaemia.

The GI explained

The GI is a physiologically based measure of the effect of carbohydrates on blood glucose levels. It provides an easy and delicious way to eat a healthy diet and at the same time control fluctuations in blood glucose. After testing hundreds of foods around the world, scientists have now found that foods with a low GI will have less of an effect on blood glucose levels than foods with a high GI.

❏ Carbohydrates that break down rapidly during digestion, releasing glucose quickly into the bloodstream have a high GI.

❏ Carbohydrates that break down slowly, releasing glucose gradually into the bloodstream, have a low GI.

The rate of carbohydrate digestion has important implications for everybody. For most people, foods with a low GI have advantages over those with a high GI. They can:

❏ Improve blood glucose control

❏ Increase satiety as they are more filling and satisfying and reduce appetite

❏ Facilitate weight loss

❏ Improve blood fat profiles

❏ Reduce risks of developing diabetes, heart disease and certain types of cancer.

A low GI diet helps people:

❑ With type 1 diabetes

❑ With type 2 diabetes

❑ With pre-diabetes (who may have been told they have 'a touch of diabetes' or impaired glucose tolerance)

❑ With gestational diabetes (diabetes during pregnancy)

❑ With hypoglycemia or low blood glucose

❑ Who are overweight or obese

❑ Who are at a normal weight but have too much fat around the middle (abdominal overweight)

❑ With higher than desirable blood glucose levels

❑ With high levels of triglycerides

❑ With low levels of HDL cholesterol ('good' cholesterol)

❑ With metabolic syndrome

❑ With polycystic ovarian syndrome (PCOS) (irregular periods, acne, facial hair)

❑ With non-alcoholic fatty liver (NAFL) disease or non-alcoholic steatohepatitis (NASH)

❑ Who want to delay or prevent age-related vision problems

❑ Who want to prevent all of the above and live a long and healthy life.

How scientists measure a food's GI value

A food's GI value must be measured in people (we call this '*in vivo* testing') according to an internationally standardised method. Currently, about 25 facilities around the world test GI values by following the standard international testing protocol.

You may hear about *in vitro* (test tube) methods, but these are shortcuts that may be useful for manufacturers developing new products, but may not reflect the true GI of a food.

Here's how we test the GI of a food following the protocol set out in the Australian Standard (*Glycemic Index of Foods AS4694-2007*).

Step 1. Ten volunteers consume a 50-gram carbohydrate portion of the reference food on three separate days (e.g. 1 cup of rice). Pure glucose dissolved in water is the usual reference food and its GI is set at 100. The test is carried out in the morning after an overnight fast. The solution is consumed within 10 to 12 minutes, and blood glucose levels are measured eight times over the next two hours (we use capillary testing as it is associated with much less variability than venous testing). The findings from those three days of testing are averaged to find each person's usual response to the reference food, glucose.

Selected GI Research Units

- The University of Sydney's Glycemic Index Research Service (SUGIRS), Sydney, Australia (www.glycemicindex.com)
- Glycaemic Index Otago, University of Otago, New Zealand (www.glycemicindex.otago.ac.nz)
- Glycemic Index Laboratories, Inc., Toronto, Canada (www.gilabs.com)
- Leatherhead Food International, Surrey, UK (www.lfra.co.uk)
- Oxford Brookes University, Oxford, UK (www.brookes.ac.uk/bms/research/nfsg/index.html)
- Hammersmith Food Research Unit, Hammersmith Hospital, London, UK (www.foodresearch.co.uk)
- Reading Scientific Services Limited (RSSL), Reading, UK (www.rssl.com)
- Biofortis, Nantes, France (www.biofortis.fr)
- NutriScience BV, Maastricht, Netherlands (www.nutriscience.nl)
- Oy Foodfiles Ltd., Kuopio, Finland (www.foodfiles.com)

Step 2. Next, we measure his or her glycemic response to a 50-gram portion of the test food (e.g. 1 cup of rice) once, using exactly the same two-hour testing protocol.

Step 3. Then we calculate each person's response to the test food as a percentage of their average response to the reference food. We do this by plotting their blood glucose response to the test food on a graph and comparing this with their response to the reference food; the response can be summarised as the **area under the curve** – the exact value of which is calculated using a computer program (Figure 1).

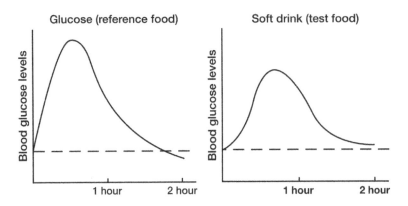

FIGURE 1. Measuring the glycemic index value of a food.

Step 4: Finally, we average the responses of all ten volunteers to the test food and this is the GI value which we publish. If the average test food response area (i.e., the area under the curve) is only 40 per cent of the reference food, then the GI of the test food is 40. Not everyone will give exactly the same number, of course, but the law of averages applies. If we tested them over and over again, people will all tend to congregate around the same number.

Because each person is his or her own control, testing foods in volunteers with diabetes or pre-diabetes gives approximately the same GI values as testing people who don't have diabetes.

In practice, the average result in the group of ten healthy people is the published GI value of the food. *At least* 240 blood glucose assays (the technical term for the test measuring the blood glucose) will have been made to generate that number. In some labs up to 640 assays are made. So there is nothing crude about GI testing.

For example, the GI value of bread (70) means that the overall fluctuation in blood glucose after eating an exchange of white bread will be about 70 per cent of the effect of pure glucose (GI value of 100).

A food's GI value cannot be predicted from its appearance, composition, carbohydrate content, or even the GI values of related foods. The only way to know a food's GI value is to test it, following the standardised methodology we've just described.

Unfortunately, there is no easy, inexpensive substitute test. Now, after nearly 30 years of GI testing, we and others around the world have determined the GI values for more than 2000 foods. The values of foods available in Australia and New Zealand appear in Part 5 of this book, as well as in annually updated editions of *The New Glucose Revolution Shopper's Guide to GI Values* and online at our website: www.glycemicindex.com.

Why is glucose used as the reference food? Pure glucose itself produces one of the greatest effects on blood glucose levels. GI testing has shown that *most* foods have less effect on blood glucose levels than glucose. For that reason, the GI value of pure glucose is set at 100, and every other food is ranked on a scale from 0 to 100 according to its actual effect on blood glucose levels.

(Note: A few foods have GI values of more than 100 – for example, jasmine rice (GI 109). The explanation is simple: glucose is a highly concentrated solution that tends to be held up briefly in the stomach. Jasmine rice, on the other hand, contains starch that leaves the stomach quickly and is then digested in a flash.)

Rice Bubbles® (GI 87) and some types of bread (e.g. white Turkish bread, GI 87) have very high GI values, meaning their effect on blood glucose levels is almost as high as that of an equal amount of pure glucose. See Figure 2.

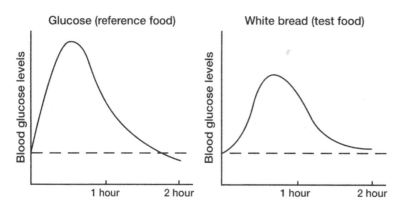

FIGURE 2. The effect of pure glucose (50 grams) and white bread (50-gram carbohydrate portion) on blood glucose levels.

Foods with a low GI value (such as lentils, GI 26–48) show a flatter blood glucose response when eaten, as shown in Figure 3. That means that the resulting peak blood glucose level is lower, and the return to baseline levels may be slower than with a high GI food.

Why do we use the 'area under the curve' in GI calculations? The area under the curve is the best way to take into account *all* the data available to us. It is preferable to taking just one or two points (e.g. the peak). It is reassuring to know, however, that the GI value is a good predictor of the actual peak level, as well as the absolute level of blood glucose at 30 minutes, 60 minutes and 90 minutes. We also know that the higher the GI the bigger the fall (ie from the peak to the trough).

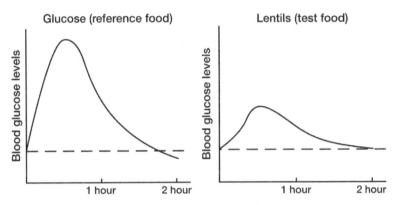

FIGURE 3. The effect of pure glucose (50 grams) and lentils (50-gram carbohydrate portion) on blood glucose levels.

Why low GI foods are a smart choice

For most people, low GI foods have advantages over high GI foods. The slow digestion and gradual increase and decrease in blood glucose responses after eating a low GI food helps control blood glucose levels. This is also particularly beneficial for people with diabetes or glucose intolerance as it reduces the secretion of the hormone insulin. Plus, slower

The only way to know a food's GI value is to test it. The GI cannot be predicted from the food's appearance, composition, carb content or even the GI values of related foods.

digestion helps to delay hunger pangs – meaning you're less likely to overeat or make poor food choices as the result of hunger, which can promote weight loss if you're overweight.

Lower glucose levels over the course of the day also improve heart health. Abnormally high insulin levels resulting from a regular diet of high GI carbs

Common questions

If testing were continued long enough, wouldn't you expect the areas under the curve to become equal, even for very high and very low GI foods?

Many people assume that if the amount of carbohydrate in two foods is the same, then the areas under the curve will ultimately be the same. This isn't the case, though, because the body is not only absorbing glucose from the gut into the bloodstream, but it is also *extracting* glucose from the blood. Just as a garden can utilise a gentle rain better than a sudden deluge, the body can metabolise slowly digested food better than quickly digested carbohydrate. Fast-release carbohydrate causes 'flooding' of the system and the body cannot extract the glucose from the blood fast enough. Just as water levels rise quickly after a torrential rain, so do glucose levels in the blood. But the same amount of rain falling over a longer period can be absorbed into the ground and water levels do not rise.

Why are glucose and white bread used as test foods in GI testing — why not only glucose?

In the past, some scientists used a 50-gram carbohydrate portion of white bread as the reference food, because it was more typical of what we actually eat. On this scale, where the GI value of white bread is set at 100, some foods will have a GI value of over 100, because their effect on blood glucose levels is higher than that of bread.

The use of two standards has caused some confusion, so the glucose = 100 scale is now recommended. It is possible to convert from the bread scale to the glucose scale using the factor 0.7 (70 ÷ 100). This factor is derived from the fact that the GI value of white bread is 70 on the glucose = 100 scale.

To avoid confusion throughout this book, we refer to all foods according to a standard whereby glucose equals 100.

promote high blood fats and high blood pressure, thus increasing the risk of heart attack. Keeping your blood glucose levels stable helps ensure that blood vessels remain elastic and supple, reducing the formation of fatty streaks and plaques that cause atherosclerosis, known more widely as hardening of the arteries. And good blood glucose management means your body is less likely to form blood clots in the arteries, which can precipitate a heart attack. Spikes in blood glucose levels also increase inflammation: a high glucose concentration stresses cells and triggers inflammatory responses.

You don't have to eat only low GI foods to benefit. Studies show that when a low and a high GI food are combined in one meal (for example, lentils and rice), the overall blood glucose response is intermediate. You can keep both your glucose and insulin levels lower over the course of the whole day if you choose at least one low GI food at each meal.

Can the GI be applied to everyday meals?

Criticism of the GI has focused on unpredictable outcomes of blood glucose measurements after meals containing variations in fat, protein and fibre levels. Most of our meals consist of a variety of foods – not just a single food. Even though GI values are derived from testing single foods in isolation, we and other scientists have found that it is possible to predict the blood glucose response for a meal that consists of several foods with different GI values.

Concerned about the methodology of recent studies showing unpredictable responses, we and our co-researchers at the University of Toronto's Department of Nutritional Sciences conducted studies with mixed meals on two groups of healthy subjects in Toronto and Sydney. We had previously done smaller studies, but we wanted to revisit the question, using more meals and variety in two different centres with judiciously selected foods. This time, 14 different test meals were used in Sydney and Toronto, and the food combinations reflected a range of typical breakfast choices.

Despite the variations in nutrient content, blood glucose responses remained consistent with GI measures. In fact, we were startled by the degree of predictability. The carbohydrate, fat and protein composition of the meals varied over a wide spectrum. The glucose responses varied over a fivefold range, and yet 90 per cent of that variation was explained by the amount of carbohydrate in the meal and the GI values of the foods as given in published GI tables. We found that the GI works just as predictably whether subjects consume a single portion of one item or a normal meal; we reported these findings in the *American Journal of Clinical Nutrition*.

How do you estimate the overall GI of a meal?

Over the years, many readers – researchers and dietitians in the nutrition field, as well as laypeople – have asked us to explain how to estimate the total GI of a meal. So for their benefit, and for the more curious among you, we take a moment to walk you through two brief examples.

First of all, the GI value of a meal or recipe is not the sum of the GI values of each food in the meal, nor is it simply an average of their GI values. The GI of a meal, menu or recipe consisting of a variety of carbohydrate foods is a weighted average of the GI values of each food. The weighting is based on the proportion of the total carbohydrate contributed by each food.

To estimate the GI of a mixed meal, you need to know the GI of the carbohydrate foods in the meal (information we provide in the tables in Part 5), plus the total carbohydrate content of the meal and the contribution of each food to the total carbohydrate. You will find this information in food-composition tables or nutrient-analysis computer programs. The following calculations may look complicated – and, in fact, in practice, you don't need to make these sorts of calculations to adopt the low GI way of eating, but dietitians and nutrition researchers sometimes have to.

Let's look at a snack of rockmelon (GI 68) and ice-cream (GI 37–49). Depending on the amounts of each food, we could calculate the total content of these carbohydrates from food-composition tables. Let's say the meal contains 60 grams of carbohydrate, with 20 grams provided by the rockmelon (that is 33 per cent) and 40 grams by the ice-cream (that is 67 per cent). For the purposes of this calculation, we're using low fat vanilla ice-cream (GI 46).

To estimate the GI value of this dish, we multiply the GI value of rockmelon by its proportion of the total carbohydrate:

$$68 \times 33\% = 22$$

and multiply the GI value of ice-cream by its proportion of the total carbohydrate:

$$46 \times 67\% = 31$$

We then add these two figures to give a GI value for this dish of 53.

Here's another scenario for the classic combination of beans and rice. If half the carbohydrate in the mixed meal comes from a food with a GI value of 30 (for example black beans) and the other half from a rice with a GI value of 80, then the mixed meal will have a GI of 55, determined as follows:

$$(50\% \text{ of } 30) + (50\% \text{ of } 80) = 55$$

Our rice and beans example demonstrates that it's not necessary to avoid all high GI foods in order to eat a low GI diet. Nor is it necessary to calculate the GI value for every meal you eat. Rather, simply choose a low GI food in place of a higher GI food. Simply including one low GI food per meal is enough.

We'll share many more helpful dietary suggestions with you throughout the rest of the book – and in Part 3 you will find our guide to low GI eating.

Glycemic index or glycemic load?

Your blood glucose rises and falls when you eat a meal containing carbohydrate. How high and how long it rises on any one occasion depends on two things: how much carbohydrate you eat and the GI of the carbohydrate you eat. The more carbohydrate you eat, the higher your blood glucose goes. The higher the GI of the food you eat, the higher your blood glucose goes. A small amount of a high GI food may raise your blood glucose as much as a large amount of a low GI food.

The glycemic load (GL), initially developed by researchers at Harvard University, takes in the amount of carbohydrate you eat *and* its GI to help predict how much a serving of food will raise blood glucose. If a serving of food has a GL of 10, that means it will raise blood glucose by as much as 10 grams of glucose.

The GL of a food is a mathematical calculation – determined by multiplying the GI of a particular food by the available carbohydrate content (meaning the carbohydrate content minus fibre) in a particular serving size (expressed in grams), divided by 100. The formula is:

$$GL = (GI \times \text{the amount of carbohydrate}) \text{ divided by } 100$$

Let's take a single apple as an example. It has a GI of 38 and it contains 15 grams of carbohydrate.

$$GL = 38 \times 15 \div 100 = 6$$

What about a small serving of French fries? Its GI is 75 and it contains 29 grams of carbohydrate.

$$GL = 75 \times 29 \div 100 = 22$$

So we can predict that our fries (GL 22) will pack nearly four times the glycemic punch of an apple (GL 6).

Proponents of the GL – both within the scientific nutrition community and beyond it – think that this concept should be used instead of the GI when comparing foods because it more fully reflects a food's glycemic potential.

But a word of caution: we don't want people *avoiding* all carbs and striving for a diet with the lowest GL possible.

The problem with GL is that it doesn't distinguish between foods that are low carb (and thus higher in fat and/or protein) or slow carb (that is, low GI carbs). Some people whose diets have an overall lower GL are consuming more saturated fat or protein and fewer carbohydrates of any kind, including healthy, low GI carbs.

Following a low GL path could mean that you're unnecessarily restricting foods, missing out on nutrients and the other proven benefits of a higher carbohydrate diet, and thus eating a less healthful diet – one that's too low in carbohydrates and full of the wrong types of fats and proteins. That's why we advocate sticking with the GI.

Research also shows that by choosing carbs by their GI value – and opting primarily for those that are low GI – you'll get a healthy, safe diet with an appropriate quantity and quality of carbohydrate. In fact, you'll be increasing your intake of nutritional powerhouse foods, including fruits and vegetables, legumes (including beans, chickpeas and lentils) and wholegrains. And by choosing moderate servings of low GI foods, you'll automatically be eating lower GL foods, too – so a low GI diet is a win–win situation, while a low GL diet is a 'mixed bag'.

You can think of GL as the amount of carbohydrate in a food 'adjusted' for its glycemic index.

Yes, a handful of high GI foods, such as watermelon, have a low GL, but we recommend that you don't limit any fruits or vegetables, other than some potatoes (see This for that in Chapter 13).

A word here about portion sizes: some carb-rich foods such as pasta have a low GI but *could* have a high GL if the serving size is very large. Portion sizes do count.

• Use the GI to identify your best carbohydrate choices.
• Keep your portion size in check to limit the overall GL.

What makes a food high or low GI?

For many years now scientists have been studying what gives one food a high GI and another one a low GI. That research has generated a huge amount of information, which can be confusing. The table following summarises the factors that influence the GI value of a food.

The physical state of the starch in a food is by far the most important factor influencing its GI value. This is why technological advances in food processing over the past 200 years have had such a profound effect on the overall GI values of the carbohydrates we eat.

The effect of starch gelatinisation on the GI

The starch in raw food is stored in hard, compact granules that make it difficult to digest. This is why potatoes would probably give you abdominal pain if you ate them raw and why most starchy foods need to be cooked. During cooking, water and heat expand the starch granules to different degrees; some granules actually burst and free the individual starch molecules. (That's what happens when you make gravy by heating flour and water until the starch granules burst and the gravy thickens.)

If most of the starch granules have swollen and burst during cooking, the starch is said to be fully gelatinised. Figure 1 below shows the difference between raw and cooked starch in potatoes.

Factors that influence the GI value of a food

Factor	Mechanism	Examples of food where the effect is seen
Starch gelatinisation	The less gelatinised (swollen) the starch, the slower the rate of digestion.	Al dente spaghetti, oats and biscuits have less gelatinised starch.
Physical entrapment	The fibrous coat around beans and seeds and plant cell walls acts as a physical barrier, slowing down access of enzymes to the starch inside.	Pumpernickel and grainy breads, legumes and barley.
High amylose to amylopectin ratio*	The more amylose a food contains, the less water the starch will absorb and the slower its rate of digestion.	Basmati rice and legumes contain more amylose and less amylopectin.
Particle size	The smaller the particle size, the easier it is for water and enzymes to penetrate.	Finely milled flours have high GI values. Stone-ground flours have larger particles and lower GIs.
Viscosity of fibre	Viscous, soluble fibres increase the viscosity of the intestinal contents, and this slows down the interaction between the starch and the enzymes. Finely milled whole-wheat and rye flours have fast rates of digestion and absorption because the fibre is not viscous.	Rolled oats, beans, lentils, apples, psyllium husks.
Sugar	The digestion of sugar produces only half as many glucose molecules as the same amount of starch (the other half is fructose). The presence of sugar also restricts gelatinisation of the starch by binding water and reducing the amount of 'available' water.	Many biscuits, raisin bread and some breakfast cereals that are high in sugar have relatively low GI values.
Acidity	Acids in foods slow down stomach emptying, thereby slowing the rate at which the starch can be digested.	Vinegar, lemon juice, lime juice, some salad dressings, pickled vegetables, classic sourdough bread.
Fat	Fat slows down the rate of stomach emptying, thereby slowing the digestion of the starch.	Potato chips have a lower GI value than boiled white potatoes.

* Amylose and amylopectin are two different types of starch. Both are found in foods, but the ratio varies.

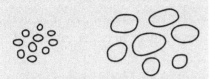

FIGURE 1. The difference between raw (compact granules, left) and cooked (swollen granules, right) starch in potatoes.

The swollen granules and free starch molecules are very easy to digest, because the starch-digesting enzymes in the small intestine have a greater surface area to attack. The quick action of the enzymes results in a rapid blood glucose increase after consumption of the food (remember that starch is nothing more than a string of glucose molecules). As a result, food containing starch that is fully gelatinised will have a very high GI value.

In foods such as biscuits, the presence of sugar and fat and very little water makes starch gelatinisation more difficult, and only about half of the granules will be fully gelatinised. For this reason, biscuits tend to have medium GI values.

The effect of particle size on the GI

The particle size of a food is another factor that influences starch gelatinisation and GI value. Grinding or milling grains reduces particle sizes and makes it easier for water to be absorbed and digestive enzymes to attack the food. This is why many foods made from fine flours tend to have a high GI value. The larger the particle size, the lower the GI value, as Figure 2 illustrates.

When starch is consumed in 'nature's packaging' – whole intact grains that have been softened by soaking and cooking – the food will have a low GI. For example, cooked pearl barley's GI value is 25 and most cooked legumes have a GI of between 30 and 40 whether homecooked or canned.

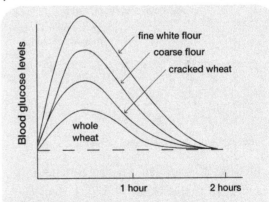

FIGURE 2. The larger the particle size, the lower the GI value.

The effect of amylose and amylopectin on the GI

There are two types of starch in food – amylose and amylopectin. Researchers have discovered that the ratio of one to the other has a powerful effect on a food's GI value.

Amylose is a straight-chain molecule, like a string of beads. These tend to line up in rows and form tight compact clumps that are harder to gelatinise and therefore harder to digest (see Figure 3, below).

Amylopectin, on the other hand, is a string of glucose molecules with lots of branching points, like you'd see in some types of seaweed or a piece of ginger root. Amylopectin molecules are therefore larger and more open, and the starch is easier to gelatinise and to digest. Foods that have little amylose and plenty of amylopectin in their starch have higher GI values – for example, jasmine rice and wheat flour.

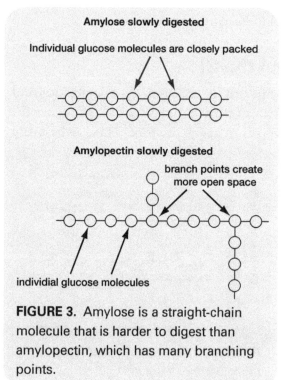

FIGURE 3. Amylose is a straight-chain molecule that is harder to digest than amylopectin, which has many branching points.

Foods with a higher ratio of amylose to amylopectin have lower GI values – for example, basmati rice and legumes.

The only whole (intact) grain food with a high GI is low-amylose rice, such as jasmine (GI 89). Low-amylose varieties of rice have starch that is very easily gelatinised during cooking and therefore easily broken down by digestive enzymes. This may help explain why we sometimes feel hungry not long after rice-based meals. However, some varieties of rice (basmati and long-grain white rice) have lower GI values, because they have a higher amylose content than normal rice. Their GI values are in the range of 50–59.

The effect of sugar on the GI

Table sugar or refined sugar (sucrose) has a GI of between 60 and 65. The reason: table sugar is a disaccharide (double sugar), composed of one glucose molecule coupled

Why does pasta have a low GI value?

Somewhat surprisingly, pasta in any shape or form has a relatively low GI value (30–60). Great news for pasta lovers, but portion size is still important. Keep it moderate to keep the GL (glycemic load) moderate. In the early days of GI research, we assumed that pasta has a low GI value because the main ingredient was semolina (durum or hard wheat flour), and not finely ground wheat flour.

Subsequent research has shown, however, that even pasta made entirely from plain wheat flour has a low GI value. The reason for the slow digestion rate and subsequent low GI value is the physical entrapment of the ungelatinised starch granules in a sponge-like network of protein (gluten) molecules in the pasta dough. Pasta and noodles too are unique in this regard.

Overcooked pasta is very soft and swollen in size and will have a higher GI value than pasta cooked al dente. Adding egg to the dough lowers the GI further by increasing the protein content. Asian noodles such as hokkien, udon, and rice vermicelli also have low to medium GI values.

with one fructose molecule. (See The GI Story for a fuller explanation of the structure of sugars.) Fructose is absorbed and taken directly to the liver, where it is immediately oxidised (burned as the source of energy). The blood glucose response to pure fructose is very modest (GI 19). Consequently, when we consume sucrose, only half of what we've eaten is actually glucose; the other half is fructose. This explains why the blood glucose response to 50 grams of sucrose is approximately half that of 50 grams of corn syrup or maltodextrin – where the molecules are all glucose ones.

Many foods containing large amounts of refined sugar (sucrose) have a GI close to 60. This is the average of glucose (GI 100) and fructose (GI 19). It's lower than that of ordinary white bread, with a GI value averaging around 70. Kellogg's Coco Pops, which contains 39 per cent sugar, has a GI value of 77, lower than that of Rice Bubbles (GI 87), which contains little sugar.

Most foods containing simple sugars do not raise blood glucose levels any more than most complex starchy foods like bread. This is one of the key findings of the GI, and it has 'liberalised' the management of diabetes.

The sugars that naturally occur in food include lactose, sucrose, glucose and fructose in variable proportions, depending on the food. On theoretical grounds, it is difficult to predict the overall blood glucose response to a food,

One of the spin-offs from research on the GI is the recognition that both sugary and starchy foods can raise your blood glucose.

because stomach emptying is slowed by increasing the concentration of the sugars. Some fruits, for example, have a low GI value (grapefruit's GI is 25), while others are relatively high (watermelon's is 76). The higher the acidity of the fruit, the lower the GI value. Consequently, it is not possible to lump all fruits together and say they will have a low GI value, because they are high in fibre. They are not all equal. (For a comparison of all fruits, take a look at the fruit section of the table in Part 4.)

Many foods containing sugars are a mixture of refined and naturally occurring sugars – sweetened yoghurt, for example. Their overall effect on blood glucose response is difficult to predict. This is why we've tested individual foods to determine their GI values rather than guessing or making generalisations about entire food groups.

The effect of fibre on the GI

The effect of fibre on a food's GI value depends on the type of fibre and its viscosity or thickness.

Dietary fibre comes from plant foods – it is found in the outer bran layers of grains (corn, oats, wheat and rice, and in foods containing these grains), fruits and vegetables and nuts and legumes (dried beans, peas and lentils). There are two types – soluble and insoluble – and there is a difference.

Soluble fibres are the gel, gum and often jellylike components of apples, oats and legumes. Psyllium, found in some breakfast cereals and dietary fibre supplements such as Metamucil®, is soluble fibre. These viscous fibres thicken the mixture of food entering the digestive tract. By slowing down the time it takes for the fibre to pass through the stomach and small intestine, foods with high levels of soluble or viscous fibre lower the glycemic response to, or glycemic impact of food, which is why legumes, oats and psyllium have a low GI.

Insoluble fibres are dry and branlike and commonly thought of as roughage. All cereal grains and products made from them that retain the outer layer of the grain

The GI was never meant to be used in isolation

At first glance you might assume that some indulgence foods such as chocolate, seem a good choice simply because they have a low GI value. Fat chance! This is absolutely not the case.

A food's GI value was never meant to offer the only criterion by which it is judged. Large amounts of fat (and protein) in food tend to slow the rate of stomach emptying and therefore the rate at which foods are digested in the small intestine. High fat foods will tend to have lower GI values than their low fat equivalents. For example, potato chips have a lower GI value (54) than potatoes baked without fat (77). Many biscuits have a lower GI value (55–65) than bread (70).

But clearly, in these instances, a lower GI value doesn't translate into a better, healthier choice. Saturated and trans fat in these foods will have adverse effects on coronary health that are far more significant than the benefit of lower blood glucose levels. These foods should be treated as indulgences, for special occasions, rather than as part of a regular diet.

We are not recommending that you avoid all fats. Just as there are differences in the nature of carbohydrates in foods (what we refer to as the quality, conveyed as the GI value), there are differences in the quality of fats. You should be just as choosy about the fats you eat as you are about carbohydrates.

Healthy fats, such as the omega-3 and omega-6 polyunsaturated fats, are not only good for you, but they also help to lower the blood glucose response to meals. On the other hand, many saturated fats increase your risk of obesity, heart disease and other serious health conditions.

are sources of insoluble fibre (for example wholegrain bread and All–Bran), but not all foods containing insoluble fibre are low GI.

Insoluble fibres will only lower the GI of a food when they exist in their original, intact form – for example, in whole grains of wheat. Here they act as a physical barrier, delaying access of digestive enzymes and water to the starch within the cereal grain. Finely ground wheat fibre, such as in wholemeal bread, has no effect whatsoever on the rate of starch digestion and subsequent blood glucose response. Breakfast cereals made with wheat flakes will also tend to have high GI values unless there are other ingredients in the food that will lower the GI.

The effect of acid on the GI

Several research findings over the last decade have indicated that a realistic amount of vinegar or lemon juice as a salad dressing eaten with a mixed meal has significant blood glucose-lowering effects.

As little as 1 tablespoon of vinegar in a vinaigrette dressing (with 2 teaspoons oil) taken with an average meal lowered blood glucose by as much as 30 per cent. Our research shows that lemon juice is just as powerful. Vinegar or lemon juice may also be used in marinades or sauces.

These findings have important implications for people with diabetes or who are at risk for diabetes, coronary heart disease, or the metabolic syndrome (see The GI and your heart in Chapter 9).

The effect appears to be related to the acidity, because some other organic acids (like lactic acid and propionic acid) also have a blood glucose-lowering effect, but the degree of reduction varies with the type of acid.

Real sourdough breads made the traditional way, in which lactic acid and propionic acid are produced by the natural fermentation of starch and sugars by the bacterial starter culture, also can reduce levels of blood glucose and insulin by up to 25 per cent compared to normal bread.

In addition, studies show that there's higher satiety – that is, people feel fuller and more satisfied – associated with breads that have decreased rates of digestion and absorption, like sourdough. There's significant potential to lower your blood glucose and insulin and increase satiety with sourdough breads, so incorporating them into your diet is a smart choice. (We discuss the concept of satiety more fully in The GI and your weight in Chapter 4.)

Low GI basics

Blood glucose is the amount of glucose, or sugar, in your blood. It changes throughout the day depending on what you eat, and it can have a profound effect on your health – your mood, how hungry you are, and whether you develop conditions such as diabetes.

- Your body's blood glucose response to a meal is primarily determined by the meal's carbohydrate content. Both the quantity and the quality of carbohydrates in food influence the rise in blood glucose that you experience.
- Carbohydrates that break down quickly during digestion have high GI values. Their blood glucose response is fast and high.
- Carbohydrates that break down slowly, releasing glucose gradually into the bloodstream, have low GI values. In comparison to foods with high GI values, these are more desirable for optimal health.
- Avoiding carbohydrate foods altogether is counterproductive. You will end up eating harmful foods and fats, and you'll miss favourite foods such as fruit, bread, and pasta.

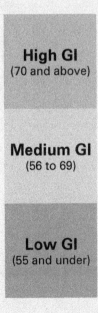

High GI
(70 and above)

Medium GI
(56 to 69)

Low GI
(55 and under)

Chapter 2

What's wrong with today's diet?

You may be wondering, 'What's wrong with the way I eat now?' It's possible that you already follow a balanced, nutrient-dense diet that emphasises whole foods and low GI carbs. But the simple truth is that the majority of Australians and New Zealanders do not; our lifestyle makes it all too easy to stray from a healthful regime. That's why it's so important to have a concrete, working knowledge of how to eat for optimum well-being.

We didn't always eat the way we do today. During the Paleolithic (Stone) Age, humans were hunter-gatherers, consuming the animals and plants found in their natural environment. Our ancestors were fussy about which parts of animals they ate. They preferred the hind legs of the largest animals and the females over the males because they contained more fat and were therefore juicier and more flavourful. They also enjoyed organ meats – liver, kidneys, brains – foods that are extremely rich sources of nutrients.

As humans evolved over time, they became more and more carnivorous. From the latest studies of modern hunter-gatherer diets, it appears that our ancestors obtained about two-thirds of their energy intake from animal foods (including fish and seafood) and only one-third from plant foods. Although they ate more protein and less carbohydrate than we do now, their fat intake, interestingly, was roughly the same as now – but the type of fat was primarily healthy unsaturated fat rather than unhealthy saturated fat (which we'll discuss shortly). This is because the fat of wild animals, including their organs, has much higher proportions of unsaturated fat than typically found in the farmed animals we consume today.

Our predecessors' carbohydrate intakes were lower, because the main plant foods they had available were fruits and vegetables rather than cereals. Wheat, rice and other cereal grains were largely absent until after the introduction of agriculture and the domestication of crops and animals (sometimes called the Neolithic revolution), which began some 10000 years ago.

So why does this matter to you? Because these findings have important implications for current dietary recommendations. Although our ancestors ate plenty of animal foods, they also ate large amounts of micronutrient-rich plant foods (leaves, berries, nuts), which would have been gathered every day, ensuring that their overall diet was both naturally low GI and low GL. It doesn't mean that we all need to be meat-eaters to be healthy, but it does imply that we need to consider carefully the types and amount of protein, carbohydrate and fat we eat.

Beginning about 10000 years ago, when we became farmers growing crops rather than hunter-gatherers, our diet changed in many ways. Starch entered the human diet, in a big way, for the first time; large quantities of harvested cereal grains tipped the human diet ratio from being more animal to more plant. Those plants were what we would now call wholegrain cereals (wheat, rye, barley, oats, corn and rice). The cultivation of legumes (beans), starchy roots and tubers and fruits and berries also contributed to the now higher carbohydrate intake of our farmer ancestors.

But food preparation was simple: grinding food between stones and cooking it over the heat of an open fire. The result was that although we were eating a high carbohydrate diet, all the carbohydrates in our food were digested and absorbed slowly; thus, the effects of these carbohydrate foods on our blood glucose were minimal.

This diet was ideal because it provided slow-release energy that helped to delay hunger pangs and provided fuel for working muscles long after a meal had been eaten. It was also easy on the insulin-producing cells in the pancreas. As far as we can tell, diabetes was rare.

Over time our ancestors developed the technology to grind flours more and

> **One of the most important ways in which our diet differs from that of our ancestors is the speed of carbohydrate digestion and the resulting effect on our blood glucose and hence every cell of the body.**

more finely, and to separate bran completely from white flour. Finally, with the advent of high-speed roller mills in the nineteenth century, it was possible to produce white flour so fine that it resembled talcum powder in appearance and texture. These fine white flours were — and are — highly prized because they make soft bread and delicious, airy cakes and flaky pastries.

As incomes grew, the foods commonly eaten by our ancestors — barley, oats and legumes — were cast aside; consumption of fatty processed meat increased. The composition of the average diet changed again. We began to eat more saturated fat, less fibre and more easily digested carbohydrates.

Then something we didn't expect happened, too — blood glucose rises after a meal became higher and more prolonged, stimulating the pancreas to produce more insulin.

As a result of these developments, we not only experienced higher blood glucose spikes after a meal, but we also experienced greater insulin secretion. As we've mentioned, our bodies require insulin to metabolise carbohydrate, but too much or too little spells trouble. Researchers believe that excessively high glucose and insulin levels are among the key factors responsible for heart disease and hypertension. And because insulin also influences the way we metabolise foods, it ultimately determines fat storage around the body.

Among the consequences of these major dietary changes, one is crucial for our discussion here: traditional diets all around the world contained slowly digested and absorbed carbohydrate — foods that we now know are low GI. On the other hand, our modern diet, with its rapidly digested carbohydrates, is based on high GI foods.

What we eat now

Today's Western diet is the product of industrialisation and many amazing inventions — pasteurisation, sterilisation, refrigeration, freezing, roller drying and spray drying, to name just a few. In the cereal-foods world, there's also high-speed roller milling, flaking, toasting, high-temperature and high-pressure extrusion, puffing guns, short-time bread fermentation — you name it, it's been invented.

Traditional diets all around the world contained slowly digested and absorbed carbohydrates.

Insulin plays critical roles in our health and well-being

One important function of the pancreas, a vital organ near the stomach, is to produce the hormone insulin. Insulin plays several critical roles in our health and well-being.

First, it regulates our blood glucose levels. When you eat a meal containing carbohydrate, your blood glucose level rises. This causes the pancreas to secrete insulin (unless you have type 1 diabetes), which pushes the glucose out of the bloodstream and into the muscles and tissues, where it provides engery for you to carry out your regular activities. The movement of glucose out of the blood and into the body's cells (particularly the muscles and liver) is finely controlled. Just the right amount of insulin takes the glucose level back to normal.

Second, insulin plays a key part in determining the fuel mix that we burn from minute to minute – and whether we burn fat or carbohydrates to meet our energy needs. It does this by switching muscle cells from fat-burning to carb-burning. The relative proportions of fat to carbohydrate in your body's fuel mix are dictated by the prevailing levels of insulin in your blood. If insulin levels are low, as they are when you wake up in the morning, then the fuel you burn is mainly fat. If insulin levels are high, as they are after you consume a high carbohydrate meal, then the fuel you burn is mainly carbohydrate.

Carbohydrates stimulate the secretion of insulin more than any other component of food. When carbohydrates are slowly absorbed by our bodies – which is the case with low GI foods – the pancreas doesn't have to work as hard and secretes less insulin. If it is overstimulated over a long period of time, which often occurs as a result of a diet rich in high GI foods, it may become 'exhausted'. Type 2 diabetes may develop in someone who is genetically susceptible and whose pancreas has been overworked. Even without diabetes, excessively high insulin levels incease the risk of heart disease in everyone.

The benefits are many: we have a plentiful, affordable, palatable (some would say too palatable) and safe food supply. Gone are the days of monotonous meals, food shortages, weevil-infested and otherwise spoiled food. Also long gone are such widespread vitamin deficiencies as scurvy and pellagra. Today's food manufacturers develop and sell delicious and safe products that satisfy just about everyone.

Many of today's low-cost foods are still based on our cereal staples – wheat, corn and oats – but the original grain has been drastically altered to produce more palatable breads, cakes, biscuits, crackers, pastries, breakfast cereals and snack foods that bear no resemblance to the original food.

Our busy lives have also driven the need for convenience food that take little time to prepare. Pre-cooked oats, rice and wheat products are now a common sight on supermarket shelves.

While these developments are easy on our time and tastebuds, people's health is being affected. Our bodies quickly digest and absorb many of the carbohydrate foods we consume the most – think cornflakes, white bread, quick-cooking rice. The resulting effect on blood glucose levels has created a problem of epidemic proportions.

With a wave of the fat wand

We've placed quite a bit of emphasis on carbohydrates, but our health is also affected by another key component in food, which often goes hand-in-hand with carbohydrates: fat.

Food manufacturers, bakers and chefs know we love to eat fat. We love its creaminess and feel in the mouth and find it easy to consume in excess. Fat makes meat more tender, vegetables and salads more palatable, and sweet foods even more desirable. And fat makes numerous carbohydrates even tastier: with a wave of the fat wand, bland high carbohydrate foods such as rice, potatoes and wheat are magically transformed into highly palatable, energy-dense foods such as fried rice, French fries and croissants. In fact, when you analyse it, much of our diet today is an undesirable but delicious combination of fat and high GI carbohydrates.

One problem with fat is the amount we eat, sometimes without knowing it. Fat provides a lot of kilojoules – more than any other nutrient per gram – and it is the least satiating nutrient. This is great for someone who's starving, but it's a real disadvantage for those of us who constantly verge on eating too much. Fat provides 37 kilojoules per gram – more than twice the energy of protein or carbohydrate. And the main form in which our bodies store those extra kilojoules is, you guessed it, fat.

Whatever the fat content of your diet, the type of fat you eat matters — monounsaturated fats, found in nuts, seeds, olive oil, avocado, etc., should dominate. Eating more fat from these sources gives you a nutritional profile more like a Mediterranean diet, which will also help you lower your triglyceride levels and increase your HDL (good) cholesterol.

For the past 25 years, health authorities have wanted people to reduce the amount of saturated fat they eat. Unfortunately, *all* fats have been lumped together as bad

Choosing the good fats and giving bad fats the flick

Emphasise the following mono- and polyunsaturated fats in your diet:

- olive and canola oils
- mustard seed oil
- margarines and spreads made with canola, sunflower or other seed oils
- avocados
- fish, shellfish, prawns, scallops, etc.
- walnuts, almonds, cashews, etc.
- olives
- muesli (not toasted)
- linseeds

Minimise saturated fats and oils including:

- fatty meats and meat products – e.g. sausages, salami
- full-fat dairy products – milk, cream, cheese, ice-cream, yoghurt
- coconut and palm oils
- potato chips, packaged snacks
- cakes, biscuits, slices, pastries, pies, pizza
- deep-fried foods – fried chicken, chips, Chiko rolls, spring rolls

A word of warning

Some high-fat foods – chocolate, nuts, sausages, pizza, potato chips and ice-cream – have low GI values. When you are choosing low GI foods, you're after low GI carbs, not high-fat foods. But they are high in saturated fat and energy-dense and are easy to over-consume. Treat yourself to these indulgences in small amounts at regular times. Avoiding them completely takes too much discipline!

Eat well, move more

One of the golden rules is to accumulate 60 minutes of physical activity every day, including incidental activity and planned exercise. This will help you control your weight for a whole host of reasons. To make a real difference to your health and energy levels, exercise has to be regular and some of it needs to be aerobic. But every little bit counts – and, best of all, any extra exercise you do is a step in the right direction.

Though some people can make a serious commitment to 30-plus minutes of planned exercise three or four times a week, most of us have a long list of excuses. We're too busy, too tired, too rushed, too stressed, too hot, too cold to go to the gym or take a walk or do a regular exercise routine. But there's good news. Research tells us that the kilojoules we burn in our everyday activities are important too, and that any amount of movement is better than none at all.

– the message 'reduce fat' was easier to give than 'reduce saturated fat'. Today, we know that this simplified message was counterproductive. People have avoided even the most essential of fats, the highly polyunsaturated, long-chain fats such as omega–3s that are fundamental to human health. Dietitians restricted fat because of its high energy content and tendency to be overeaten – only to replace it with large quantities of high GI carbs that have adverse effects of their own. We fooled ourselves into thinking that *any* low-fat diet – especially one formulated with the help of a sophisticated food industry – was automatically a healthy diet. But it's not.

A healthy weight is not about dieting

We need to balance our food intake with the rate our bodies use it – that is, to eat the amount of kilojoules from food that our bodies need. Consuming more kilojoules than we use is a cause for gaining weight and experiencing health problems. That balance, as many of us know, is difficult to achieve.

Why? It's extremely easy to overeat in our modern world. Refined foods, convenience foods and fast foods are often soft and delicious (well, to many of us!) and tend to lack fibre and chewiness; as a result, we often overdose on kilojoules long before we realise we're full.

It's even easier not to exercise; it takes longer to walk somewhere than it does to drive, and our schedules are often so full that making time for physical activity seems impossible. That means we burn even fewer kilojoules than we should, even as we're eating more. Our appetite meter no longer works properly and the more we try to ignore hunger, the more we end up over-eating. The result: our kilojoule intake exceeds our energy needs on a regular basis, and we gain weight.

Despite what many would have you believe, the answer to maintaining a healthy weight is not about 'dieting' – reducing your food intake to a low level that matches a low level of energy expenditure. Nutritionists and public health experts are beginning to appreciate that a healthy diet comes in many different forms that may differ greatly in terms of proportions of fat, protein and carbohydrate. As a result, finding a solution that works for you has never been easier or more viable. Aim to choose nutritious foods that suit your lifestyle and cultural and ethnic origins, as these are the ones you are most likely to stick with for life.

Combining a healthy, flexible diet you can live with long-term with an active lifestyle is the best way to stay healthy and fit. That doesn't mean spending an hour at the gym six days a week. It means grabbing the opportunity for physical activity wherever you can. It means using the stairs instead of lifts and escalators, taking in the sun at lunchtime, using a treadmill while you watch the news, reading on an exercise bike, working in the garden, walking to school, parking a little extra distance from the office, or taking the dog for a walk each day. Be creative with whatever works for you, just *do it*. Even housework burns kilojoules. Small bursts of activity accumulate to increase fat burning. You don't have to take exercise too strenuously – just do it regularly in a way you enjoy.

There are two fundamental principles to eating well: the carbohydrates are slow-release and the fat is relatively unsaturated (even when the intake is high). But no diet plan will work in the long term if it eliminates your favourite foods, whether these are bread or potatoes, ice-cream or chocolate. We will show you how you can eat a balanced and healthy diet – one tailored to *your* tastes and *your* needs – without feeling deprived. Part 3, Your Guide to a Low GI Diet for Life, is an easy way to make the switch to low GI eating for lifelong health and well-being.

Common questions

Isn't the insulin response more important than the GI value?
Wouldn't it be better to have an insulin index of foods?

The insulin demand exerted by foods is indeed important for long-term health, but it doesn't necessarily follow that we need an insulin index of foods instead of a glycemic index. When they have been tested together, the glycemic index is extremely good at predicting a food's insulin index. (In other words, a low GI food has a low insulin index value and a high GI food has a high insulin index value.) There are some instances, however, in which a food has a low GI but a high insulin index value. This applies to dairy foods and to some highly palatable, energy-dense 'indulgence foods'. Some foods (such as meat, fish and eggs) that contain no carbohydrate, just protein and fat (and have a GI of essentially zero), still stimulate significant increases in blood insulin.

We don't currently know how to interpret a low GI-high insulin response for long-term health. It may be a good outcome, because the increase in insulin has contributed to the low level of glycaemia. On the other hand, it may be less than ideal, because the increased demand for insulin contributes to beta-cell 'exhaustion' and the development of type 2 diabetes. Until studies are carried out to answer these types of questions, the glycemic index remains the best dietary tool for predicting the effects of carbohydrates on health.

Chapter 3

Carbohydrate
– what it is, why we need it, how we digest it

Besides water, carbohydrate is the most widely consumed substance in the world. One of three main macronutrients (protein and fat are the other two), carbohydrate is the main source of energy found in plants – including fruit, vegetables, cereals and grains. There is virtually none in animal foods apart from dairy foods. The simplest form of carbohydrate is glucose, which is:

- a universal fuel for most organs and tissues in our bodies
- the primary fuel source for our brain, red blood cells and a growing foetus, and
- the main source of energy for our muscles during strenuous exercise.

Some plant foods contain large amounts of carbohydrate (rice, corn and potato, for instance), while others, such as beans, broccoli and carrots, have much smaller amounts of carbohydrate. Breast milk, cow's milk and milk products (but not cheese) contain carbohydrate in the form of milk sugar or lactose.

Just as a car runs on petrol, your body uses fuel (the food you eat). The fuel your body burns comes from a mixture of the macronutrients – protein, fat, carbohydrates and alcohol – that you consume. If you want to function well, be healthy and feel your best, you need to fill your fuel tank – your body – with the right amount and the right kind of fuel every day.

Your body burns the macronutrients in a specific order. Because your body has no place to store unused alcohol, it tops the list. Excess protein comes second, followed by carbohydrate; fat comes in last. Your body's fuel is usually a mix – a combination of carbohydrate and fat, in varying proportions. After meals, it's predominantly carbohydrate and between meals, it's mainly fat.

Your body's ability to burn all the fat you eat is the key to weight control. If fat burning is inhibited, fat stores gradually accumulate. Because of this, the relative proportions of fat to carbohydrate in your body's fuel mix are critical.

What is carbohydrate?

Carbohydrate is a part of food. Starch is a carbohydrate; so, too, are sugars and nearly all dietary fibre. Starches and sugars are nature's reserves created by energy from the sun, carbon dioxide and water.

The simplest form of carbohydrate is a single-sugar molecule called a **monosaccharide** (*mono* meaning one, saccharide meaning sweet). **Glucose** is a monosaccharide that occurs in food (as glucose itself and as the building block of starch) and is the most common source of fuel for the cells of the human body. **Fructose** and **galactose** are also monosaccharides.

If two monosaccharides are joined together, the result is a **disaccharide** (*di* meaning two). **Sucrose**, or common table sugar, is a disaccharide, as is **lactose**, the sugar in milk, and **maltose**. As the number of monosaccharides in the chain increases, the carbohydrate becomes less sweet. Maltodextrins are **oligosaccharides** (*oligo* meaning a few). They taste only a little sweet and are commonly used as a food ingredient.

Starches are long chains of sugar molecules joined together like the beads in a string of pearls. They are called **polysaccharides** (*poly* meaning many). Starches are not sweet-tasting at all.

Dietary fibres are large carbohydrate molecules containing many sorts of monosaccharides. They are different from starches and sugars because they are not broken down by human digestive enzymes. Dietary fibre is not digested in the small intestine; it reaches the large intestine without changing its form. Once there, bacteria begin to ferment and break it down. Different fibres have different physical and chemical properties. **Soluble fibres** are those that can be dissolved in water; some soluble fibres are very thick and therefore slow the speed of digestion. **Insoluble fibres**, such as cellulose, are not soluble in water and do not directly affect the speed of digestion.

The sources of carbohydrate

The carbohydrate in our diet come primarily from plant foods – cereal grains, fruits, vegetables and legumes (dried beans, chickpeas and lentils). Milk and foods made from milk (yoghurt and ice-cream, for example) also contain carbohydrate in the form of milk sugar, or lactose. Lactose is the first carbohydrate we encounter as infants; human milk contains more lactose than the milk of any other mammal, and it accounts for nearly half the energy that an infant will use.

Foods that are high in carbohydrate include:

- **Cereal grains:** rice, wheat, maize (corn), oats, barley, rye and anything made from them – bread, pasta, noodles, flour, breakfast cereal
- **Fruits:** apples, bananas, grapes, apricots, peaches, plums, cherries, pears, mango, kiwifruit
- **Starchy vegetables:** potatoes, sweet potatoes, sweet corn, yams
- **Legumes:** all dried beans (kidney, black, cannellini), lentils, chickpeas, split peas
- **Dairy products:** milk, yoghurt, ice–cream

Turning food into fuel

To be able to use the carbohydrate in foods, your body has to break it down into a form that it can absorb and the cells can use; that process is digestion. An example of how your body does this can be seen in the process of eating and digesting a piece of bread.

1. When you chew the bread, it combines with saliva. Amylase, an enzyme in saliva, starts the process of chopping up the long-chain starch molecules into smaller-chain ones, such as maltose and maltodextrins (see What is carbohydrate in this chapter).
2. When you swallow the bread, it lands in your stomach; there it gets pummelled and churned, much like clothes in a washing machine. The stomach's job is to deliver its load, bit by bit, to the small intestine. If the bread has viscous fibres in it (such as oats and flax) or is acidic (like sourdough), mixing takes longer and the stomach empties more slowly.
3. Once the bread is in your small intestine, an avalanche of digestive juices does the majority of the work involved in digestion. Starch is broken down into smaller and smaller chains of glucose. Many starches are rapidly digested, while others are more resistant, and thus the process is slower. The starch inside any whole kernels in the bread will be protected from attack and take longer to be broken down to glucose.

If the mixture of food and enzymes is highly viscous or sticky, owing to the presence of viscous fibre, mixing slows down, and the enzymes and starch take longer to make contact. The products of starch digestion will also take longer to move toward the wall of the intestine, where the last steps in digestion take place.

4. At the intestinal wall, the short-chain starch products, together with the sugars in foods, are broken down by specific enzymes. The monosaccharides that finally result from starch and sugar digestion include glucose, fructose and galactose. These are absorbed from the small intestine into the bloodstream, where they are available to the cells as a source of energy.

5. Within minutes of eating, glucose appears in the bloodstream. The rate at which it appears (either in a big gush or a little trickle), is determined by the rate of digestion, as well as the rate at which food is emptied from the stomach. Together, these factors influence the GI of the food.

Taste test

Try this simple test for yourself. Take a bite of fluffy white bread and keep it in your mouth for 2 minutes. What's left? Virtually nothing – the enzymes in your mouth have made short work of it. Now take a cooked (al dente) pasta shell (or other shape) and hold it in your mouth. After 2 minutes, you'll find you still have a clearly defined piece of pasta left. That's because the carbohydrates in the pasta are resistant to enzyme action. So it is with all the starches in low GI foods.

Carbohydrate is brain food

Carbohydrate (glucose) is your brain's primary fuel source. If you are starving or deliberately avoiding carbs, under some circumstances the brain will make up the shortfall by burning compounds called 'ketones'.

Your brain is the most energy-demanding organ in your body, responsible for about one-quarter of your obligatory energy requirements that keep your body functioning. Unlike muscle cells, which can burn either fat or carbohydrate, the brain does not have the metabolic machinery to burn fat. If you fast for 24 hours, or decide not to eat carbohydrates, your brain will initially rely on small stores of carbohydrate in your liver; but within hours, these are depleted, and the liver begins synthesising glucose from non-carbohydrate sources, including your muscle tissue. It has only a limited ability to do this, however, and any shortfall in glucose availability has consequences for brain function.

The benefits of carbohydrate on mental performance are well documented. Medical research shows us that people's intellectual performance dramatically improves after they eat carbohydrate-rich foods (or a glucose load). In recent studies, subjects were tested on various measures of 'cognitive function', including word recall, maze learning, arithmetic, short-term memory, rapid information processing and reasoning. All types of people – young people, university students, people with diabetes, healthy elderly people and those with Alzheimer's disease – showed an improvement in mental ability after they ate glucose or a carbohydrate meal. Interestingly, research shows that low GI carbohydrates enhance learning and memory more than high GI carbs, probably because there is no rebound fall in blood glucose.

Too little glucose can also have serious physical consequences. In Chapter 5 we discuss hypoglycaemia, which results from low blood glucose.

What's wrong with a low carbohydrate diet?

Low carbohydrate diets are nothing new: a low carb diet to lose weight was first published in 1864. Low carb diets are either high in protein or high in fat or both. They cannot be anything else, because we have to get our energy from something (and alcohol, the only other macronutrient, won't keep you alive for long).

There are several variations of a low carbohydrate diet; we'll confine our discussion to those where the reduction of carbohydrate is steep. This includes those that are low in carbohydrate, containing less than 100 grams of carbohydrate per day and others that are *very low*, with reductions to as little as 20 to 30 grams of carbohydrate per day (ketogenic diets). The latter is the case with the first phase or 'kick start' of various popular diet books and is not recommended by us or most health authorities.

Without enough carbohydrate in your diet you may experience in the short term:

- muscle fatigue, causing even moderate exercise to be an exceptional effort
- insufficient fibre intake and therefore constipation
- headaches and tiredness due to low blood glucose levels

- bad breath due to the breakdown products of fat (ketones), and
- bad moods and even clinical depression.

A recent review of low carb diets has concluded that they are relatively safe and effective for weight loss in the short term, but there were potential risks in the long term (longer than six months).

One major concern is high saturated fat intake and the repercussions. Even a single meal high in saturated fat can have an adverse effect on blood vessels by inhibiting vasodilation, the normal increase in the diameter of blood vessels that occurs after a meal. A short-term and long-term effect of a low carb diet includes an increase in LDL cholesterol. Compounding this, there may be a low intake of micronutrients that are protective against disease. For this reason, a vitamin and mineral supplement is an essential accompaniment to a low carb diet.

Low carb diets are often high in protein (although not all high protein diets are low in carbohydrate). In people with diabetes, higher long-term protein loads (over six months) may accelerate decline in kidney function and increase calcium loss in urine, potentially increasing the risk of osteoporosis and kidney stones.

To ensure that blood glucose levels can be maintained between meals, your body draws on the glucose stored in the liver; that form of glucose is called glycogen. Supplies of glycogen are strictly limited and must be replenished from meal to meal. If your diet is low in carbohydrate, your glycogen stores will be low and easily depleted.

Once your body has used up its glycogen stores, which occurs 12 to 24 hours after you begin a low–carb diet, it will start breaking down muscle protein to create glucose for your brain and nervous system to use. However, this process can't supply all of the brain's needs. As mentioned earlier, under these circumstances, the brain will make use of ketones, which are a by-product of the breakdown of fat. The level of ketones in the blood rises as the fast continues. You can even smell the ketones on the breath.

In people who are losing weight on a low carb diet, the level of ketones in the blood rises markedly, and this state, called ketosis, is taken as a sign of success. But the brain may not be at its best, and one result is that mental judgement is impaired. In low carb diet studies, volunteers complained of headaches and physical and mental lethargy. Researchers from Tufts University found that low carb dieters had slower reaction times in tests performed two days and one week after starting the diet and a gradual decline in memory recall. In Australia, scientists found poorer mood and even depression after one year from the start, even though the dieters had achieved significant weight loss. Finally, since your muscle stores of glycogen will have been depleted, you'll also find strenuous exercise hard going, and you may tire easily. See The GI and your weight in Chapter 4 for more information on low carb diets.

Ketosis and pregnancy

Ketosis is a serious concern for pregnant women. The foetus can be harmed and its brain development impaired by high levels of ketones crossing from the mother's blood via the placenta. Because being overweight is often a cause of infertility, women who are losing weight may fall pregnant unexpectedly. One of the primary reasons we advocate a healthy low GI diet for pregnant women is that there are absolutely no safety concerns for mother and baby. Indeed, there is some evidence that a low GI diet will help the mother control excessive weight gain during pregnancy.

How much carbohydrate do you need?

Most of the world's population eats a high carb diet based on staples such as rice, corn, millet and wheat-based foods, including bread or noodles. In some African and Asian countries, carbohydrates may form as much as 70 to 80 per cent of a person's energy intake – though this is probably too high for optimum health. In contrast, most people in industrialised countries eat less than half their energy as carbs. Our diets typically contain about 45 per cent of energy in carbohydrate form. Is this too low, too high, or just right?

How much carbohydrate should you be eating?

Doctors and public health nutritionists now agree that your carbohydrate intake can vary over quite a large range. They specify that the *type* and *source* of the carbohydrate and fat are more important than the proportions.

The actual range shouldn't be lower than 40 per cent or higher than 65 per cent of energy as carbohydrate, i.e., moderate to high. This is a long way from a low or very low carbohydrate diet, which may contain as little as 10–25 per cent of energy in the form of carbs.

If you look carefully at diets all around the world, it's clear that both high and moderate intakes of carbohydrate are commensurate with good health; the choice is ultimately up to you. Both types of diets, however, need to emphasise low GI carbs and healthy fats. The way of eating that you'll enjoy and tend to follow over the long term is the one that is closest to your usual diet. Our low GI approach has built-in flexibility when it comes to the amount of carbohydrate you eat.

In 2002 the US National Institutes of Health (NIH) published new nutritional guidelines suggesting a range of carbohydrate intakes that could adequately meet the body's needs while minimising your disease risk. We like the NIH's figures in part because they allow for individual tailoring. Specifically, they advise the following ranges:

- **Carbohydrate:** 45–65 per cent of energy
- **Fat:** 25–35 per cent of energy
- **Protein:** 15–35 per cent of energy
[source: www.health.gov/dietaryguidelines]

If you have diabetes, carbohydrate can be as low as 40 per cent, according to the newest guidelines of the prestigious Joslin Clinic in the United States. Chances are your diet already falls within these flexible ranges; if so, we encourage you to stick with what you have. If your preference is for more protein or more fat and fewer carbs, then go ahead – just be choosy about the quality. (For more about protein, see Chapter 13.) We believe that you are the best judge of what you can live with.

However, we do recommend that you consume at least 125 grams of carbohydrate a day, even if you are on a weight-loss program. Whatever the amount, the type of carbohydrate is important and that's where the GI, wholegrains and fibre come into the story.

Is a high carbohydrate, low-fat diet for you?

Is consuming 50 per cent or more of your kilojoules from carbohydrates and less than 30 per cent from fats (the remaining 15 per cent or more should come from protein) realistic for you? That depends. If you have always been health conscious and avoided high-fat foods, or if you follow an Asian or Middle Eastern diet, then chances are you're already eating a high carbohydrate diet, and it's a good choice for you.

Of course, the number of kilojoules and the amount of carbohydrate varies with your weight and activity levels. If you're an active person – as we hope you are! – with average energy requirements who is not trying to lose weight (that is, with an average intake of 8500 kilojoules per day), you'll be eating 275 grams of carbohydrate. If you are trying to lose weight and are consuming a low-kilojoule diet (in other words, you're a small eater on 5000 kilojoules per day), that means you would be eating about 150 grams of carbohydrate a day.

Is a moderate carbohydrate diet for you?

Many Australians and New Zealanders prefer more moderate carbohydrate intakes. A Mediterranean-type diet is higher in fat and provides only 45 per cent of energy as carbohydrate. In the past, most nutritionists would have frowned upon this, but that's no longer the case, as research has shown that this type of diet can have important health benefits. As long as you carefully consider the types of fat and the types of carbohydrate you're eating, then this level of carbohydrate intake is perfectly commensurate with good health. At this level, you'll consume at least 125 grams of carbohydrate a day if you are a small eater and 225 grams if you are an average eater. See Part 3 for an idea of how many servings of bread, cereal, pasta or rice will provide these amounts of carbohydrate.

For specific information about your own energy and exact carbohydrate needs, you should consult an accredited practising dietitian (APD). Your primary care GP or a medical specialist you see for a specific condition may have one or more dietitians in their practice. Alternatively, look in the Yellow Pages under Dietitians, contact the Dietitians Association of Australia (DAA) in your home state.

The real deal on protein and health

Adding more protein to your diet makes good sense for weight control. In comparison with carbohydrate and fat, protein makes us feel more satisfied immediately after eating it and reduces hunger between meals. In addition, protein increases our metabolic rate for 1 to 3 hours after eating. This means we burn more energy by the minute compared with

If you look carefully at diets all around the world, it's clear that both high and moderate intakes of carbohydrates are commensurate with good health; the choice is ultimately up to you.

the increase that occurs after eating carbs or fats. Protein foods are also excellent sources of micronutrients, such as iron, zinc, vitamin B12 and omega-3 fats.

As your body can't stockpile extra protein from one day to use up the next, you need to eat it everyday.

Which foods are high in protein?

The best sources of protein are meats (beef, pork, lamb), chicken, fish and shellfish. As long as these are trimmed of fat and not served with creamy sauces, you can basically eat sensibly to suit your appetite, though you'll find your appetite for lean protein will have a natural limit. When buying protein foods, choose the leanest cuts, remove all the visible fat and grill, bake, braise, stir-fry or pan-fry.

Another excellent source of protein is any type of legume (beans, chickpeas or lentils) – a low GI food that is easy on the budget, versatile, filling, nutritious and low in kilojoules. Legumes are high in fibre, too – both soluble and insoluble – and are packed with nutrients, providing a valuable source (in addition to protein) of carbohydrate, B vitamins, iron, zinc, magnesium and phytochemicals (natural plant chemicals that possess antiviral, antifungal, antibacterial and anticancer properties). Whether you buy dried beans, lentils and chickpeas and cook them yourself at home, or opt for the very convenient, time-saving canned varieties, you are choosing one of nature's lowest GI foods.

Dairy products are also good sources of protein – and the combination of protein and calcium that is unique to dairy foods can aid weight management. Research has shown that the more calcium or dairy foods (it's hard to separate the two) people eat, the lower their weight and fat mass. Calcium is intimately involved in burning fat – a process we want to encourage. Choose low-fat dairy products, including milk, yoghurt and cottage cheese. Go easy on high-fat cheeses such as cheddar, feta, camembert and brie – though you don't have to cut them out entirely. It's better to have a small serving of one of these cheeses than a giant serving of a reduced-fat version that doesn't taste anywhere near as good.

Nuts are excellent sources of protein, dietary fibre and micronutrients – and they contain very little saturated fat (the fats are predominantly mono- or polyunsaturated). With nuts, take care not to overeat them, because they're energy dense – meaning they pack a lot of kilojoules into a small weight. Any nut will do, but research shows that eating 30 grams of walnuts every day can help lower cholesterol and reduce heart attack risk. If you eat them as a snack, put a small handful in a bowl; don't eat them straight from the package.

Eggs have been shedding their undeservedly bad reputation brought on because of their cholesterol content; in fact, they are a great source of protein and several essential vitamins and minerals. We now know that high blood cholesterol results from eating large amounts of saturated fat (rather than cholesterol) in foods. And if you select omega-3-enriched eggs, you will increase your intake of this valuable fat as well as your protein intake.

Common questions

How low should a low GI diet go?

We believe there's a real need to define the difference between a low GI *diet* and a low GI *food*. Because a low GI food is defined as 55 or less, people have made the reasonable assumption that a whole diet that averages less than 55 is 'low enough'. In fact the average Australian and American diet already has a GI of 56 to 58 because we all eat low GI fruits and dairy products and of course sugar has a medium GI (68). To reduce the risk of chronic disease, we believe that a low GI eating pattern/diet must have a much lower number.

What we now know from observational/cohort studies is that the GI of the diet of people in the lowest quintile (20 per cent of the population) is about 40–45. Since this reduces the risk of chronic diseases like diabetes and heart disease and people can achieve it in real life, we think it's a reasonable definition of a low GI diet or low GI meal (that is 45 or less).

Low GI basics

- The glycemic index (GI) is the measure of carbohydrate quality, a ranking that describes how much the carbohydrate (sugars and starches) in foods affects blood glucose levels.
- Slow digestion and gradual rise and fall in blood glucose after eating low GI foods controls blood glucose levels and delays hunger.
- The ranking from 0 to 100 reflects how fast the carbohydrate in foods hit the bloodstream. Fast (a high scale) is not so good for the body, slow (a low scale) is more sustaining.
- Low GI eating is flexible and fits in with your lifestyle and food likes and dislikes.
- Low GI eating is not just about the food. It also incorporates healthy living and advocates incorporating physical activity during the day. Not a strict regime of going to the gym six days a week, but encourages 'real world' activity that will fit into whatever busy schedule you may have.
- Not all carbohydrates are created equal as they behave differently in our bodies – some release glucose into the bloodstream quickly whereas others are 'slow release' which is more beneficial to our bodies.
- How much carbohydrate you include in your diet depends on your choice – just make sure you include plenty of low GI foods and healthy fats in moderation.
- When you switch to eating low GI carbs that have less 'glycemic punch', you help to keep your blood glucose on an even keel and your energy levels perfectly balanced, and you'll feel fuller for longer periods between meals.

Part 2

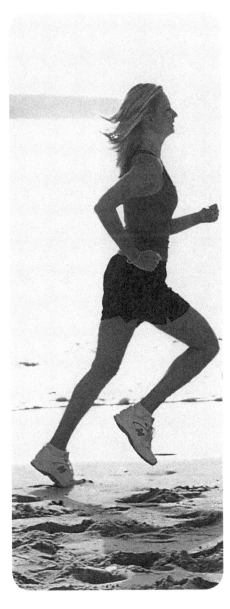

The GI for your health

- Weight control
- Diabetes
- Pre-diabetes
- Pregnancy
- Hypoglycaemia
- Heart health
- PCOS
- Children
- Exercise

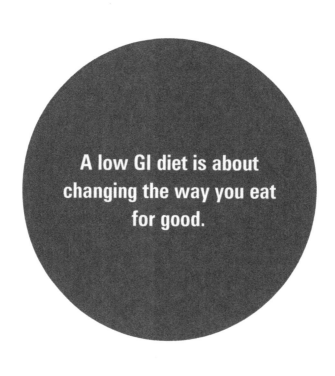

A low GI diet is about changing the way you eat for good.

Chapter 4

The GI and weight control

It is sad but true that 19 out of 20 people who lose weight by dieting will regain the lost weight. Those who succeed are those who adopt a lifestyle solution to weight concerns, not a temporary fix. A low GI diet is about changing the way you eat for good. One of the loudest messages in this chapter is 'don't diet'. *Don't* severely restrict food intake, *don't* skip breakfast, *don't* skip meals, *don't* follow fad diets – you are just asking for trouble. Instead, one by one adopt simple lifestyle 'manoeuvres', only some of which are specific to food. The focus is on eating *well* and moving *more*. The aim is to maximise your muscle mass (increase your engine size), minimise your body fat (decrease the cushioning), and keep you burning the optimal fuel mix for lifelong weight control (high-octane energy with built-in engine 'protectants').

Being slim or normal weight is no longer the norm. Between half and two-thirds of adults in Australia and New Zealand are classed as overweight or obese. Men are worse off than women, and our children are affected, too – approximately one in four weigh much more than they should for their age and height.

The role our genes play in weight control

There are many overweight people who say, 'Well, my mother's the same', 'I've always been overweight', or 'It must be in my genes'. These comments do have some truth behind them.

There is plenty of evidence to back up the idea that our body weight and shape is at least partially determined by our genes. A child born to overweight parents is much more likely to be overweight than one whose parents are not overweight. Most of this knowledge comes from studies of twins. Identical twins tend to be similar in body weight even if they are raised apart. Twins adopted out as infants show the body-fat profile of their biological parents rather than that of their adoptive parents.

We also know that when naturally lean people are fed 10 per cent more energy than they need, they increase their metabolic rate and their body *resists* the opportunity to gain weight, while overweight people, fed the same excess energy, pile on the kilos. The information stored in our genes governs our tendency to burn off or store excess kilojoules.

The importance of resting metabolic rate

Our genetic make-up underlies our metabolic rate – how many kilojoules we burn per minute. Bodies, like cars, differ in this regard. An eight-cylinder car consumes more fuel than a small four-cylinder one. A bigger body requires more kilojoules than a smaller one. When a car is stationary, the engine idles – using just enough fuel to keep the motor running. When we are asleep, the 'revs' are even lower and we use a minimum number of kilojoules. Our resting metabolic rate (RMR) – the kilojoules we burn by just lying completely at rest – is fuelling our large brain, heart and other important organs. When we start exercising, or even just moving around, the number of kilojoules (the amount of fuel we use) increases. But the greatest proportion of the kilojoules used in a 24-hour period are those used to maintain our RMR.

Since our RMR is where most kilojoules are used, it is a significant determinant of body weight. The lower your RMR, the greater your risk of gaining weight, and vice versa. Whether you have a high or low RMR is genetically determined and runs in families. We all know someone who appears to eat like a horse but is positively thin. Almost in awe we comment on their fast metabolism, and we may not be far off the mark.

Men have a higher RMR than women because their bodies contain more muscle mass and are more expensive to run; body fat, on the other hand, gets a free ride. These days, too many men and women have undersized muscles that hardly ever get a workout. Increasing muscle mass with weight-bearing (resistance) exercise will raise your RMR and is one of the secrets to lifelong weight control.

Interestingly, our genes dictate the fuel mix we burn in the fasting state (overnight). Some of us burn more carbohydrate and less fat even though the total energy used is the same. Scientists believe that subtle deficiencies in the ability to burn fat (as opposed to carbs) lie behind most states of being overweight and obese.

Indeed, in their latest research, if you have one copy of a high risk gene called FTO, geneticists have found you are 30 per cent more likely to become overweight. If you have two copies, then you are 67 per cent more likely! That is the strongest association yet of a common gene with obesity. Unfortunately, one in six people of European descent carry two copies and are therefore more prone to gain weight in the current environment.

This doesn't mean that if your genes are to blame you should resign yourself to being overweight. But it may help you understand why you have to watch what you eat while other people don't. Furthermore, the current epidemic of being overweight and obesity can't be blamed on our genes – our genes haven't mutated in a space of 25 years, but our environment has. So while genetics writes the code, environment presses the buttons. Our current sedentary lifestyles and food choices press all the wrong buttons!

If you were born with a tendency to be overweight, what you eat matters more. Genes can be switched on or off. By being choosy about carbohydrates and fats you will maximise your insulin sensitivity, *up*-regulate the genes involved in burning fat and *down*-regulate those involved in burning carbs. By moving your fuel 'currency exchange' from a 'carbohydrate economy' to a 'fat economy', you increase the opportunity of depleting fat stores over carbohydrate stores. This is exactly what will happen when you begin to eat a nutritious, low GI diet.

> **If your genes are to blame you shouldn't resign yourself to being overweight too. But it may help you understand why you have to watch what you eat while other people don't.**

Food choices affect your appetite

Foods affect your appetite; they dictate when and how much you eat. If digestion takes time and involves lower parts of your intestine, you stimulate natural appetite suppressants. Consequently, both quality and quantity of food are important for weight control.

Among all four major sources of kilojoules in food (protein, fat, carbohydrate and alcohol), fat has the highest energy content per unit of weight, twice that of carbohydrate and protein. A high-fat food is therefore said to be 'energy dense', meaning there are a lot of kilojoules in a standard weight of food. A typical croissant made with wafer-thin layers of buttery pastry contains about 2000 kilojoules – a whacking 20 per cent of total energy needs for most people for 24 hours! To eat the same amount of energy in the form of apples, you have to eat about six large apples. So, getting more energy – kilojoules – than your body needs is relatively easy when eating a high-fat food. That's why there has been so much emphasis on low-fat diets for weight control.

What really matters is not the fat content but a food's 'energy density' (kilojoules per gram). Some diets, such as traditional Mediterranean diets, contain quite a lot of fat (mainly from olive oil), but are not so energy dense because the oil comes with a large volume of watery fruits and vegetables. On the other hand, many new low-fat foods on the market are energy dense. Indeed, some have much the same energy density as the original high-fat food because 2 grams of carbohydrate have replaced every gram of fat. If a low-fat food has the same kilojoules per serving as a high-fat food, then it's just as easy to overeat. Nutritionists have therefore had to fine-tune the message about fat and weight control.

- Higher fat intake is compatible with healthy weight loss.
- The type of fat is more critical than the amount.
- Only saturated fat and trans fat need to be limited.
- Think energy density per serving – not high fat or low fat.

Insulin plays critical roles in our health and well-being

One important function of the pancreas, a vital organ near the stomach, is to produce the hormone insulin. Insulin plays several critical roles in our health and well-being.

First, it **regulates our blood glucose levels**. When you eat a meal containing carbohydrate, your blood glucose level rises. This causes the pancreas to secrete insulin (unless you have type 1 diabetes), which pushes the glucose out of the bloodstream and into the muscles and tissues, where it provides energy for you to carry out your regular activities. The movement of glucose out of the blood and into the body's cells (particularly the muscles and liver) is finely controlled. Just the right amount of insulin takes the glucose level back to normal.

Secondly, insulin **plays a key part in determining the fuel mix that we burn** from minute to minute – and whether we burn fat or carbohydrate to meet our energy needs. It does this by switching muscle cells from fat-burning to carb-burning. The relative proportions of fat to carbohydrate in your body's fuel mix are dictated by the prevailing levels of insulin in your blood. If insulin levels are low, as they are when you wake up in the morning, then the fuel you burn is mainly fat. If insulin levels are high, as they are after you consume a high carbohydrate meal, then the fuel you burn is mainly carbohydrate.

Carbohydrates stimulate the secretion of insulin more than any other component of food. When carbohydrates are slowly absorbed by our bodies – which is the case with low GI foods – the pancreas doesn't have to work as hard and secretes less insulin. If it is overstimulated over a long period of time, which often occurs as a result of a diet rich in high GI foods, it may become 'exhausted'. Type 2 diabetes may develop in someone who is genetically susceptible and whose pancreas has been overworked. Even without diabetes, excessively high insulin levels increase the risk of heart disease in everyone.

Why insulin resistance is a big deal

Many overweight people, but not all, are insulin resistant (see Chapter 6). This condition has genetic underpinnings and results in high insulin secretion after every meal. In time even fasting insulin levels tend to rise. Having persistently high insulin levels is likely to make you fatter and fatter, undermining all your efforts at weight control. It is the very reason why people with diabetes and polycystic ovarian syndrome (PCOS) find it so hard to lose weight.

The higher your insulin levels, the more carbohydrate you burn at the expense of fat. This is because insulin has two powerful actions: one is to 'open the gates' so that glucose can move into the muscle cells and be used as the source of energy. The second role of insulin is to *inhibit* the release of fat from fat stores. Unfortunately, the burning of glucose inhibits the burning of fat (and vice versa).

These actions persist even in the face of insulin resistance because the body overcomes the hurdle by just pumping out more insulin into the blood. Unfortunately, the level that finally drives glucose into the cells is many times more than is needed to switch off the use of fat as a source of fuel. If insulin is high all day long, as it is in insulin-resistant and many overweight people, then the cells are being forced to use

A healthy low GI diet plus physical activity is the most powerful way of optimising insulin sensitivity and decreasing insulin levels over the course of the whole day.

glucose as their fuel source, drawing it from either the blood or stored glycogen. Blood glucose therefore swings from low to high and back again, playing havoc with our appetite and triggering the release of stress hormones. Our limited stores of carbohydrate in the liver and muscles also undergo major fluctuations over the course of the day. When you don't get much chance to use fat as a source of fuel, it is not surprising that fat stores accumulate around different parts of the body.

Low GI smart carbs help you lose weight

Based on good scientific evidence, the GI helps people lose weight, specifically that dangerous fat around the belly. There is concrete evidence that a low GI diet increases the rate of weight loss compared to a conventional low-fat diet. The confirmation comes from our own weight loss studies at the University of Sydney, as well as research from the Children's Hospital in Boston and Hotel Dieu Hospital in Paris.

What's more, well-designed studies published in major medical journals have confirmed that the fat loss is maintained long term. This was especially evident in those overweight volunteers who secreted more insulin during meals. That is a critically important point because it is where other diets have failed. Let's take a close look at all the facts supporting a healthy low GI diet.

The filling power of low GI carbs

One of the biggest challenges to losing weight is ignoring that gnawing feeling in your gut: hunger. Indeed, it is impossible to deny extreme hunger – food-seeking behaviour is wired into our brains to ensure we survive when energy intake is too low. Extreme hunger followed by binge eating can develop into a vicious cycle – and that is one reason rapid weight loss is discouraged.

The low GI diet is based on an important scientifically proven fact – that foods with low GI values are more filling than their high GI counterparts. They not only give you a greater feeling of fullness instantly, but delay hunger pangs for longer and reduce food intake during the remainder of the day. In contrast, foods with a high GI can actually stimulate appetite sooner, increasing consumption at the next meal.

Some foods and nutrients are simply more satiating than others, kilojoule for kilojoule. In general, protein packs the greatest punch, followed by carbohydrate and then fat. Most of us can relate to the fact that a good steak has greater filling power than a croissant, despite the fact that they provide an equal number of kilojoules.

There are also foods that are 'more-ish' – corn chips and potato chips, for example. Fatty foods, in particular, have only a weak effect on satisfying appetite relative to the number of kilojoules they provide. This has been demonstrated clearly in experiments where volunteers were asked to eat until their appetite was satisfied. They ate far more kilojoules if the foods were high in fat than when they were starchy or sugary foods. Even when the fat and carbohydrate were disguised in yoghurts and milk puddings, people consumed more energy from the high fat option. A gram of fat contains twice as many kilojoules as a gram of protein, starch or sugar.

In our laboratory at the University of Sydney, we developed the world's first satiety index of foods. Volunteers were given a range of individual foods that contained equal numbers of kilojoules, and then their satiety responses and subsequent food intake were compared. We found that the most important determinant of satiety was the actual weight or volume of the food – the higher the weight per 1000 kilojoules, the higher the filling power. So foods that were high in water (and therefore the least energy dense), such as porridge, apples and potatoes, were the most satiating. When water contents were equal, however, protein and carbohydrate were the best predictors of satiating power.

Then, if carbohydrate contents were similar, the GI became the most important determinant – low GI foods being more satiating than high GI foods. (It is true that potatoes, despite their high GI, are high on the satiety index scale, but in theory a low GI potato would be even more satiating.)

> **Eating to lose weight with low GI smart carbs gives you freedom, flexibility and security. What's more, it's sustainable.**

Invariably, foods that provided a lot of kilojoules per gram (energy-dense foods such as croissants, chocolate and peanuts) were the least satisfying. These foods are more likely to leave us wanting more and to lead to what scientists call 'passive overeating' without realising it. In developing our low GI diet, we made good use of these findings, encouraging food choices that will keep you feeling fuller for longer.

In addition to our own research, at least 20 other studies from around the world have confirmed that low GI foods, in comparison to their nutrient-matched high GI counterparts, are more filling, delay hunger pangs for longer and/or reduce energy intake during the remainder of the day. There are several explanations: low GI foods remain longer in the gut and reach much lower parts of the small intestine, triggering receptors that produce natural appetite suppressants. Many of these receptors are present only in the lower gut. It doesn't take a genius to appreciate that a food that dissolves and disappears from the gut quickly won't satisfy for hours on end.

We now know that low GI meals are associated with higher levels of two helpful hormones, known by their abbreviations CCK and GLP-1. Both produce feelings of pleasant fullness after eating and reduce food intake over the course of the day. GLP-1 has a further beneficial effect – it improves insulin sensitivity, a factor that helps facilitate weight control over the long term.

Here's the deal on GI and appetite.

- Low GI foods are more filling because they remain longer in the gut.

Test for yourself and feel the difference

You can experience one benefit of low GI carbs with this simple breakfast challenge. Try out each of the following breakfasts on consecutive mornings, one high GI and one low GI, and feel the difference yourself. By mid-morning you'll be thinking better, feeling better and have more insight into your natural hunger and satiety cues with Breakfast 1.

Breakfast 1 – a low GI option
½ cup natural muesli
with ½ cup low-fat milk
and ½ a banana

Breakfast 2 – a high GI option
1 cup cornflakes
with 1 cup low-fat milk
and 2 slices of rockmelon

- High GI foods may stimulate hunger because the precipitous fall in blood glucose levels stimulates counter-regulatory responses.
- Stress hormones such as adrenalin and cortisol are released when glucose levels rebound after a high GI food. Both stimulate appetite.
- Low GI foods may be more satiating simply because they are often less energy dense than their high GI counterparts. The naturally high water and fibre content of many low GI foods increases their bulk without increasing their energy content.

Fat loss is faster with low GI foods

There are now a dozen or more studies showing that people who eat low GI foods lose more body fat than those eating high GI foods. In one study conducted by Harvard scientists, overweight adults were instructed to follow either a conventional high fibre, low-fat diet or a low GI diet containing more good fats and and low GI carbs. The low GI group's diet emphasised foods such as porridge, eggs, low-fat dairy produce and pasta. In contrast, the low-fat diet emphasised high fibre cereal products, potatoes and rice. Both diets contained the same number of kilojoules and were followed for 18 months (6 months of intense intervention and 12 months of follow-up). At the end changes in weight were similar in both groups. But, among the subjects who had high insulin levels (half of them), those on the low GI diet lost nearly 6 kilograms of weight compared to only 1 kilogram on the conventional low-fat diet. Moreover, they lost three times more body fat and had greater improvements in cardiovascular risk factors.

In our own research unit at the University of Sydney, we have made similar findings in a group of young overweight adults who followed one of the four popular diets. To ensure dietary compliance, we gave them most of the food they needed for the whole 12-week period. At the end, we found that weight and body fat loss were over 50 per cent greater in those following our low GI diet than those following the conventional low fat approach. Those instructed to follow a high protein diet also lost more body fat but showed adverse effects on blood lipids. Fortunately, the cholesterol-raising effect of the high protein diet could be prevented by simultaneous consumption of low GI carbs.

Why do low GI diets work so well for weight loss? The most important reason is likely to be the effect on day-long insulin levels – low GI foods result in lower levels of insulin over the course of the whole day.

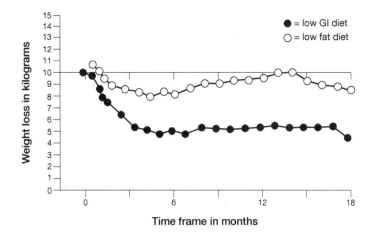

Figure 4: Overweight adults with relatively high insulin levels lost more weight and sustained that weight loss over time on a diet that was low GI rather than a conventional low-fat diet.

The hormone insulin is not only involved in regulating blood glucose levels, but also plays a key part in fat storage. High levels of insulin mean the body is forced to burn carbohydrate rather than fat. Thus, over the day, even if the total energy burned is the same, the proportions of fat to carbohydrate are different. Oxidising carbohydrate won't really help you lose weight, but burning fat will.

These are not idle claims. Dr Emma Stevenson's research with Loughborough University in the UK demonstrated over and over that, compared with healthy conventional meals, low GI meals were associated with greater fat oxidation during episodes of moderate exercise in overweight volunteers.

People who are overweight have been shown to have high glycogen (carbohydrate) stores that undergo major fluctuations during the day. This suggests that glycogen is a more important source of fuel for them. If glycogen is being depleted and replenished on a regular basis (before and after each meal, for example), it is displacing fat from the engine. Each meal restores glycogen (especially if the food has a high GI value) and the cycle repeats itself. Carbohydrate 'balance', as it's called, is turning out to be one of the best predictors of future weight gain.

The benefits of a low GI diet for weight control go beyond appetite and fat burning. When you first begin a diet, your metabolic rate drops in response to the reduction in food intake, which makes weight loss slower and slower. Research shows your metabolic rate drops much less, however, on a low GI diet

The 'famine reaction'

The invisible enemy of any dieting effort is a natural physiological phenomenon that makes it progressively more difficult for dieters to keep losing weight, and even more difficult for them to keep it off. Dr Amanda Sainsbury-Salis, obesity researcher at the Garvan Institute in Sydney, calls this the 'famine reaction'; it's a survival mechanism that's been helping the human race to survive famines and food shortages for millions of years. The famine reaction is the reason why after each dieting effort, you end up doing battle with ravenous hunger, craving for fattening foods, guilt-ridden binge-eating, lethargy, weight plateauing and rapid rebound weight gain. These are all classic signs of the famine reaction in full swing. It has nothing to do with lack of commitment or willpower. It's why conventional dieting advice fails.

In her book *The Don't Go Hungry Diet*, Dr Sainsbury-Salis explains the origin of these tell-tale symptoms – a naturally occurring hormone called neuropeptide Y. Its secretion causes irrepressible increases in hunger, the hallmark feature of the famine reaction, but also acts to prevent further weight loss and promote fat accumulation, regardless of whether or not the person continues to follow a program of diet and physical activity. Neuropeptide Y is just one of a whole army of hormones and brain chemicals that bring on the famine reaction. All conspire to make sure you hit the wall of resistance to further weight loss. Drinking water, moving more and eating more fibre only serve to make the famine reaction stronger: more hunger, more cravings, more lethargy, an even slower metabolic rate and longer plateau.

How do you switch off the famine reaction? Simple. It can be switched off by *eating freely*, eating sensibly to appetite. In other words, eating enough to satisfy your physical hunger, including your favourite foods. Nothing more complicated than that. The science behind this concept is brand new but rock solid. And it provides another explanation for the long-term success of our low GI diet, that is, a diet underpinned by sensible *eating to appetite*, enjoying foods that make you feel fuller for longer, because they take many more hours to be digested and absorbed.

The fat brake

Here is another crucial piece of scientific research with the potential to change your life for the better. According to Dr Amanda Sainsbury-Salis, not only does your body have the potential to mount a famine reaction to stop you losing weight, it also possesses a remarkable system that protects you from gaining weight. She calls it the 'fat brake'. If you can pick up the fat brake signals, it it will actually be difficult for you to get fat. Just as there are brain chemical and hormones that control the famine reaction, there is an opposing army of brain chemicals controlling the fat brake. The commander is a hormone called leptin that has the opposite effects to neuropeptide Y. It acts to blunt the appetite, increase the tendency to be active and boost the metabolic rate. So not only should you heed signals that say 'eat more' but also those that say 'eat less' and 'don't eat yet'.

than a conventional diet. If your engine revs are higher, you'll not only lose weight faster, you'll also be much less likely to regain it.

The fall in metabolic rate that occurs whenever we restrict our energy intake is part of our body's natural response to food scarcity. This brings us to two new and profound concepts in the obesity research field, described in lay terms as the 'famine reaction' and the 'fat brake'.

Low GI and weight re-gain

Many people who successfully lose weight find themselves gradually putting the weight back on. Scientists are now focusing on this critical period, trying to determine the optimal dietary strategy for maintaining weight loss, and preventing weight re-gain. The findings of the largest study of its kind, the Diogenes Study, led by Professor Arne Astrup at the University of Copenhagen, are now available. This collaborative project from eight countries in the European Union included approximately 800 overweight or obese individuals, all of them parents of young children. One or two parents in each family underwent an eight-week weight loss diet using a low-calorie diet formula, which was designed to achieve a weight loss of a certain percentage of their original starting weight (11 kilos or about 24 pounds). If the parents were successful in meeting this target, they were offered the opportunity to participate in the next stage of the study, which investigated the problem of weight re-gain. In this part of the study, volunteers were assigned to one of five different dietary regimes, designed to test the relative effectiveness of the GI as well as protein content in weight control.

The diets were:

Low protein, low glycemic index: Group 1
Low protein, high glycemic index: Group 2
High protein, low glycemic index: Group 3
High protein, high glycemic index: Group 4
Control diet, medium protein and medium glycemic index: Group 5

Over the course of 26 weeks, the investigators found that both low GI diets AND high protein diets were equally effective in preventing weight re-gain (see Figure 5). But they also found something that took them by complete surprise. The third diet group that combined both low GI and high protein strategies together, continued to lose weight throughout the one year follow up. This was something never seen before in any study of weight maintenance after weight loss. Furthermore, this group had the lowest drop-out rate of any of the groups, a testament to the fact that this diet was not only effective, it was acceptable to the volunteers and their families – not too difficult, complex or hard to sustain. Interestingly, the Diogenes Study achieved only a moderately small reduction in GI (from about 58 to 50) yet it was sufficient to produce these outstanding results.

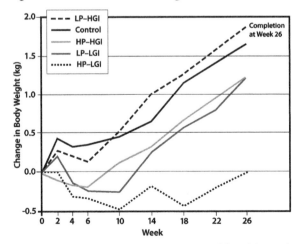

Figure 5. This chart shows changes in body weight. All subjects in the Diogenes Study (www.diogenes-eu.org) underwent an 8-week period of fast weight loss before starting on one of five dietary strategies to prevent weight re-gain.

Low GI carbs and lifelong weight control

One of the best reasons to adopt a low GI diet is the value-added benefits you get for long-term weight control. People who *naturally* eat a diet with a low GI have been found to be at lower risk of being overweight and gaining weight in the future. Studies in the United States, Denmark and Japan tell us that low GI diets *are* sustainable and have distinct advantages over other types of diets. There is no evidence that high protein intake, for example, benefits weight in the long term.

These types of studies (called epidemiological or observational) control or adjust for all the known confounding factors associated with weight gain: age, family history, physical activity, alcohol intake, fibre intake and so on. Hence it is highly unlikely that a low GI diet is just a coincidental marker of a group of people at low risk of weight gain. The remarkable fact is that GI and GL are often showing strong relationships with disease while total carbohydrate, sugar, protein and total fat are not.

Epidemiological studies also prove to us that many people are already eating a diet that has a low GI. In other words, it is practical and feasible to select low GI foods from the vast array of foods currently on supermarket shelves. You don't have to jump through a hoop or turn yourself inside out to adopt a diet that gives you the benefits of lifelong health and weight control.

Part 3, Your Guide to a Low GI Diet for Life, provides all the information you need to make the change to a low GI diet along with the low GI food menu ideas, food finder and delicious recipes making the most of low GI ingredients.

Low GI basics

There is no doubt that reducing portion sizes and eating fewer kilojoules will lead to weight loss. Just how you do this is the name of the game. These days, we are eating less but getting fatter. Instead of eating fewer kilojoules we are eating more, especially in the form of high GI refined starches and sugars. Cutting out the carbs is not the answer. The real solution to both weight loss and weight maintenance is to be choosy about the type of carbohydrates you eat.

Tips for long-term weight loss

1. Choose low GI carbs. Eat regularly and try to include low GI carbs at every meal. This will stave off hunger and strengthen your resolve against temptation.
2. Reduce your fat intake by cutting out saturated fat in foods such as chocolate, biscuits and chips.
3. Snack smarter, snack low GI and say 'no thanks' to high GI biscuits, crackers, lollies and soft drinks.
4. Think balance and moderation. Eat a little less. Do a little more.

Make healthy eating a habit. Motivation is what gets you started. Habit is what helps to keep you going. Here are some key tips.

- Make breakfast a priority.
- If it's healthy keep it handy.
- Don't buy food you want to avoid.
- Eat small portions regularly. Eat when you are hungry and stop when you are full (you don't have to leave a clean plate).

Chapter 5

The GI and diabetes

Diabetes is on its way to becoming one of the most serious and most common health problems in the world. A type 2 diabetes epidemic is gaining momentum in many developed and newly industrialised nations. Worldwide the total number of people with diabetes is 246 million, and the International Diabetes Federation predicts it will affect 380 million people by 2025. In some developing countries, half of the adult population already has type 2 diabetes. Even in developed countries, the rate of type 2 diabetes is increasing at an alarming rate. It is estimated that in Australia there are 1.5 million people with diabetes and, in New Zealand, 250 000.

The prediction is that one out of every three people in the United States born in the year 2000 will develop type 2 diabetes. Australia and New Zealand are not lagging too far behind in statistics like these. In the absence of any sort of preventive intervention, a high proportion of people with pre-diabetes will eventually develop diabetes. The GI has far-reaching implications for diabetes and pre-diabetes (see Chapter 6). Not only is it important in treating people with diabetes, but it may also help prevent people from developing type 2 diabetes in the first place, and possibly even prevent some of the complications of diabetes.

What is diabetes?

Diabetes is a chronic condition in which there is too much glucose in the blood. Keeping your blood glucose levels normal requires the right amount of a hormone called insulin (see Chapter 4). If there is no insulin, not enough insulin, or if the insulin does not do its job properly, diabetes develops.

Type 1 diabetes (formerly referred to as insulin-dependent diabetes, or juvenile onset diabetes) is an autoimmune disease triggered by as yet unknown environmental factors (possibly a virus) that usually develops in childhood or early adulthood. In type 1 diabetes the pancreas cannot produce any insulin, because the body's immune system has attacked and destroyed its insulin-producing beta cells. About 10 per cent of people with diabetes have type 1 diabetes. To survive, everyone with type 1 diabetes requires insulin, delivered through injections or an insulin pump.

Type 2 diabetes (formerly known as non-insulin-dependent diabetes or maturity onset diabetes) has a large genetic component, but overeating, being overweight and not exercising enough are important lifestyle factors that can contribute to its development, particularly in people who have a family history of diabetes. Eighty-five to 90 per cent of people with diabetes have type 2 diabetes.

Typically, type 2 diabetes develops after the age of 40. However, our society's increasing physical inactivity and obesity has led to the diagnosis in younger and younger people. Even children less than ten years of age are developing type 2 diabetes.

People develop type 2 diabetes because they have developed insulin resistance. As type 2 diabetes progresses, the body may struggle to make the extra insulin needed and then may ultimately develop a shortage of insulin. Treatments for type 2 diabetes aim to help people make the best use of the insulin their bodies produce and to try to make it last as long as possible. In some cases, oral medications and insulin injections may be necessary to treat this type of diabetes.

What is insulin resistance?

Insulin resistance means that your body is insensitive, or 'partially deaf', to insulin. The organs and tissues that ought to respond to even a small increase in insulin remain unresponsive. So your body tries harder by secreting more insulin to achieve the same effect. This is why high insulin levels are found in people with type 2 diabetes who are insulin resistant.

Why do people get type 2 diabetes?

As our ancestors settled down and became farmers and began to grow food crops 10 000 years ago, their diet was no longer protein-based. It was more carbohydrate-based, in the form of whole cereal grains, vegetables and beans. Such a dietary change would also have changed the glucose levels in their blood. While they ate a high protein diet, the glucose levels in their blood would not have risen significantly after a meal.

When they started eating carbohydrate regularly, their blood glucose levels would have increased after meals. The amount by which the glucose levels in the blood increased after a meal would have depended on the GI of the carbohydrate. Crops such as spelt wheat grain, which our ancestors grew, had a low GI value. These foods would have had a minimal effect on glucose levels in the blood and the demand for insulin would have been similarly low.

The second major change in our diet came with industrialisation and the advent of new milling procedures that produced highly refined carbohydrate, instead of

Are you at risk of type 2 diabetes?

More than four million Australians and New Zealanders have diabetes or pre-diabetes and are at risk of heart disease and stroke. To find out if you're at risk of type 2 diabetes, answer the following questions.

☐ 1. Tick the box if you have a family history of any of the following:
- diabetes
- heart disease
- high blood pressure
- polycystic ovarian syndrome

☐ 2. Tick the box if you are:
- overweight
- over 55
- of Chinese, Indian, Maori or Pacific Islander heritage
- an Aboriginal or Torres Strait Islander
- had diabetes in pregnancy

If you have ticked either or both boxes above you are at risk of developing type 2 diabetes and should discuss screening tests for this condition with your doctor.

wholegrain products, which we now know increases the GI value of a food. When this highly refined food is eaten, it causes a greater increase in blood glucose levels. To keep blood glucose levels normal, the body has to make large amounts of insulin. The vast majority of the commercially packaged foods and drinks that most people eat today have a high GI value. All of this strains the body's insulin-making capabilities.

Our bodies adapt to such major changes in diet over long periods of time. Because our European ancestors had thousands of years to adapt to a diet with a lot of carbohydrate, they were in a better position to cope with the changes in the GI values of foods. We believe that's why people of European descent have a lower prevalence of type 2 diabetes than people whose diets have recently changed to include lots of high GI foods. There is, however, only so much that our bodies can take. As we continue to consume increasing quantities of foods with high GI values, plus excessive amounts of saturated fats, our bodies are coping less well. The result can be seen in the significant increase of people developing diabetes.

Large-scale studies at Harvard University, in which thousands of men and women have been studied over many years, have shown that people who ate large amounts of refined, high GI foods were two to three times more likely to develop type 2 diabetes or heart disease. The most dramatic increases in diabetes, however, have occurred in populations that have been exposed to these lifestyle changes over a much shorter period of time. In some groups of Native Americans and populations within the Pacific region, up to one adult in two has diabetes because of the rapid dietary and lifestyle changes they have undergone in the twentieth and twenty-first centuries.

Latest findings on diabetes testing

Following a study in the UK led by Professor Kamlesh Khunti and an international consensus statement, European authorities are considering changing the diagnostic criteria for diabetes. The recommendation is to use HbA1c testing instead of the traditional oral glucose tolerance test, which could almost double the number of people classed as having the disease. The American Diabetes Association formally opted for this form of diagnosis for type 2 diabetes in 2010.

(HbA1c is a form of haemoglobin used primarily to identify the average plasma glucose concentration over prolonged periods of time.)

Treating diabetes

Watching what you eat is essential if you have diabetes. For some people with type 2 diabetes, diet, along with exercise, is *the* most critical way to keep their blood glucose levels in the normal range (4–6 mmol/L). Others also need to take tablets or insulin. Everyone with type 1 diabetes must receive insulin, no matter what their diet. Regardless of the type or degree of their diabetes and their doctor-approved treatment, everyone with diabetes must carefully consider what they eat in order to keep their blood glucose levels under control. There's no question about it, research shows that good (also called 'tight') blood glucose control helps to prevent the dire complications that can arise: heart attacks, strokes, blindness, kidney failure and leg amputations.

It wasn't until the 1970s that carbohydrate was considered to be a valuable part of the diabetic diet. Researchers found that a higher carbohydrate intake brought both improved nutritional status and insulin sensitivity. In the early 1980s, with Dr David Jenkins's development of the glycemic index, the foundations were established for our present-day understanding of the real effect of those carbohydrates on blood glucose levels.

Some people think that because carbohydrate raises blood glucose levels, people who have diabetes shouldn't eat it at all. We cannot stress enough that this is simply not correct. Carbohydrate is a useful component of a healthy diet and helps maintain insulin sensitivity and provides physical endurance. Mental performance is also better when meals contain carbohydrate rather than just protein and fat. (See Carbohydrate is brain food in Chapter 3).

Fundamentally, the GI shows that the way for people with diabetes to incorporate more carbohydrates into their diet – while keeping tight control on their blood glucose levels – is to choose low GI carbs.

Lowering the GI of your diet is not as hard as it seems, because nearly every carbohydrate food that we typically consume has an equivalent food with a low or lower GI value. Our research has shown that blood glucose levels in people with diabetes are greatly improved if foods with a low GI value are substituted for high GI foods – the This for that approach we talk about in Chapter 13, Getting started.

We showed a group of people with type 2 diabetes how to replace the high GI foods they normally ate with low GI foods. After three months we found a significant drop in their average blood glucose levels. They did not find the diet at all difficult; rather, they commented on how easy it had been to make the change and how much more variety had been introduced into their diet.

Similar results have been reported by other researchers studying both type 1 and type 2 diabetes. For example, large studies in Australia, Europe and Canada of people with type 1 diabetes have shown that the lower the GI of the diet, the better the diabetes control.

The improvement in diabetes management seen after changing to a low GI diet is often better than that achieved with some of the newer, expensive diabetes medications and insulins. Making this type of change in your everyday diet does not mean that your diet has to be restrictive or unpalatable.

The menus and recipes in Part 3, Your Guide to a Low GI Diet for Life, will show you how to reduce the overall GI value of your diet.

Many people with type 2 diabetes end up taking oral medication and/or insulin to control blood glucose levels. An increased intake of low GI carbs can sometimes make these drugs unnecessary. Sometimes, however, despite your best efforts with diet, medication will be necessary to obtain good blood glucose control. This is eventually the case for most people with type 2 diabetes as they grow older and their insulin-secreting capacity declines further.

Diabetes complications

Heart attacks, leg amputations, strokes, blindness and kidney failure are more common in people with diabetes. The reason: poor blood glucose control can damage the blood vessels in the heart, legs, brain, eyes and kidneys – all parts of the body that are susceptible to vascular damage. Poor blood glucose control can also damage the nerves in the feet, leading to pain and irritation, numbness and loss of sensation.

In addition to high blood glucose levels, many researchers believe that high levels of insulin also contribute to the damage of the blood vessels of the heart, legs and brain. High insulin levels are thought to be one of the factors that might stimulate muscle in the wall of blood vessels to thicken. Thickening of this muscle wall causes the blood vessels to narrow and can slow the flow of blood to the point that a clot can form

Lowering the GI of your diet is not as hard as it seems, because nearly every carbohydrate food has an equivalent food with a low or lower GI.

and stop blood flow altogether. This is what happens to cause a heart attack or stroke.

We know that high GI foods cause the body to produce larger amounts of insulin, which results in higher levels of insulin in the blood. Eating low GI foods not only helps to control blood glucose levels, but it also does so with lower levels of insulin. Lower levels of both blood glucose and insulin may have the added benefit of reducing large-vessel damage, which accounts for many of the problems that people with diabetes tend to experience.

Diabetes and snacks

The GI is especially important when you eat carbohydrate by itself and not as part of a mixed meal. Carbohydrate tends to have a stronger effect on blood glucose levels when it is eaten alone rather than as part of a meal with protein foods, for example. This is the case with between-meal snacks, which most people with diabetes eat.

Many people taking insulin or oral medications need to eat some form of carbohydrate between meals to prevent their blood glucose from dropping too low (although newer forms of medication have lessened the likelihood of your needing to do this).

Snacks, when chosen wisely, can make a significant nutrient contribution even if you're not taking any diabetes medication. We recommend them especially for small children, to ensure a sufficient energy intake. Even for adults, regular snacks can prevent extreme hunger and help to reduce the amount of food eaten at a single sitting, which can help manage blood glucose levels.

Studies that have looked at the effects of small, frequent meals (rather like grazing) versus two or three large meals each day have found that in people with type 2 diabetes, blood glucose and blood fat levels improve when meal frequency increases. There's also evidence that you will reap metabolic benefits by eating at regular set times rather than haphazardly.

Snacking isn't a licence to eat more food. Rather, it is a way to spread the same amount of food over more frequent and smaller meals. Research indicates that if you spread your nutrient load more evenly over the course of a day, you may reduce the need for insulin in the disposal and uptake of carbohydrates. Researchers have seen this effect in people without diabetes, too. Although it has not been proven by controlled trials, it may also be that small, frequent meals could reduce your risk of developing diabetes by reducing the periodic surges in insulin that follow large meals.

Choose low GI foods for a between-meal snack

An apple, with a GI of 38, is better than a slice of white toast, with a GI of around 70, and will result in a smaller jump in the blood glucose level. Other low fat, low GI snack ideas include:

- a fruit smoothie
- a low-fat milkshake
- low-fat fruit yoghurt
- 5 or 6 dried apricot halves
- small banana

- 1 or 2 oatmeal biscuits
- an orange
- a scoop of low-fat ice-cream in a cone, and
- a glass of low-fat milk

> Symptoms of hypoglycaemia differ from person to person, but can include feeling hungry (even ravenous), feeling shaky, sweating, having a rapid heart beat, and being unable to think clearly.

Hypoglycaemia – exception to the low GI rule

We discuss hypoglycaemia in greater detail in Chapter 8, but we want to mention it here briefly because people with diabetes who use insulin or oral medication may sometimes experience hypos, which occur when blood glucose levels drop below 4 mmol/L, the lower end of the normal range.

Hypoglycaemia (or low blood sugar) is a potentially dangerous situation that must be treated immediately by eating approximately 15 grams of an easily absorbed source of carbohydrate to quickly raise blood glucose levels. This could include glucose tablets or gels, regular soft drink or cordial, jelly beans, or sugar. If you aren't about to eat your next meal or snack, follow up with another 15 grams of lower GI carbohydrates, like an apple or banana, or a slice of low GI bread, unsweetened yoghurt or sweetened yoghurt or a glass of low-fat milk to keep your blood glucose from falling again until you next eat.

If you're having trouble controlling your blood glucose levels ...

Many factors can affect your blood glucose levels – what you eat and drink, your weight, your stress levels, how much exercise you're getting, and the medications you're taking. So if you have diabetes and you're finding it hard to achieve 'tight control' of your blood glucose levels, we cannot stress strongly enough how important it is to seek help. Treating diabetes really is a team effort. Ideally, on your team there will be a doctor (and possibly an endocrinologist or specialist physician), a diabetes educator, a dietitian, a podiatrist, an exercise specialist, an eye doctor and a dentist. There may also be a counsellor (psychologist or psychiatrist) to help you cope with living with a chronic disease. Working with a healthcare team like this is the best way you can avoid the serious complications that diabetes can cause. That's the clear message from numerous studies of people with diabetes in recent years.

> The most important member of your team is you, and knowledge is your best defence. Only you can make sure you know as much as possible about your diabetes and only you can act on the advice you are given.

Common questions

Does sugar cause diabetes?

No. There is absolute consensus that sugar in food does not cause diabetes. Type 1 diabetes (insulin-dependent diabetes) is an autoimmune condition triggered by unknown environmental factors, such as viruses. Type 2 diabetes (non-insulin-dependent diabetes) is strongly inherited, but lifestyle factors, such as lack of exercise and being overweight, increase the risk of developing it. In the past, when the dietary treatment of diabetes involved strict avoidance of sugar, many people wrongly believed that sugar was in some way implicated as a cause of the disease. While sugar is off the hook, high GI foods are not. Population studies have shown that high GI diets increase the risk of developing both type 2 diabetes and gestational diabetes (diabetes during pregnancy).

Why are people with diabetes now allowed sugar?

Research has proved that people with diabetes can eat the same amount of sugar as the average person – without compromising diabetes control.

It's important, however, to remember that 'empty kilojoules' – whatever the source, be it sugar, starch, fat, or alcohol – won't keep your body operating optimally. The clichéd expression 'moderation in all things' has withstood the test of time for obvious reasons. Research shows that moderate daily consumption of refined sugar (30–50 grams or 6–10 teaspoons) doesn't compromise blood glucose management. Keep in mind that this refers not only to the sugar you add to coffee or cereal but also to the sugar already contained in the foods you eat – jams, ice-cream, yoghurt, and so on.

Can GI values obtained from tests on healthy people be applied to people with diabetes?

Yes. Several studies show a strong correlation between values obtained in healthy people and people with diabetes (type 1 and type 2). By its very nature, GI testing takes into account differences in glucose tolerance between people. High GI foods are still digested quickly, and low GI foods are still digested slowly. Some people with diabetes have *gastroparesis*, a disorder in which the emptying of the stomach slows down. The ranking of foods according to their GI values is still applicable.

Some vegetables, such as pumpkin, appear to have higher GI values. Does this mean people with diabetes shouldn't eat them?

People with diabetes can eat pumpkin (GI 66), parsnip (GI 52), turnip and swedes (GI 72), whatever their GI value. Unlike potatoes and cereal products, these vegetables are low in carbohydrate. So their glycemic load is low. Other low carbohydrate vegetables are carrots, broccoli, tomatoes, onions and salad greens, which contain only a small amount of carbohydrate but are packed with micronutrients. They should be considered 'free' foods for everyone. Eat them to your heart's content. See the Vegetables section in the tables in Part 4.

If additional fat and protein cause lower glycemic responses, shouldn't you advocate higher protein or higher fat diets for people with diabetes?

Yes and no. It's a matter of degree and quality, rather than quantity. This type of diet shouldn't be taken to extremes because very low carb diets have little to recommend them – they are difficult to sustain and they don't reduce the risk of chronic disease. If your preference is to eat more protein and fat and moderately reduce carbohydrate intake, then go ahead. The US-based Joslin Clinic for people with diabetes recommends a diet with 40 per cent of energy from carbohydrates (that's lower than is typical), with a greater proportion of protein and good fats. The emphasis should be on quality – good fats, low GI carbs and nutritious protein sources such as fish, poultry, lean red meat, tofu and legumes. If your preference is for higher carbohydrate intake, then that's OK too, but the quality of those carbs is of paramount importance.

I have diabetes, but I enjoy an occasional drink. Is that a problem?

Enjoying a small amount of alcohol with food will have little effect on your blood glucose levels. Indeed recent research from the University of Sydney suggests that a glass or two of wine with or before a meal may reduce glucose levels by 25 per cent. But the amount and kind of carbohydrate you eat with the alcohol is much more important than the alcohol itself. This is because there's very little carbohydrate in most alcoholic drinks: on average, a 285 ml glass of regular beer contains only 5 grams (or 1 teaspoon) of sugars; low alcohol beer has 4 grams; a 100 ml glass of wine has a mere 2 grams; and a standard shot of spirits has less than 1 gram of sugars.

Moderate drinking is the amount that has been linked with the least risk and greatest benefits. The good news is that research indicates that in general, the level of alcohol consumption associated with the least risk for people with diabetes is the same as that for the rest of the adult population. That is, men are advised to drink no more than two standard drinks on any day, women no more than one, and both men and women should aim to have at least two alcohol-free days each week.

However, if you are overweight, have poorly managed blood glucose levels, high blood pressure, high triglycerides or other diabetic complications, your diabetes healthcare team may advise you to drink less or not to drink at all.

Would someone with diabetes need to reduce their insulin dose if they changed to low GI foods?

In theory yes, but in practice no. Most studies have not shown a need for a significantly reduced insulin dose when consuming a low GI diet. This is probably because the insulin dose is dictated not just by carbohydrates in the diet but by protein and fat as well. Preliminary studies of people using insulin pumps have suggested that they could reduce their insulin dosage and maintain the same blood glucose levels, but further research is needed to confirm this.

Low GI basics

When it comes to diabetes, following a low GI diet can be as effective at lowering your blood glucose levels as taking diabetes tablets. On a day-to-day basis, low GI foods can minimise the peaks and troughs in blood glucose that makes life so difficult when you have diabetes. There isn't any optimum diet for all people with diabetes. Whether you eat higher fat, low fat, high protein, high carbohydrate, certain characteristics are desirable

If you have diabetes you should be eating:

- A low GI diet containing wholegrain breads (made with intact kernels); cereals like oats, pearl barley, couscous, cracked wheat, legumes like kidney beans and lentils, and all types of fruit and vegetables.
- Only small amounts of saturated fat. Limit cookies, cakes, butter, potato chips, take-away fried foods, full-fat dairy products, fatty meats and sausages, which are all high in saturated fat. The poly- and mono-unsaturated olive, canola, and peanut oils are healthier types of fats that can be eaten in moderation.
- A moderate amount of sugar and sugar-containing foods. It's OK to include your favourite sweetener or sweet food – small quantities of sugar, honey, maple syrup, jam – to make meals more palatable and pleasurable.
- Only a small quantity of alcohol (see Step 10 in Chapter 13 for guidelines)
- Only a small amount of salt and salted foods. Try lemon juice, freshly ground black pepper, garlic, chilli, herbs, and other flavours instead of relying on salt.

Chapter 6

The GI and pre-diabetes

If you have pre-diabetes (the term used to describe impaired glucose tolerance and/ or impaired fasting glucose), it means that you have blood glucose levels somewhere between normal and diabetes. It's diagnosed by either a fasting blood glucose test or an oral glucose tolerance test.

- Impaired fasting glucose (IFG) is diagnosed if the fasting glucose is 6.1–6.9 mmol/L.
- Impaired glucose tolerance (IGT) is diagnosed after a glucose tolerance test if the 2-hour glucose level is 7.8–11.0 mmol/L.

Studies around the world show that there are twice as many people with pre-diabetes as with diabetes – in fact it is currently estimated that there are about 300 million people worldwide with pre-diabetes. So it is a major public health problem that's only going to get worse unless something is done.

Left untreated, pre-diabetes can develop into type 2 diabetes. It also puts you at risk of some of the complications associated with diabetes, such as heart attacks and stroke. That's why, as well as making lifestyle changes to deal with pre-diabetes, you could also benefit from advice on how to prevent heart disease and stroke.

The good news is that there is very strong evidence that you can prevent, or at the very least delay, getting type 2 diabetes – and all of its complications.

In fact several large studies have shown that three out of five people with pre-diabetes can prevent the development of type 2 diabetes – very good odds indeed.

Be well, know your BGL
(blood glucose level)

Normal ranges for:

Fasting glucose	3.5–6.0 mmol/L
Non-fasting glucose	less than 11.1 mmol/L
Glycated haemoglobin	4.0–6.0 per cent

Risk factors for developing pre-diabetes

If there's type 2 diabetes in your family you probably already know that you have an increased chance of getting it too. But genes alone don't account for the current diabetes/pre-diabetes epidemic. Instead, it's what's being called our 'diabetogenic environment' – the food we eat and our sedentary lifestyle. The most obvious trigger is that we're all getting heavier; and carrying extra body fat goes hand in hand with pre-diabetes and type 2 diabetes. People who are overweight, particularly around their middle, have up to three times more chance of developing type 2 diabetes than people who are in the healthy weight range.

Risk factors you cannot change:
- A family history of diabetes
- Your ethnic background (people of Asian, Indian, Aboriginal, Torres Strait Island, Maori and Pacific Island background have a greater risk)
- Having polycystic ovarian syndrome (PCOS)
- Having diabetes in pregnancy or giving birth to a big baby (more than 4 kilograms), or
- Having heart disease, angina, or having had a heart attack.

Risk factors you can do something about:
- Being overweight, especially if that weight is around your middle
- Being sedentary
- Smoking

- Having high blood pressure
- Having high triglycerides
- Having low HDL (good) cholesterol
- Having high total LDL cholesterol, and
- Unhealthy eating.

Of course not every overweight person is going to develop pre-diabetes or type 2 diabetes (many don't), but the underlying metabolic problem in pre-diabetes and type 2 diabetes – that is, insulin resistance – is exacerbated by being overweight.

As we explain in The GI and diabetes in Chapter 5, insulin resistance means your body cells are resistant to the action of insulin. They don't let glucose in as easily as normal, so the blood glucose level tends to rise. To compensate, the pancreas makes more and more insulin. This eventually moves the glucose into the cells, but the blood insulin levels stay high. Having high insulin levels all the time spells trouble.

Being overweight makes this situation worse because the excess fat 'blocks' the action of the insulin, putting added pressure on the body's ability to maintain optimal blood glucose levels.

Six steps to delay or prevent pre-diabetes

Several studies around the world (in China, Finland, the United States, Japan and India, for example) have shown conclusively that people with pre-diabetes can delay or prevent the development of diabetes. All of these studies were based on people who made lifestyle changes. People increased their level of activity, ate a healthier diet and achieved modest weight loss (about 5–10 kilograms). All these changes are achievable with a little effort, and the long-term benefit is enormous – not having to live with diabetes and reducing your risk of heart attack and stroke.

There's nothing you can do about the inherited risk factors or family history. But you can do something about your weight, the food you eat and a sedentary lifestyle. And if you smoke, you can quit.

1. Aim for moderate weight loss

For most people with pre-diabetes, the first priority has to be reducing body weight. You don't have to lose a lot of weight for it to help. Research has shown that people with pre-diabetes who lose 5–10 per cent of their body weight at diagnosis can prevent or delay the onset of type 2 diabetes.

2. Lower your saturated fat intake

We know that people who develop type 2 diabetes are more likely to have a high saturated fat intake. Saturated fat promotes insulin resistance, making it harder for insulin to do its job of regulating your blood glucose levels. To eat less saturated fat:

Use low-fat dairy products – Routinely purchase low-fat milk, cheese, custard, ice-cream and yoghurt rather than their regular forms.

Choose your snack foods wisely – Don't buy chocolates, biscuits, potato chips, cereal bars, muffin bars, etc.

Cook with the good oils – The healthier oils to use are olive, canola and mustard seed oils.

Take care when you are eating away from home – Give up the French fries and potato wedges with sour cream along with other deep-fried foods, pizza and pies.

Eat lean meats – such as chicken, turkey, red meat trimmed of excess fat.

3. Boost your omega-3 intake

While high fat intakes are associated with diabetes there is one type of fat that's the exception – the very long chain omega-3 fatty acids. Dietary trials in animals and people have shown that increased omega-3 intake can improve insulin sensitivity and therefore could reduce diabetes risk.

Our bodies only make small amounts of these unique fatty acids, so we rely on dietary sources, especially fish and seafood, for them. Aim to include fish in your diet at least twice a week such as a main meal of fresh fish *not* cooked in saturated fat, plus at least one sandwich-sized serving of, say, canned salmon or tuna.

As well as eating these great sources of long-chain omega-3s, you can also increase your total omega-3 intake by eating short-chain omega-3s, which are found in canola oil and margarine, nuts and seeds (particularly walnuts and linseeds), and legumes such as baked beans and soybeans.

4. Lower the GI of your diet

Studies show that people who base their diet on carbohydrates with a low GI are the least likely to develop type 2 diabetes. The findings of some studies suggest that simply changing the bread you eat can make a difference.

5. Increase your fibre intake

Higher fibre intakes are also associated with a lower incidence of type 2 diabetes. Specifically, higher intakes of wholegrain cereals and fruit and vegetables are recommended.

Get the benefit of wholegrains (grains that are eaten in nature's packaging or close to it) with foods such as:

- Barley – try pearl barley in soup, or in recipes such as barley risotto or a barley salad
- Whole-wheat or cracked wheat such as bulgur in tabbouli
- Traditional rolled oats (not instant) for breakfast in porridge or muesli, and
- Wholegrain breads – (low GI versions are best).

If you don't eat much fruit or vegetables at the moment, aim for at least one piece of fruit and two servings of vegetables each day then build up gradually by eating one extra piece of fruit and one extra serving of vegetables each week.

Increase your intake until you reach two servings of fruit and five servings of vegetables every day.

6. Get regular physical activity

All the studies that have proven that a healthy lifestyle can prevent the development of type 2 diabetes have included a comprehensive exercise program in their definition of a healthy lifestyle. You need 150–210 minutes of moderate level physical activity each week, which is of course around 30 minutes of activity each day. The kinds of activities that proved most useful to people with pre-diabetes included walking, jogging, cycling, swimming, dancing and ball games – activities that are suitable for most Australians and New Zealanders.

Physical activity has many benefits, including increasing your lean body mass (giving you more muscles) and decreasing your body fat stores, which lead to lower insulin resistance and better insulin sensitivity. You get these benefits with regular exercise even if you don't lose weight.

And being physically active is not just about playing sport. 'Be more active in as many ways as you can. Think of a movement as an opportunity, not an inconvenience, and make it part of your day,' urge Australia's National Physical Activity Guidelines, as do similar guidelines in many countries around the world.

Low GI basics

Pre-diabetes can develop into type 2 diabetes if left untreated and also increase the risk of complications associated with diabetes such as heart attacks and stroke. Despite 'genetic' factors, there are risk factors that can be addressed by looking at diet and lifestyle.

Tips for managing pre-diabetes

1. Aim for moderate weight loss by adopting a low GI approach to food and swapping high GI foods for low GI, such as more wholegrains, fruits and vegetables.
2. Increase the activity in your day. This doesn't mean big workouts but looking at increasing the incidental exercise in your day such as taking the stairs, walking or cycling to work. If it involves movement of any kind – just do it.
3. On the days that it seems difficult to reach for healthy food or push yourself to exercise – think about the benefits to your heart health and waistline.
4. Encourage your children to exercise. Type 2 diabetes is increasing in young people, so encouraging your children to be more active is a very important part of reducing their risk of later developing pre-diabetes or diabetes. Turning off the TV and computer and getting kids outside to play may be one of the most health-promoting things you can do as a parent.

Chapter 7

The GI and pregnancy

During pregnancy a woman's need for almost all nutrients increases and, while her ability to absorb them also increases appreciably, the key is the food she selects. Most people are aware of the importance of nutrients such as iron, calcium, folate and iodine, but what might not be so clear is that the quality of carbohydrate in the diet can also have a significant impact on the growth and development of the baby. There's even evidence that the type of carbohydrate a woman eats can play a role in increasing her fertility.

To understand the connection between the GI of carbohydrate and pregnancy we need to have a closer look at the importance of glucose to babies.

Babies and blood glucose

A woman's body changes during pregnancy to ensure a steady supply of glucose to her baby. Glucose is the main fuel the baby uses to grow and it crosses freely from mother to baby through the placenta. How much glucose the baby receives depends directly on the mother's blood glucose level and the rate of placental blood flow. The higher the glucose concentration in the mother's blood, the more glucose is transferred to the baby.

In any pregnancy, insulin resistance and increased insulin secretion are normal, as insulin requirements increase by two to three times her normal needs. But for women with a predisposition to diabetes, problems can arise. For example, if the degree of insulin resistance in the mother is too great or if she is unable to make enough extra insulin to meet the demand, her glucose levels will remain elevated. What's more they will become more elevated as her pregnancy progresses, with insulin demand increasing markedly from 28 weeks' gestation – the stage when gestational diabetes is most commonly diagnosed.

Gestational diabetes

Gestational diabetes is the name given to the diagnosis of elevated blood glucose levels during pregnancy. Gestational diabetes occurs in about 7 per cent of all pregnancies in Australia. It is more likely if a woman has risk factors such as:

- A family history of diabetes
- Overweight
- Older in age, or
- Of certain ethnic origin (particularly Southern European, Middle Eastern or Southeast Asian).

The problem with high blood glucose during pregnancy

Although gestational diabetes doesn't usually develop until 28 weeks' gestation, higher than normal blood glucose levels are a concern whenever they occur in pregnancy. Increased glucose is associated with an increased rate of high blood pressure, pre-eclampsia and infection of the placenta (chorioamnionitis).

Furthermore, if a woman's blood glucose level is high, then higher levels of glucose will also be transferred to her baby. Babies make their own insulin from about 15 weeks to handle glucose. So extra glucose stimulates the baby's pancreas to make extra insulin. The extra glucose is metabolised and stored, making the baby grow bigger and fatter than normal.

An overfat baby can present problems for labour and delivery and the newborn infant is also at risk of low blood glucose (hypoglycaemia), low blood calcium (hypocalcaemia), jaundice (hyperbilirubinaemia), respiratory distress and a high red blood cell count (polycythaemia). Any of these conditions may necessitate special medical intervention.

A baby's exposure to high blood glucose also has serious longer term consequences. Children of women who have had gestational diabetes are at greatly increased risk of obesity and glucose intolerance as they grow up. The risk of children becoming overweight adults rises in step with the levels of blood glucose they were exposed to during pregnancy. Untreated gestational diabetes, for example, doubles a child's risk of being overweight or obese by five to seven years of age.

The good news for pregnant women is that by treating elevated glucose levels during pregnancy, the risk of any problems drops considerably. And this is where the GI comes to the fore. Foods with a low GI typically evoke a lower rise in blood glucose levels, making maintenance of normal glucose levels easier. Lower blood glucose rises after meals means a lower demand for insulin, too, which can lessen the load when the mother's pancreas is struggling.

A recent study in just over 1000 pregnant women confirmed a relationship between the GI of the women's diets and their glucose levels. The researchers found that the lower the GI of the mum-to-be's diet, the lower her average blood glucose (HbA1c) and the lower her response to a glucose load. So the good news is that following a low GI diet means lower blood glucose levels during pregnancy.

The benefit of a low GI diet in pregnancy has been further demonstrated by an Australian study. The researchers led by endocrinologist Dr Robert Moses compared the outcomes of pregnant women eating either low or high GI diets. Both types of diet were equally nutritious. The babies of mothers eating a low GI diet were of normal size, but were smaller and had less body fat than the babies of mothers eating the moderate to high GI high fibre, low sugar diet. This study showed that the GI appears to have a more important effect on birthweight than any single dietary factor, including the amount of protein, fat or carbohydrate.

The future impact of gestational diabetes

If you've had gestational diabetes in one pregnancy you are likely to get it in subsequent pregnancies. You also have a high risk of of developing type 2 diabetes at some point later in life. Depending on your risk factors such as your age, ethnic background, weight and your glucose levels during pregnancy, that point could be closer than you think. A recent study found one-third of women had developed type 2 diabetes within five years of having gestational diabetes. It is important to see your doctor every year to be screened for diabetes too.

Diabetes before pregnancy

When diabetes exists before pregnancy, it greatly increases the risk of birth defects. However, this risk depends almost entirely on a mother's glycemic control before and during her pregnancy. One of the most critical times for good glucose control is during the first seven to eight weeks' gestation because this is when the baby's major organs are formed.

One of the major events at this time is the formation of the neural tube (the baby's future brain and spinal cord). At this early stage the baby's pancreas hasn't started working so its concentration of glucose is a direct reflection of the mum-to-be's blood glucose. When the mother's blood glucose levels are high, the baby is flooded with extra glucose at a rate much greater than normal. Breaking down this glucose requires oxygen, but so much glucose means the baby uses oxygen faster than it can be delivered. The resulting shortage of oxygen is one of the reasons that cells die and malformations occur.

With careful management of blood glucose levels a woman with diabetes can have a perfectly healthy pregnancy. But, as you might imagine, an unplanned pregnancy along with poor glycemic control could have serious consequences for the unborn child. If it's unexpected, a woman can be eight weeks or more into a pregnancy before she knows about it and if her blood glucose levels are high, damage can already be done.

The message should be clear: if you have diabetes and could get pregnant, make sure you have good blood glucose control first.

If you have diabetes, pre-diabetes or even a risk of diabetes, plan pregnancy with good blood glucose levels in mind. Following a low GI diet could help you achieve this. Neural tube defects are linked to poor glycemic control and US research has suggested a link between the GI of a woman's diet during early pregnancy and the risk of her baby developing a neural tube defect.

Reducing your risk of gestational diabetes

Although pregnancy can unmask a predisposition to diabetes, developing gestational diabetes may not be inevitable even if you are at risk. Gestational diabetes is the result of a combination of factors – your genetic susceptibility plus risk factors such as a high-fat diet and sedentary lifestyle. Living a healthy lifestyle could reduce your risk.

We know, for example, that being overweight increases your risk of gestational diabetes, but research suggests that eating a diet with a high glycemic load is just as risky.

In a US study of more than 10 000, predominantly Caucasian, women, those who had a high-glycemic-load diet with low fibre content were twice as likely to develop gestational diabetes as other, similar women, independent of their body mass index.

Getting pregnant

If you're having difficulty getting pregnant due to problems with ovulation, a low GI diet could help. Glucose control and insulin sensitivity are important determinants of ovulation and fertility and a study published in *Obstetrics & Gynecology* in 2007 suggested that modifications to diet and lifestyle could prevent most cases of ovulatory infertility. Key dietary aspects favouring fertility were higher consumption of monounsaturated fat rather than trans fat, vegetable rather than animal protein sources, and low GI carbohydrates.

Common questions

Is there a GI plan for breastfeeding mothers?

A low GI diet is ideal while you are breastfeeding. Breastfeeding requires a lot of energy and theoretically this additional energy comes from the body fat laid down during pregnancy. Of course in reality it often doesn't all get used up and many new mothers have to make a concerted effort to work off the baby weight. To do this, though, it is important that you don't go on a low kilojoule diet or any sort of extreme measure such as the low carb diets popular in the media. Since breastfeeding tends to increase your appetite (the body's way of ensuring you have the energy required to produce milk) this is good news, as staying on such a diet would be a nightmare! This is what makes the low GI approach so successful – forget about trying to count kilojoules or even your portions of food.

First and foremost focus on the sorts of foods you are eating. Low GI foods are the wholegrains, fresh fruit and vegetables and legumes. By eating these foods as the mainstay of your meals you can trust your appetite and eat to satisfaction while you are breastfeeding. Also get back to some exercise – even if it's just a daily walk with the pram. You should then find that the weight slowly starts to shift – realistically give yourself at least that first six months to get back to your pre-pregnancy weight.

Your daily food guide for healthy eating during pregnancy

A healthy, low GI diet during pregnancy includes:

- 6–10 servings of low GI breads, cereals and other starchy carbs
- 2–3 servings of fruit
- 2–3 servings of low-fat milk products or alternatives
- 3 servings of lean meat or alternatives
- 3 servings of healthy fats, and
- 5–6 servings or more of vegetables.

A menu for the day might look something like this:

Breakfast	*Example*
1 serving of fruit	150 ml fruit juice
2 servings of low GI bread	2 slices of low GI toast, each spread with
1 serving of healthy fats	1 teaspoon of canola margarine
1 serving of vegetables	1 large grilled tomato
½ serve of lean meat or alternative	1 poached egg

Snack	*Example*
1 serving of fruit	3 fresh apricots
1 serving of healthy fats	10 almonds

Lunch	*Example*
2 servings of low GI carbs	1 cup of steamed basmati rice
1 serving of lean meat or alternative	100 g canned tuna or salmon
1 serving of vegetables	1 cup of salad vegetables such as strips of red capsicum, shallots, cucumber and carrot dressed with
1 serving of fat	1 tablespoon of oil/vinegar dressing
1 serving of milk or milk product	1 glass of low-fat milk

Snack   *Example*
1 serving of milk or milk product   A cup of low-fat fruit yoghurt

Dinner   *Example*
1½ servings of lean meat   150 g lean beef steak or chicken
   or alternative   1½ cups of steamed broccoli, snow
3 servings of vegetables   peas, carrot and baby squash
                                              dressed with lemon juice
3 servings of low GI carbs   3 baby new potatoes and 1 fresh cob
                                              of sweet corn

Snack   *Example*
1 serving milk product or fruit   A cup of low-fat milk with Milo® or a
                                              cup of fresh fruit salad

Eating well during pregnancy

To eat for optimum health for you and your baby plus maintain a
healthy weight, make a switch to a low GI eating plan. Take a look at
the 10 step guide to low GI eating in Chapter 13 to get you started.
Of course, there are additional requirements for what to include in
your diet when pregnant, including good sources of protein,
increasing calcium and iron intake, limiting foods high in saturated
fats and holding back on the refined sugar found in soft drinks,
confectionery, chips and highly processed food.

Low GI basics

Controlling blood glucose with a low GI diet combined with regular exercise and a healthy eating plan can reduce the risk of gestational diabetes by reducing high blood glucose levels that can be detrimental to both the baby and the mother.

Tips for managing your diet through pregnancy

- Eat small, frequent meals.
- Choose low GI breads, breakfast cereals and rice, and include pasta, fruit, legumes and low-fat milk and milk products as low GI sources of carbohydrate.
- Include good sources of protein in meals – such as lean meat, poultry, fish and seafood, eggs, nuts, low-fat cheese and cottage cheese.
- Eat plenty of vegetables and salads.
- Limit foods high in saturated fat such as cakes, biscuits, pastries, sausage, salami, chips, takeaway foods, butter, cream – high saturated fat diets are linked with the development of insulin resistance.
- Limit food and drinks containing large amounts of refined or added sugar or starch with low nutritive value, such as soft drink, confectionery, chips and other packet snacks.
- Avoid alcohol. Drink plenty of water.
- Use iodised salt – sparingly – in cooking to help prevent iodine deficiency.

Chapter 8

The GI and hypoglycaemia

Your body needs to maintain a minimum threshold level of glucose in the blood at all times to keep the brain and central nervous system functioning. If for some reason blood glucose levels fall below this threshold (specifically, below 4 mmol/L, the low end of the normal range), you experience hypoglycaemia. It comes from the Greek words 'hypo' (meaning under) and 'glycaemia' (meaning blood glucose) – hence *blood glucose level below normal.*

If you already have diabetes and are treating it with medication, you probably already know all about hypoglycaemia. If you don't have diabetes but you have vague health problems, including fatigue and depression, and you think you may have hypoglycaemia or someone tells you that you probably have 'low blood sugar', you need to see your doctor and get a proper diagnosis.

Hypoglycaemia has a variety of unpleasant consequences. Many of these are stress-like symptoms such as anxiety, trembling, sweating, palpitations, dizziness and nausea. Poor concentration, drowsiness and lack of coordination may also be experienced. For people with type 1 diabetes, treatment with readily absorbed carbohydrate is essential. Without this, coma and even death may ensue.

This is not the case, however, for people without diabetes who experience 'reactive' hypoglycaemia, which occurs after eating and is the most common form of hypoglycaemia. When blood glucose levels rise too quickly after eating, they cause an excessive amount of insulin to be released. This draws too much glucose out of the blood and causes the blood glucose level to fall below normal. The result is hypoglycaemia.

The diagnosis of reactive hypoglycaemia *cannot* be made simply on the basis of symptoms. Instead, it requires the detection of low blood glucose levels when the symptoms are actually being experienced. A blood test is required to do this – a home blood glucose meter is not considered precise enough for the diagnosis of hypoglycaemia in people without diabetes. Because it may be difficult – or almost impossible – for someone to be in the right place at the right time to have a blood sample taken while experiencing the symptoms, a glucose tolerance test (GTT) is sometimes used to try to make the diagnosis. This involves drinking pure glucose, which causes the blood glucose levels to rise. If too much insulin is produced in response, a person with reactive hypoglycaemia will experience an excessive fall in their blood glucose level. Sounds simple enough, but there are pitfalls.

Testing must be done under strictly controlled conditions; low blood glucose is best demonstrated by measuring properly collected blood samples. If your doctor uses an oral glucose tolerance test to diagnose hypoglycaemia, you have to continue it for at least three to four hours (the normal time is two hours). Your insulin levels would be measured at the same time.

- Hypoglycaemia is far less common than once was thought (unless you have diabetes).
- Hypoglycaemia due to a serious medical problem is rare.

Treating hypoglycaemia

The aim of treating reactive hypoglycaemia is to prevent sudden, large increases in blood glucose levels. If the blood glucose level can be prevented from rising quickly, then excessive, unnecessary amounts of insulin will not be produced and the blood glucose levels will not plunge to abnormally low levels.

Smooth, steady blood glucose levels can readily be achieved by switching from high GI foods to low GI foods. This is particularly important when you eat foods that contain carbohydrates by themselves. Low GI foods such as wholegrain bread, low-fat yoghurt and low GI fruits are best for snacks.

If you can stop the big swings in blood glucose levels, then you will not get the symptoms of reactive hypoglycaemia, and chances are you will feel a lot better.

Notably, hypoglycaemia due to a serious medical problem is rare. Such conditions require in-depth investigation and treatment of the underlying medical problem causing hypoglycaemia. But having an irregular eating pattern is the most common dietary habit seen in people who have hypoglycaemia.

How to treat hypoglycaemia

Raise your blood glucose levels quickly with rapid-acting carbohydrate such as:

- Glucose tablets or gels (10–20 grams), or
- ½ cup regular (not diet) soft drink, fruit juice, or sweetened fruit beverage
- 4 large jelly beans or 7 small jelly beans, or
- 2–3 teaspoons of sugar

Follow within 15–20 minutes with carbohydrate foods that will maintain blood glucose levels:

- 1 slice of low GI bread, or
- 1 banana or apple, or
- A container of unsweetened yoghurt (170–227 grams) or ½ a container (85–113 grams) of sweetened yoghurt, or
- 1 glass of low-fat milk

Low GI basics

The aim of treating hypoglycaemia is to prevent sudden, large increases in blood glucose levels. Smooth, steady blood glucose levels can be achieved by switching from high GI foods to low GI foods.

Tips for managing hypoglycaemia

- Eat regular meals and snacks – plan to eat every 3 hours.
- Include low GI carbohydrate foods at every meal and for snacks.
- Mix high GI foods with low GI foods in your meals – the combination will give an overall intermediate or medium GI.
- Avoid eating high GI foods on their own for snacks – this can trigger reactive hypoglycaemia.
- Having an irregular eating pattern is the most common dietary habit seen in people who have hypoglycaemia.

Chapter 9

The GI and heart health

According to the National Heart Foundation, heart disease kills one Australian every 10 minutes. For New Zealanders the figure is one death every hour. It is the single biggest killer of Australians and New Zealanders.

Most heart disease is caused by atherosclerosis, also referred to as 'hardening of the arteries'. Most people develop atherosclerosis gradually during their lifetime. If it occurs slowly it may not cause any problems at all, even into old age. But if its development is accelerated by one or more of many processes (such as high cholesterol or high blood glucose levels), it can develop faster and cause trouble sooner.

Atherosclerosis leads to reduced blood flow through the affected arteries. In the heart, this can mean that the heart muscle does not receive enough oxygen to provide the power for pumping blood, and it changes in such a way that it causes pain (particularly, central chest pain, or angina pectoris).

Knowing your blood glucose level is just as important as knowing your cholesterol level to help prevent heart disease.

96 LOW GI DIET handbook

Elsewhere in the body, atherosclerosis has a similar blood-flow-reducing effect: in the legs it can cause muscle pains during exercise; in the brain it can cause a variety of problems, from irregular gait to strokes.

An even more serious consequence of atherosclerosis occurs when a blood clot forms over the surface of a patch of atherosclerosis on an artery. This process, called thrombosis, can result in a complete blockage of the artery, with consequences ranging from sudden death to a small heart attack from which the patient recovers quickly.

Thrombosis can happen elsewhere in the body, and the extent of it determines how serious it is. The probability of developing thrombosis depends on the tendency of the blood to clot versus the natural ability of the blood to break down clots (fibrinolysis). These two counteracting tendencies are influenced by a number of factors, including the level of glucose in the blood.

People who have gradually developed atherosclerosis of the arteries to the heart (which are called the coronary arteries) may gradually develop reduced heart function. For a while the heart may be able to compensate for the problem, so there are no symptoms, but eventually it begins to fail. It might start with shortness of breath, initially on exercise, and there may sometimes be swelling of the ankles.

Modern medicine has many effective drug treatments for heart failure, so this consequence of atherosclerosis does not now have quite the same serious implications it had in the past.

Risk factors for heart disease

Risk factors you cannot change:
- Being male
- Being older
- Your ethnic background
- Having a family history of heart disease, and
- Being postmenopausal

Risk factors you can do something about:
- Smoking
- High blood pressure
- Having diabetes or pre-diabetes
- Having high blood cholesterol, high triglycerides and low levels of the 'good' (HDL) cholesterol
- Having elevated CRP (C-reactive protein) levels (a marker of low-grade chronic inflammation somewhere in the body)
- Being overweight or obese, or having extra fat around your abdomen, and
- Being sedentary

Why do people get heart disease?

Atherosclerotic heart disease develops early in life when the many factors that cause it have a strong influence. Over many decades doctors and scientists have identified the risk factors (what we call red flags) in healthy people as well as in those with established heart disease. Your risk of developing heart disease is determined by things you cannot change, such as genetic (inherited) factors, and things you can do something about.

When heart disease is detected, two types of treatment are typically given. First, the effects of the disease are treated (for example, medical treatment with drugs and surgical treatment to bypass blocked arteries); and, second, the risk factors are treated in order to slow down further progression of the disease.

Treatment of risk factors after the disease has already developed is secondary prevention. In people who have not yet developed the disease, addressing risk factors that contribute to heart disease is primary prevention.

The risk factors you can do something about:

Smoking

Smokers have more than twice the risk of heart attack as non-smokers and are much more likely to die if they suffer a heart attack. Smoking is also the most preventable risk factor for heart disease. Smokers tend to eat fewer fruits and vegetables compared with non-smokers (and thus miss out on vital protective anti-oxidant plant compounds). Smokers also tend to eat more fat and more salt than non-smokers. While these dietary differences may put the smoker at greater risk of heart disease, there is only one piece of advice for anyone who smokes: quit.

High blood pressure

High blood pressure is the most common heart disease risk factor. High blood pressure (hypertension) is harmful because it demands that your heart work harder and it damages your arteries.

An artery is a muscular tube. Healthy arteries can change their size to control the flow of blood. High blood pressure causes changes in the walls of arteries, which makes atherosclerosis more likely to develop. Blood clots can then form and the weakened blood vessels can easily develop a thrombosis (clot) or rupture and bleed.

Having diabetes and pre-diabetes

Diabetes and pre-diabetes cause inflammation and hardening of the arteries. High levels of glucose in the blood, even short-term spikes after a meal, can have many undesirable effects and are a predictor of future heart disease. A high level of glucose in the blood means:

- The cells lining the arteries take up excessive amounts of glucose.
- Highly reactive charged particles called 'free radicals' are formed, which gradually destroy the machinery inside the cell, eventually causing the cell's death.
- Glucose adheres to cholesterol in the blood, which promotes the formation of fatty plaque and prevents the body from breaking down cholesterol.
- Higher levels of insulin develop, which in turn raise blood pressure and blood fats, while suppressing 'good' (HDL) cholesterol levels. This cholesterol seems to protect against heart disease because it clears cholesterol from our arteries and helps its removal from our bodies. Having low levels of HDL in the blood is one of the most important markers of heart disease.

High insulin levels also increase the tendency for blood clots to form. This is why so much effort is put into helping people with diabetes achieve normal control of blood glucose levels. Even when cholesterol levels appear to be normal, other risk factors, such as triglycerides, can be highly abnormal.

Even moderately raised blood glucose levels before or after a meal have been associated with increased risk of heart disease in normal 'healthy' people. (For more information on diabetes complications see The GI and diabetes in Chapter 5.)

High blood cholesterol

Cholesterol is vital for healthy cells. Our bodies can make most of the cholesterol we need – about 1000 mg per day – but in certain circumstances, we make more than necessary. This causes the level of cholesterol in our blood to build up, and that's when problems occur. When the body accumulates too much cholesterol, it can be deposited on the walls of the arteries, which become bloated and damaged and may become blocked. 'Bad' or LDL cholesterol does the most damage to the blood vessels and is a risk factor for heart disease.

The blood also contains triglycerides, another type of fat linked to increased risk of heart disease. Having too much triglyceride is often linked with having too little HDL cholesterol. Although people can inherit having excess levels of triglycerides, it's most often associated with being overweight or obese.

Having high blood cholesterol is partly determined by our genes, which can 'set' the cholesterol level slightly high and which we cannot change; and partly by lifestyle or dietary factors, which push it up further – which we can do something about.

A diet high in saturated fat is the biggest contributor. Diets recommended for lowering blood cholesterol are low in saturated fat, high in good carbohydrate (particularly wholegrains) and high in fibre.

There are some relatively rare genetic conditions in which particularly high blood cholesterol levels occur. People who have inherited these conditions need a thorough examination by a specialist doctor followed by a rigorous cholesterol-lowering eating plan combined with drug treatment to reduce and control the risk of heart disease.

C-reactive protein (CRP)

Scientists have recently established that CRP in the blood is a powerful risk factor for heart disease. It is a measure of chronic low-grade inflammation anywhere in the body and shows the damaging effect of high glucose levels and other factors on the blood vessel walls.

Studies at Harvard have shown that CRP levels are higher in women consuming high GI/high GL diets. That's one more good reason to choose low GI!

Being overweight or obese, or having extra fat around your abdomen

Overweight and obese people are more likely to have high blood pressure and diabetes. They are also at increased risk of developing heart disease. Some of that increased risk is due to high blood pressure and the tendency to diabetes, but there is a separate, 'independent' effect of obesity.

When increased fatness develops, it can be distributed evenly all over the body or it may occur centrally – in and around the abdomen. The latter is strongly associated with heart disease. In fact, you can have 'middle-age spread' – a potbelly or a 'muffin midriff' – and still be within a normal weight range. But that extra fat around the middle is playing havoc with your metabolism. Abdominal fat increases our risk of heart disease, high blood pressure and diabetes. In contrast, fat on the lower part of the body, such as hips and thighs, doesn't carry the same health risk.

The International Diabetes Federation has established new criteria for defining metabolic syndrome that reduce waist circumference thresholds to make it easier for doctors to identify people who have the condition. (A person with metabolic syndrome will have abdominal obesity plus at least two of the following other risk factors: high triglycerides, low HDL cholesterol, elevated blood pressure and/or increased blood glucose.) The recommended limits of waist measurement are:

For people of European origin
- Men 94 cm
- Women 88 cm

For people from South Asia and China
- Men 90 cm
- Women 80 cm

More information is available at www.idf.org/home/

Being sedentary

People who aren't active or don't exercise have higher rates of death and heart disease compared to people who perform even mild to moderate amounts of physical activity. Even gardening or going for a walk can lower your risk of heart disease.

Exercise and activity speed up your metabolic rate (increasing the amount of energy you use), which helps to balance your food intake and control your weight. Exercise and activity also make your muscles more sensitive to insulin (you'll need less to get the job done) and increase the amount of fat you burn.

The effect of exercise doesn't end when you stop moving. People who exercise have higher metabolic rates, and their bodies burn more kilojoules per minute even when they are asleep.

Preventing heart disease

Thankfully, more and more people have their blood pressure tested and are checked for diabetes regularly. Increasingly, blood-fat tests are done to check people's risk factors for heart disease as well. If you haven't been checked recently, ask your doctor for these tests.

A good health professional will offer lifestyle advice that can reduce your risk of heart disease, including stopping smoking, regular exercise and eating a healthy diet. But often, people find it difficult to follow this advice for long. This is especially true if heart disease isn't an immediate and life-threatening problem. But remember that it's better to take steps to be healthy today than to wait until heart disease has dramatically impaired your health.

Metabolic syndrome and insulin resistance increase the risk of heart attacks

Surveys show that one in two adults over the age of 25 has at least two features of what is seen to be a silent disease: the metabolic syndrome, or insulin resistance syndrome. This syndrome (sometimes called Syndrome X) is a collection of metabolic abnormalities that can 'silently' increase your risk of heart attack. The list of features is getting longer and longer, and the number of diseases linked to insulin resistance is growing.

People with metabolic syndrome are three times as likely to have a heart attack or stroke compared with people without the syndrome and they have a fivefold greater risk of developing type 2 diabetes (if it's not already present).

The metabolic syndrome is a cluster of risk factors for a serious heart attack, recognised as a 'cardiovascular time bomb'. In 2005, the International Diabetes Federation agreed on a definition of metabolic syndrome to make it easier for doctors to identify people who are at risk. A person with metabolic syndrome will have extra fat around the abdomen plus two of the following risk factors:

- High triglycerides
- Low HDL cholesterol
- Raised blood glucose, and
- Raised blood pressure.

The key to understanding metabolic syndrome is insulin resistance, which is discussed in The GI and diabetes in Chapter 5. Tests on people with the metabolic syndrome show that insulin resistance is very common. If your doctor has told you that you have high blood pressure and pre-diabetes (formerly you might have been advised you have 'a touch of sugar' or 'impaired glucose tolerance'), then you probably have metabolic syndrome.

The GI and heart health

The GI is vitally important for coronary health and the prevention of heart disease. First, it has benefits for weight control (see The GI and Weight Control), helping to satisfy appetite and preventing overeating. Secondly it helps reduce post-meal blood glucose levels, which improves the elasticity of the walls of the arteries, making dilation easier and improving blood flow. Thirdly, blood fats and clotting factors can also be improved by low GI diets. Studies have shown that HDL levels

> **By working on several fronts at once, a low GI diet has a distinct advantage over other types of diet or drugs that target only one risk factor at a time.**

are correlated with the GI and GL of the diet. People with the lowest GI diets have the highest and best levels of HDL – the good cholesterol.

Furthermore, research studies in people with diabetes have shown that low GI diets reduce triglycerides in the blood, a factor strongly linked to heart disease. Last, low GI diets have been shown to improve insulin sensitivity in people at high risk of heart disease, thereby helping to reduce the increase in blood glucose and insulin levels after eating.

Research shows that low GI diets not only improve blood glucose in people with diabetes, but they also improve the sensitivity of the body to insulin.

In a recent study, patients with serious disease of the coronary arteries were given either low or high GI diets before surgery for coronary bypass grafts. They were given blood tests before their diets and just before surgery and during surgery small pieces of fat tissue were removed for testing. The tests on the fat showed that the low GI diets made the tissues of these 'insulin insensitive' patients more sensitive – in fact, they were back in the same range as normal control patients after just a few weeks on the low GI diet.

In another study, young women in their thirties were divided into those who did and those who did not have a family history of heart disease and had not yet developed the condition. They had blood tests followed by low or high GI diets for four weeks, after which they had more blood tests. When they had surgery (for conditions unrelated to heart disease), pieces of fat were removed and tested for insulin sensitivity. The young women with a family history of heart disease were insensitive to insulin originally (those without the family history of heart disease were normal), but after four weeks on the low GI diet, their insulin sensitivity was back within the normal range.

In both studies, the diets were designed to try to ensure that all the other variables (total energy, total carbohydrates) were not different, so that the change in insulin sensitivity was likely to have been due to the low GI diet rather than any other factor.

Work on these exciting findings continues, but what is known so far strongly suggests that a low GI diet not only improves body weight and blood glucose in people with diabetes, but it also improves the body's sensitivity to insulin.

One major study provides the strongest evidence in support of the role of GI in heart disease. Conducted by Harvard University and commonly referred to as the Nurses' Health Study, this ongoing, long-term study follows over 100 000 nurses, who every few years provide their personal health and diet information to researchers at Harvard School of Public Health.

Recent research reported in the *British Journal of Nutrition* found that eating just one extra low GI item per meal can lower blood glucose levels and reduce the risk of metabolic syndrome.

The Nurses' Health Study found that those who ate more high GI foods had nearly twice the risk of having a heart attack over a ten-year period of follow-up compared to those eating low GI diets. This association was independent of dietary fibre and other known risk factors, such as age and body mass index, or BMI. In other words, even if fibre intake was high, there was still an adverse effect of high

The importance of low GI wholegrains

We've all heard the advice to increase our intake of wholegrain foods to improve heart health, but a recent study from Professor Susan Jebb in Cambridge in the United Kingdom suggests that high GI wholegrains may not be as helpful as we thought. In her study, she required volunteers to consume 60 grams or 120 grams of wholegrain foods such as bread and breakfast cereal every day for two to four months. Disappointingly, not one single risk factor for heart disease improved. It's possible that wholegrains that produce blood sugar spikes are countering any positive effects of all the goodness found in wholegrains. So make sure that any wholegrains you choose also come with a low GI.

GI diets on risk. Importantly, neither sugar nor total carbohydrate intake showed any association with risk of heart attack. That means there was no evidence that lower carbohydrate or sugar intake was helpful.

One of the most important findings of the Nurses' Health Study was that the increased risk associated with high GI diets was largely seen in those with a BMI over 23. There was no increased risk in those under 23. The great majority of adults, however, have a BMI greater than 23; indeed, a BMI of 23 to 25 is considered normal weight. The implication therefore is that the insulin resistance that comes with increasing weight is an integral part of the disease process.

If you are very lean and insulin sensitive, high GI diets won't make you more prone to heart attack. This might explain why traditional-living Asian populations, such as the Chinese, who eat high GI rice as a staple food, do not show increased risk of heart disease. Their low BMI and their high level of physical activity work together to keep them insulin sensitive and extremely carbohydrate tolerant.

It will take many years of further research to show that this simple dietary change to a low GI diet will definitely slow the progress of atherosclerotic heart disease. In the meantime, it is already clear that risk factors for heart disease are improved by a low GI diet.

Common questions

I understand that low GI foods help keep blood glucose stable. What's wrong with high blood glucose levels?

High blood glucose levels pose a threat to your health even if you don't have diabetes. In fact, elevated blood glucose levels within the 'normal' range can damage the blood vessels and circulatory system, increasing the risk of a heart attack, type 2 diabetes, weight gain and even certain types of cancer. It does so by increasing the production of damaging free radicals and creating oxidative stress and inflammation.

Over time, the effects of high blood glucose levels become even more noticeable. In people with diabetes in poor control, problems may occur with the skin, leading to bacterial infections, fungal infections and itching. Nerves may be damaged, causing numbness, prickling, tingling, burning and aching sensations. There may even be a loss of nerve function so that a process like digestion is impaired. The narrowing of large blood vessels will slow blood flow and cause heart disease, stroke and the loss of circulation, which can lead to amputation. Small blood vessels may become damaged, which can cause problems that may include blurry vision, blindness and kidney disease.

For all of these reasons, we advise that eating a diet rich in low GI foods helps to control blood glucose levels in people with and without diabetes, and can ward off both short- and long-term health problems.

Low GI basics

Low GI diets are consistent with the other required dietary changes needed for prevention of heart disease.

Heart disease is the single biggest killer of Australians and New Zealanders. There are risk factors for heart disease that cannot be changed, such as genetics, but risk factors such as smoking, high blood pressure, diabetes and pre-diabetes, high blood cholesterol and being overweight or obese can be changed through lifestyle and dietary changes.

Metabolic syndrome or insulin resistance syndrome dramatically increases the risk of having a heart attack or stroke.

By working on several fronts (lowering blood glucose levels, encouraging a healthy range of foods, improving body weight), a low GI diet has a distinct advantage over other types of diets or drugs that target only one risk factor at a time.

Tips for managing your risk of heart disease and metabolic syndrome

- Reduce the risk factors by stopping smoking, exercising more, losing a little extra weight and working on lowering blood pressure and cholesterol levels.
- Work towards a diet that is rich in slowly digested, low GI carbohydrates.
- Choose fruits and vegetables and wholegrain breads over high salt or sugary pre-prepared snacks.

Chapter 10

The GI and PCOS

Polycystic ovarian syndrome, or PCOS, often goes unrecognised, yet it is very common. Elements of the disease are believed to affect one in four women in developed nations; the severe form affects one in 20. It is a health condition linked with hormone imbalance and insulin resistance.

The signs range from subtle symptoms, such as faint facial hair, to a 'full house' of symptoms – lack of periods, heavy body-hair growth, obstinate central body fat and infertility. They can occur at any age, and can even be seen in girls as young as 10 or women as old as 70. (Contrary to popular belief, PCOS does not suddenly disappear at menopause.)

Not only are the symptoms distressing, but PCOS has also been tied to an increased risk of heart disease and type 2 diabetes. You may also see it referred to as polycystic ovarian disease, Stein-Leventhal syndrome or functional ovarian hyperandrogenism.

Only a doctor can diagnose PCOS. If you have any of the following symptoms, you should see your GP and ask him or her to refer you to an endocrinologist for proper diagnosis and treatment.

- Delayed (or early) puberty
- Irregular or no periods
- Acne
- Excess body or facial hair

- Unexplained fatigue
- Excess weight around the waistline
- Infertility
- Mood swings
- Hot flashes in young women
- Sleep disorders such as sleep apnoea or insomnia
- Recurrent spontaneous miscarriages
- Inappropriate lactation
- Drop in blood pressure on standing up or with exercise
- Rough, dark skin in the neck folds and armpits, a mark of severe insulin resistance from any cause, and
- Hypoglycaemia (low blood glucose) after meals. The most common symptoms are light-headedness, sweating, sudden fatigue and a 'butterflies in the stomach' feeling.

It is vital to diagnose and treat PCOS as early as possible to prevent it from developing to the 'full-blown' syndrome. Keep in mind that some women do not show the 'classic' signs at all, which is why consulting a doctor who knows the many facets of PCOS is so important.

Insulin resistance and PCOS

Most women with PCOS have severe insulin resistance and as a result, high insulin levels. The problem is that insulin stimulates the growth and multiplication of cells in the ovary – in particular, those that make up the bulk of the ovary in which the eggs are embedded, causing them to become cystic (forms cysts). This flood of insulin leads to a vicious cycle of hormonal imbalance that creates the symptoms of PCOS.

The receptors for insulin in the ovaries are different from those in other tissues; when blood insulin levels are high, the ovary does not turn down insulin receptor numbers or reduce their activity. As a result, the action of insulin continues unabated, and ovarian cells grow and multiply and increase their metabolic activity. The result is excessive production of both male sex hormone (testosterone) and female sex hormone (oestrogen).

High testosterone levels in women bring about 'male' characteristics in women, such as weight gain and excessive hair on the face and in other areas. Excess insulin and sex hormones also stimulate an area in the brain called the hypothalamus, making it more sensitive and causing it to secrete more luteinizing hormone. This stimulates the ovaries' hormone production even more, causing a vicious cycle. Breaking that cycle is the key to managing PCOS successfully.

Insulin resistance is more common in some people than others, for example, people of Asian descent have been found to be more resistant than Caucasians. Native American, Australian Aboriginals and Pacific Islanders are more insulin resistant than most. Not surprisingly, PCOS also runs in families and may have a genetic link.

Environmental factors such as diet and a lack of physical exercise may also play a role. We also know that weight gain can trigger insulin resistance and PCOS, as can certain steroid medications. While being overweight or obese increases the degree of insulin resistance, you can be lean and still have PCOS.

Managing PCOS

Although there's no cure as such for PCOS, keeping the symptoms under control is well within your grasp by making some diet and lifestyle changes that will encourage hormonal stabilisation.

When you see your doctor, you'll find that any medical management is usually tailored to your symptoms and to some extent your priorities – regular periods, a much-wanted pregnancy, or simply a reduction in facial hair. It usually involves lifestyle changes such as eating well and exercising more, along with insulin-sensitising medication, such as metformin, to:

- Improve your PCOS symptoms – regulating menstrual cycles, reducing acne and excess hair growth
- Achieve and maintain a healthy weight
- Control your blood glucose and insulin levels
- Stabilise your hormone levels
- Boost fertility, and
- Give you more control and quality of life.

The one thing women with PCOS say again and again is that they feel 'out of control'

Insulin resistance leads to a vicious cycle of hormonal imbalance that creates the symptoms of PCOS

– gaining weight, being unable to get pregnant, growing an excessive amount of body hair in areas where it shouldn't be, and so on. The good news is that by making some basic lifestyle changes – like choosing the right kinds of foods and exercising more – you'll find yourself back in the driver's seat again. An additional benefit of making these changes is that you will reduce your future risk of developing diabetes and heart disease. Here are some steps towards taking charge.

Step 1: Manage your weight

Managing your weight is essential if you have PCOS. That's because being overweight increases insulin resistance and worsens the symptoms of PCOS. You don't need to lose a lot of weight – or body fat – to improve your symptoms. Studies show that losing as little as 5 per cent of body weight can help improve menstrual function, reduce testosterone levels, reduce excess hair growth and lessen acne. How much weight does this actually mean? Well, if you weigh 100 kilograms, this means losing about 5 kilograms of body fat can make a difference; if you're 80 kilograms, losing just 4 kilograms would bring about a change.

So what's the healthiest way to lose weight? First of all, aim to lose body *fat* rather than simply *weight*. Put the scales away and get out the tape measure, or even go by how your clothes fit. Remember, muscle weighs more than fat – so as you begin to exercise more, you may be shedding fat but adding muscle, meaning the scale might not reflect just how much you're changing.

Second, don't think about going on a restrictive diet, as it will only make you feel deprived and lead to a blow-out. Instead, incorporate low GI foods into a healthy diet.

Third, be patient; it takes time to lose body fat.

And last, get moving. Regular physical activity every day will not only help you get fit and trim, but will also improve your heart and bone health, reduce your risk of diabetes and help you manage stress.

Step 2: Eat the healthy, low GI way

The GI plays a key role in helping you beat PCOS symptoms, because it focuses on carbohydrates – their quantity and quality, and their overall effect on your blood glucose. Controlling your blood glucose levels is the first step to increasing your insulin sensitivity. If you base your diet on eating balanced low GI meals, you will make it easier for your body to burn fat and less likely for the fat to be stored in places where you don't want it. If you find it hard to get started, get help from a registered dietitian. In our most recent study, we found that women with PCOS showed greater improvements in insulin sensitivity than those following a high fibre wholegrain diet, even when weight loss was equivalent. They also showed more normal menstrual cycles and less tendency to form blood clots.

A healthy, low GI eating plan should include the following foods every day:

- Fresh vegetables and salads
- Fresh fruit
- Low GI wholegrain breads (with lots of grainy bits and/or made with intact kernels) and cereals
- Low-fat dairy products or non-dairy alternatives like soy
- Fish, lean meat, chicken, eggs, legumes and soy products, and
- Small amounts of healthy fats such as nuts, seeds, avocado, olives, olive oil, canola oil or peanut oil.

Step 3: Move more

Activity and exercise are crucial if you want to manage PCOS, as they help you control your weight, manage your insulin and make a real difference in your health and energy levels. Exercise improves insulin sensitivity so that your body needs to secrete less insulin each time you eat. Ideally, you should try to fit in activity on most days.

Research shows that just 30 minutes of moderate intensity exercise each day can help improve your health, lowering your risk of heart disease and diabetes, among numerous other health problems. Busy schedule? Break the 30 minutes down into two sessions of 15 minutes or even three sessions of 10 minutes, and you'll still enjoy the same benefits. That said, if you're trying to lose weight, the more you can exercise, the better.

A balanced exercise program, including aerobic, resistance or strength training and flexibility/stretching exercises will give you the best results. And don't forget to vary your activities – the body becomes efficient at anything it does repeatedly, so after a while, you won't see results unless you vary the type of activity or intensity.

Step 4: Take care of yourself

Eating well and being active are the cornerstones of managing PCOS, but there are a few other things you can do to help yourself. Stress reduction is at the top of the list.

Stress is a part of life for most of us and can't be avoided. The key is to be able to manage it effectively – which is absolutely crucial for women with PCOS, because too much stress can affect hormonal balance, increase blood glucose levels and lead to overeating. You can get a handle on the stress in your life by starting a stress reduction program, regular exercise, taking time out for activities you enjoy, and finding someone to talk to about your feelings. If need be, talk to a counsellor or therapist.

Enough good-quality sleep is also important. A lack of sleep – that means less than eight hours for the average person – can reduce immunity, increase stress hormones and worsen insulin resistance. If you've cut down on stress, started exercising regularly and don't drink alcohol or caffeinated beverages before bed but still have difficulty sleeping, see your doctor to find out if you may have a sleep disorder, or if medication and/or cognitive behavioural therapy may help.

Common questions

Which is more important: a low GI diet or a low carb diet?

When you have PCOS, reducing insulin levels is important. When it comes to the food you eat, the key to reducing insulin levels is reducing the glycemic load (GL) of your diet. There are two ways to do this: reduce the GI of your diet overall or reduce your carbohydrate intake. Many of the women we see try the second option first because it sounds easy to cut carbohydrate foods out of their diet. While this may help in the short-term, it is not the answer for long-term good health and management of their PCOS. This is because low carbohydrate diets can worsen insulin resistance and they eliminate many of the foods we know are important for good health and reducing risk of diseases such as cancer, heart disease and type 2 diabetes. Low carbohydrate diets also tend to lower energy levels, making exercise more difficult. A diet based on low GI foods, on the other hand, gives you the best of both worlds – enough carbohydrate for optimum insulin sensitivity, nutrition and energy levels without an excessive GL. If weight loss is a goal, high carbohydrate diets are probably not the answer for you either – as with most things, moderation is key. Whether you have a high or moderate carbohydrate intake, however, you should choose mostly healthy low GI carbs.

The good news is that eating the low GI way will mean that you feel fuller and will be less likely to over-eat. This means that measuring, counting, and weighing your food can be a thing of the past. You will also find that when you are choosy about your carbohydrates, your insulin levels will be lower and you will therefore burn more fat. Over time, and combined with some regular exercise, this will result in weight loss.

Low GI basics

Although there is no cure for PCOS, there are ways of keeping the myriad debilitating symptoms under control. These include managing weight, eating a low GI diet to help control blood glucose levels and increase insulin sensitivity, more physical exercise, learning to handle stress and getting enough sleep.

Tips for managing PCOS

- Eat small regular meals and snacks spread across the day with a focus on low GI carboydrates.
- Include plenty of fresh vegetables and salads with your meals.
- Reach for seasonal fresh fruit to steer you away from sugary treats.
- Wholegrain breads and cereals will hold the hunger pangs at bay and can be topped with jams or nut butters for extra flavour.
- Choose fish, lean meat, skinless chicken, eggs, legumes and soy products as the main protein part of your meals.
- Healthy fats such as nuts, seeds, avocados, olives, olive oil, canola oil or peanut oil can be used in moderation for cooking and salad dressings.

Chapter 11

The GI for children

If children learn to combine regular physical activity with healthy low GI eating, they will be in top condition throughout their lives. It's never too late to start. The importance of teaching children about good nutrition by providing healthy nutritious foods and by setting a good example cannot be over-emphasised. It's a win–win situation, too: if you set a good example by eating well and being active, you will also feel fitter and healthier.

Children growing up in Australia and New Zealand today face very different challenges and health concerns from those of any previous generation. On average, one child in four is overweight or obese. But today's diet and lifestyle isn't just creating obesity.

- School children are showing signs of risk factors for heart disease.
- Type 2 diabetes, once known as 'maturity onset diabetes', is appearing in children as young as eight.

Children need our guidance to learn how to respect their health and look after their bodies. Helping them develop good eating habits and being active every day is part of this.

- A US study found that one in five teenagers (15–16 year olds) has raised insulin levels, putting them at risk of type 2 diabetes, and 9 per cent of boys of this age group had signs of liver damage and 10 per cent had raised blood fats.

The increasing proportion of kilojoules children consume from high GI carbs like doughnuts, waffles, white bread and burger buns, cornflakes, biscuits, pastries, potato chips and snacks, corn chips and French fries is a key aspect of today's diet linked to increasing their risk of diabetes, heart disease and obesity. Managing these lifestyle diseases requires a holistic approach.

Healthy low GI eating has benefits for all children just as it does for adults, and it can make a difference to your family's long-term well-being.

How can the GI help children who are overweight or obese?

It's no fun being fat in a world that equates attractiveness with body shape. Maintaining high self-esteem can be very difficult for overweight or obese children. They need support, acceptance and encouragement from their parents. They need to know that they are OK whatever their weight. If you have a child who is overweight or obese, the best approach is to get the whole family living a healthier lifestyle.

There's no simple solution to this problem, but part of any management plan for school children and teenagers who are overweight or obese is about altering the balance.

First of all, we can't stress enough the importance of physical activity and we discuss the active side of the equation later in this chapter. Remember, your kids may not always hear what you tell them to do, but they sure notice what you do (or don't do) when it comes to activity and healthy eating.

Secondly, don't put your child on a diet unless this is under the guidance of a qualified health professional who has experience in managing childhood obesity. An overweight child may not need to lose a lot of weight, but their weight gain may need to slow down while they grow into their existing weight.

The proportion of overweight or obese children in the population has doubled in the last 20 years. In Australia, on average, one in five children is overweight or obese, but in some areas it is as high as one in three. And high GI diets could be making things worse. When we eat foods with a high GI the peaking glucose and insulin levels can stimulate a sequence of hormonal changes that can trigger overeating.

Dr David Ludwig, Director of the Optimal Weight for Life Program at the Children's Hospital in Boston in the US, demonstrated this effect by asking obese teenage boys to eat high, medium or low GI breakfasts and then observing their food intake for the rest of the day. As expected, after the high GI breakfast of instant porridge the boys' blood glucose and insulin levels rose the highest, then crashed back down.

When their first meal had been high GI the boys then consumed almost twice as many kilojoules with the food they chose in the later part of the day.

Falling blood glucose levels and other hormones send us in search of something else to eat. To make matters worse, the high insulin levels after a high GI meal temporarily switch off the release of fatty acids from fat tissue, making it even harder to burn off those extra kilojoules.

In a study from the UK, researchers confirmed that a low GI breakfast is more satiating for children than a high GI breakfast. On days when children ate a low GI breakfast they ate a significantly smaller lunch and vice versa – when breakfast was high GI they reported feeling significantly more hungry at lunchtime.

A low GI vs high GI breakfast

Giving children a low GI breakfast can reduce their food intake for the rest of the day and it's as simple as changing their cereal.

The following examples are the actual breakfast choices offered to children in the UK study.

Low GI	High GI
All-Bran®	Corn Flakes®
Natural muesli	Coco Pops®
Traditional rolled oats porridge	Rice Krispies®
Soy and linseed bread	Regular white bread

And in his outpatient obesity management program, David Ludwig has confirmed that children eating a low GI diet lose significantly more weight than those on a standard reduced-fat diet. On a low GI diet, the children feel less hungry and decrease their food intake naturally without being told to restrict kilojoules deliberately.

The GI and children with fatty liver

Another condition linked to obesity is the increasing prevalence of fatty liver in children. Non-alcoholic fatty liver disease (so named because it is liver disease in the absence of regular alcohol consumption), or NAFL, is estimated to affect one in three obese children.

The build-up of fat in the liver can progress to hepatitis, scarring of the liver, cirrhosis and liver failure. Researchers have speculated that our high GI diet may be contributing to this condition. By boosting insulin levels a high GI diet signals the liver to make fat from food energy and store it – insulin levels are far higher in obese children than in non-obese and there is evidence from animal studies that a high GI diet increases fat deposits throughout the body, including the liver.

Trials are currently underway in children to investigate whether a low GI diet can reverse fatty liver. By improving insulin sensitivity, a low GI diet could, at the very least, improve the metabolic conditions that contribute to this condition.

The GI and children with type 2 diabetes

Along with obesity in children comes escalating numbers with type 2 diabetes. The link between type 2 diabetes in children and obesity is very strong, with around 80 per cent of children with the condition being obese.

Because the development of type 2 diabetes lags several years behind that of obesity, we are just experiencing the beginning of the type 2 diabetes epidemic in children and adolescents. Given the current obesity rates, it is almost inevitable that there will be an epidemic of type 2 diabetes if we don't start doing something about it – right now!

Children with type 2 diabetes are believed to face the same risk of heart attack, stroke, impotence, blindness and kidney disease as adults. These diseases are usually associated with health problems in older people. The shocking thing is children with type 2 diabetes will be developing these complications at the peak of their adult life when their working and earning capacity is greatest. The implications for an individual are shocking and the public health burden overwhelming.

If you have type 2 diabetes then your children are at risk as there is a strong family link.

The GI and children with type 1 diabetes

At present, half the people with type 1 diabetes are diagnosed before they are 16 years old. For young people who are still growing and developing, it's vital to do everything possible to achieve and maintain optimal blood glucose levels. Poorly managed diabetes, particularly before puberty, can mean that children don't achieve their full growth potential. And they don't get a chance to go back and try again!

It's no mean feat keeping blood glucose levels within the recommended range without too many episodes of hypoglycaemia or hyperglycaemia. But studies here in Australia and elsewhere show that the quality of the carbohydrate consumed can be particularly relevant to glycemic control in children with type 1 diabetes.

For example, in Heather Gilbertson's study of almost 100 children with type 1 diabetes at the Royal Children's Hospital, Melbourne, the children and their parents reported that a low GI eating plan was more flexible and family friendly than the traditional carbohydrate exchange regime, and the researchers found it achieved significantly lower HbA1c levels.

For children with type 1 diabetes, their blood glucose response to foods can vary dramatically depending on the GI of the food (of course it can vary depending on lots of other factors as well). For example, regular white bread will result in two and a half times the increase in blood glucose compared to eating the same amount of carbohydrate from barley or chickpeas.

In theory, lowering the GI of the diet in type 1 diabetes could be useful to:

- reduce blood glucose levels after meals
- decrease the chance of hypoglycaemia (low blood glucose)
- reduce insulin requirements, and
- reduce the risk of diabetes complications.

The active side of the healthy kids equation

Of course what children eat is only one half of the equation to a healthy lifestyle. Regular physical activity is important for adults and no less so for children. Although they tend to run around and move a lot naturally, influences of modern society such as electronic games, computers and DVDs can have an insidious effect on decreasing children's exercise. Reduced physical activity is a major contributor to obesity, and children who are less physically active are also more insulin resistant (increasing their risk of type 2 diabetes).

When looking at your child's lifestyle, think about ways to decrease sedentary behaviour and increase both planned and incidental activity.

Decreasing the sedentary side of the equation usually means limiting TV (and other small or big screen) time. There is very good evidence relating TV viewing to obesity. An Australian study found that children who watched TV for more than 2 hours per day were more likely to consume high-energy snacks and drinks and less likely to participate in organised sports. The current viewing average in Australia is about 3 hours per day, which doesn't paint a very good picture for the future of obesity in our children!

To successfully increase incidental and planned activity in your children, you need to exercise yourself. Parental activity is a strong predictor of a child's activity so take a look at your own lifestyle and how you could be more active.

In relation to incidental activity, get your children involved in helping with household tasks, including dressing themselves and ironing their own clothes once they are old enough, and active family activities such as shopping, maintaining the garden and walking the dog.

Planned activity can mean participating in organised sports such as basketball, football, netball, T ball, etc … but if your child is not interested there are plenty of other things they can do, like riding a bike, going for a swim, or a walk, dancing or practising a martial art. Whatever they choose, make sure they enjoy it; if they don't, try something else.

Like adults, children need to do at least 30 minutes of some kind of physical activity most days of the week just to maintain good health. To lose weight, they need to do at least double that.

To keep children thinking better for longer during the school morning, make sure they eat a low GI breakfast!

Helping kids keep thinking

When you realise that our brains require a steady supply of glucose to function properly, it makes sense that the GI of a meal and the ensuing blood glucose levels can affect our ability to think. Studies in adults have suggested that low GI meals resulted in better mental performance, so to investigate this in children, researchers gave 6 to 11 year olds either a low GI breakfast (All-Bran®, GI 42) or a high GI breakfast (Coco Pops®, GI 77). Following breakfast the children were asked to complete a number of computerised tests of attention and memory for the next 3 hours.

The results indicated, perhaps not surprisingly, that the children's thinking skills declined across the morning but the rate of the decline was significantly slower following the low GI cereal breakfast, compared to the high GI cereal.

Putting the GI to work in children's diets

A low GI diet is safe and adaptable for everyone, including children. It is adaptable to different cultural backgrounds and is, by nature, packed with nutrients essential to good health.

To put the GI to work in your family, all you really need to focus on are your children's carbohydrate choices – choose low GI breads, cereals, biscuits, rice, potato, etc. The low GI options are listed in the tables at the back of this book. However, it's difficult, even for us, to talk about using low GI foods without looking at how they fit in to the rest of the diet.

The foods children eat are very much a factor of their age and stage, their family and peer group and what is available to them.

On the whole, children can eat only what we make available to them. As adults we know, or have the ability to learn, what foods are necessary for good health and as parents we have a responsibility to expose our children to a wide variety of nutritious foods. This happens naturally when a mother breastfeeds her baby because the flavours of the foods she eats are transferred through her breastmilk (so if you want baby to eat vegetables in a few months' time, eat lots of them yourself). When we do begin introducing solid foods it's important that we don't give the responsibility of food choice to our toddlers. Just because he or she relishes a biscuit, this doesn't make it an appropriate food for them.

A healthy diet for children:

- allows for good health and growth
- satisfies the appetite
- establishes good eating habits
- allows for varied and interesting meals and snacks
- accommodates the child's usual routines and activities, and
- maintains a healthy body weight.

It's never too soon to start a low GI diet

A critical time for parents to prevent problems such as obesity in their children may be before birth and possibly before conception. By starting pregnancy at a healthy body weight and eating a low GI diet during pregnancy, studies suggest you are more likely to give birth to a baby with a healthier body weight and a lower risk of obesity and diabetes later in life.

Newborns

All you really need to know at this stage is that breastmilk and infant formula are low GI! The World Health Organization recommends this as the sole source of nourishment for babies for the first six months of life, with continuation of breastfeeding for the first 12 months.

Infants and toddlers

From six months of age the world of food is just opening up and it's time for your little one to explore. Take it slowly and keep it simple. Their key need is for an increasing dietary source of iron, available from commercial iron-fortified cereals and baby foods to which you can add single vegetables, fruits and, later, meats. Dr Heather Gilbertson, a dietitian and educator with many years' experience in management of children with diabetes advises that the 'introduction of rice cereal for infants should not cause any problems. I would generally recommend mixing it with expressed breast milk to reduce its glycemic effect. Keep the foods real – fruit, vegetables, milk, pasta, oatmeal, meat, etc, *not* commercial biscuits, chips, deep-fried foods, confectionery or other junk food. Deliberately avoiding or limiting carbohydrate-containing foods will also cause blood glucose levels to drop in an infant diagnosed with a metabolic disorder. Mothers need to encourage their babies to try a wide range of tastes and textures of the fruit and vegetable variety (focusing on either low GI or a combination of low with high to modify the effect).

Low GI serving suggestions:

- Give them a slice of low GI bread rather than a biscuit.
- Offer a range of cut up pieces of fruit every day.
- Include full-fat dairy products up to age two and reduced-fat products up to age five. Milk, yoghurt and custards are calcium-rich low GI snacks.

- Try oatmeal as a low GI cereal but mix it with some iron-fortified cereal such as a wheat biscuit or rice cereal to help meet iron requirements.
- Plain cooked pasta is a low GI meal accompaniment or snack that is easily eaten hot or cold with fingers.

'As parents we have the responsibility of choosing when, where, and what is available to eat. Children have the responsibility of choosing how much and whether they eat it.' – Ellyn Satter, nutritionist

As children get older, introduce dairy foods, which all have a low GI, plus baked beans, porridge and other low GI breads and cereals. Children are naturally 'neophobic', meaning it is normal for them to refuse new foods and vegetables! This is believed to be a protective instinct but it can be excruciatingly frustrating for parents.

The tendency to reject new foods can be overcome with frequent exposure to the food so the new food is no longer new and unfamiliar. Offer a new food five to ten times in small amounts without pressuring the child to eat it and gradually you should see some acceptance. Praise any efforts at tasting new foods.

Make sure you are a good role model. Eat the same foods that you would like your children to eat. Avoid classifying foods as 'good' or 'bad' or forbidding certain foods. Instead, teach kids the concept that all foods can be eaten, some every day, others sometimes.

Avoid using food, for example dessert, as a reward. Withholding a child's favoured food can make them feel powerless and is likely to increase their desire for it. Pushing a child to eat everything on their plate with the temptation of a treat afterwards can condition children, who have an excellent in-built ability to sense when they are full, to overeat.

Schoolchildren

Children, especially younger ones, eat mostly what's available at home. That's why it's important to control the supply lines – the foods that you serve for meals and have on hand for snacks. You can influence the GI of their diet here with your choice of bread, breakfast cereal, noodles, dairy desserts and the inclusion of fruit every day.

Low GI serving suggestions:

- Make their sandwiches with low GI white or grainy bread.
- Give them fruit at least twice a day washed, cut up and looking attractive without competition (such as biscuits).
- Make or buy some healthy muesli bars.
- Give them fruit-filled, rather than cream-filled, biscuits.
- Avoid packet snacks such as crisps, savoury shape biscuits and cereal and muffin bars as much as possible. Low-fat varieties of these are not filling and not a good alternative.
- Don't completely ban your children's favourite snacks – make them one of the 'keep for a treat' foods.
- Limit fruit juice, cordial and soft drinks. Offer water and plain, low-fat milk instead.

Involve your children with food, teach them how to cook and help them grow some of their own vegetables. Little cherry tomatoes, strawberries or lettuce can easily be grown in pots and they taste delicious. Take them to a farm or orchard when it's picking season. Let them select a new fruit or vegetable to try in the greengrocer's. Have them shop for food with you (sometimes). Get to know local shopkeepers at the butcher or greengrocer, bakery or deli. If you're a regular, many shopkeepers are only too pleased to give a little one a taste of something.

Teenagers

Teenagers are going to eat lots so if you can make even half their carbs low GI you'll be doing really well. Low GI teenager basics:

- Expect them to eat what you eat, so set a good example.
- Invite them into the kitchen and ask them to do something so that they learn how to cook.
- Keep a range of packaged low GI cereals available – a bowl of cereal is an excellent snack any time of day.

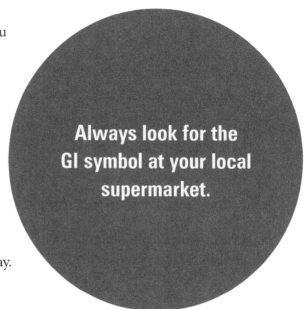

Always look for the GI symbol at your local supermarket.

- Make sure there's always a loaf of low GI bread in the cupboard, plus plenty of tempting spreads, from jams to nut butters, Vegemite to honey.
- Buy low-fat milk for everyone over five years of age in the house.
- Keep cartons of low-fat custard, flavoured yoghurt and low-fat ice-cream alongside a bowl of fruit salad or canned fruit in the fridge.
- Instant noodles or pasta topped with some grated cheese are filling low GI snacks that most teens will prepare for themselves.

At this stage it may be a good idea to think about family meals. Independent teenagers may turn up their noses at the prospect of a family meal but studies have found that the predictability of family meals makes them a comforting ritual in the often tumultuous life of a teenager. They also offer parents a chance to catch up with their children. You might be able to tempt a reluctant teen by suggesting they invite a friend to dinner or involving them in planning the menu and cooking.

Kids who take part in regular family meals are:

- more likely to eat fruit, vegetables and wholegrains
- less likely to snack on unhealthy foods, and
- less likely to smoke, use marijuana or drink alcohol.

What counts as a family meal?

Any time you and your family eat together – whether it's takeaway food or a home-cooked meal. Maybe this means you have to eat a little later to wait until someone gets home from work or perhaps you set aside breakfast on the weekend as a leisurely family affair. Whenever it is, strive for nutritious food and a pleasant atmosphere (without the TV on!).

Common questions

How can I feed a big family with cost-effective, no-hassle, low GI foods?

Feeding a big family on a budget can be hard. But low GI eating often means making a move back to the inexpensive, filling and healthy staple foods that your parents and grandparents may have enjoyed: traditional oats in porridge for breakfast; legumes such as beans, chickpeas and lentils (all available dry or, for expediency, in cans); cereal grains like barley, and plenty of fresh fruits and vegetables, which have a naturally low GI.

Some of these foods may take a little more time to prepare than high GI processed, packaged and more expensive convenience foods, but you will save money and reap immeasurable health benefits, and many of these foods will keep you and your family firing with energy all day. In the GI tables in Part 5, you'll find plenty of low GI foods to choose from that won't break your budget. Your diabetes dietitian or educator will also have plenty of ideas for low-cost, low GI meals that the whole family will enjoy.

Some soft drinks have a low GI. How often should children be allowed them?

Sweetened drinks (including soft drinks and cordials), even if they have a low GI, should not be an everyday beverage. Liquid kilojoules may be a little sneakier than most, in that they tend to bypass the satiety centre in your brain which would normally help stop you from overeating. This isn't to say that everyone should avoid soft drinks all the time, but consumption ought to rank as occasional or keep for a treat if you're trying to lose weight.

An increase in soft drink intake is contributing to the child obesity problem. Our children are drinking more of these sweetened drinks than we did when we were children. And of course the increase in serving size from the old-fashioned 240 ml bottle and 375 ml can to the widely available 500 ml bottle doesn't help. Soft drinks aren't the only problem, either. Too much fruit juice, sweetened or unsweetened, is an easy way for us to gulp down extra kilojoules.

Low GI basics

Regular physical activity combined with healthy low GI eating will minimise any health problems associated with obesity or poor diet further down the track. Switching to low GI food alternatives will satisfy your child's appetite, establish good eating habits and boost energy levels and concentration. And remember, the child is part of a family – it's better for the child, eases food preparation and benefits the entire family's health if everyone eats the same way.

Tips for managing a GI diet for children

- Lead by example and expose your children to good GI foods that are nutritious and tasty.
- Engage your children with the growing and cooking of food so that they feel part of the 'food chain' and become more willing to try a range of different foods.
- Offer children plenty of breads, cereals, vegetables and fruits to eat.
- Include lean meats, fish and dairy foods in their daily diet
- Encourage children to drink plenty of water.
- Try to include a minimum of one low GI food per meal.
- Include sugar in moderation. Adding sugar to a well-balanced low GI diet can make foods more palatable without compromising their nutritional intake.

For more information:

If you need individualised dietary guidance on managing any of the disorders in children discussed in this chapter we suggest you seek out the services of an accredited practising dietitian. There are no quick-fix pills or potions that are going to remedy these conditions; they are generally lifelong and require a holistic approach.

Chapter 12

The GI and exercise

Whether you are a professional athlete, exercising for health and fitness or aiming to lose some weight, having a good nutrition program – the type, timing and amount of food you eat before and after exercise – will help you achieve your goals whatever they are.

And that's where the GI comes in. It's a scientifically proven tool in sport and exercise nutrition that can help you to select the best carbs for your training or exercise program. We worked closely with Dr Emma Stevenson of the School of Psychology and Sports Sciences at Northumbria University to bring you the very latest research on the GI and exercise.

However, if the GI is to make any difference at all, your training diet needs to contain sufficient carbohydrate to start with.

Fuelling exercise

When you are exercising, your muscles rely on carbohydrate and fat as their main sources of fuel.

- Carbohydrate is stored in your muscles as glycogen, but the stores are limited and about 90 minutes of high-intensity exercise will deplete them.
- Fat, which provides the largest nutrient store in the body, can fuel 100–200 hours of exertion, but at a lower intensity.

In high-intensity sports, it is generally the availability of carbohydrate stores that limits performance.

The relative contribution of carbohydrate and fat as fuel while you are exercising depends on both the intensity and length of your exercise session. Generally, your body's use of carbohydrate as fuel increases as your exercise intensity increases, and decreases the longer your exercise session lasts.

Aerobic training and fitness increases your body's ability to use fat as a fuel source. This is a plus, as it conserves your limited carbohydrate stores, allowing you to exercise for longer or at a higher intensity.

What you eat affects your muscle glycogen reserves and the amount of fat and carbohydrate you use up during exercise. If you are training on a regular basis, then every meal you eat becomes an important part of your cycle of recovery and preparing for the next exercise session. That's why you need to plan carefully to boost glycogen stores and promote fat burning during exercise. And this is where you can use GI to your advantage as a useful tool to plan your pre- and post-workout meals.

GI and pre-exercise carb intake

The carbs you eat in the hours before exercise top up your muscle and liver glycogen stores so you can perform at your best during your exercise session. The findings of a number of studies show that eating low GI foods in the hours before exercise help extend endurance in athletes.

In one Australian study, cyclists ate a pre-event meal of low GI lentils on one occasion and high GI potatoes on another, 1 hour before cycling at 65 per cent of their maximum capacity. After the low GI meal, the athletes could cycle for 20 minutes longer than after the high GI meal. During exercise after the low GI meal, they also maintained their blood glucose concentrations at a higher level and used more fat.

Many other studies with male athletes support the findings of this study. Although not all studies have shown improvements in performance after a low GI pre-exercise meal or single food, they do consistently show differences in the ratio of carbohydrate and fat in the athletes' fuel mix. A high GI pre-exercise meal increases the carbohydrate used and thus reduces the amount of fat burned. It is also likely that the body's limited glycogen stores will be used up faster, leading to earlier fatigue.

Research in recent years by Dr Emma Stevenson and Professor Clyde Williams at Loughborough University in the UK has come up with a couple of important findings about low GI foods and exercise. First, the benefits of low GI foods on exercise metabolism don't just apply to male endurance athletes like cyclists exercising at high intensity. Secondly, the effects of the GI aren't restricted to single foods, they also apply to having mixed meals in the hour before exercising.

In their study, they gave women recreational exercisers (doing it for health and fitness) a high GI or low GI breakfast 3 hours before exercise. The meals were made up of a variety of foods in the typical combinations that people eat at breakfast time.

- The high GI breakfast consisted of cornflakes and milk, toast and jam and a carbohydrate-based sports drink (GI 78).
- The low GI breakfast included muesli and milk, apple, canned peaches and yoghurt and apple juice (GI 44).

After a low GI breakfast, the women's post-meal glucose and insulin response was noticeably lower than after a high GI breakfast. And when they jogged on a treadmill for 60 minutes 3 hours later, they used up significantly more fat as a source of fuel after a low GI breakfast than after a high GI breakfast.

Whether you are exercising for health and fitness, for weight loss or control, or you are training for competition, it's a real plus to use more fat as your fuel source during exercise.

What if you simply walk for exercise?

Low GI pre-exercise meals can still work for you even if you aren't an athlete, jogger or cyclist. The Loughborough team found that women will use up an average of 7.5 grams of fat and 42 grams of carbohydrate walking on a treadmill for 60 minutes after a low GI breakfast (similar to the one described previously) compared with only 3.7 grams of fat and 52 grams of carbohydrate after a high GI one.

So, if you are counting the kilojoules, the women used up twice as many from fat in the low GI trial compared with the high GI one.

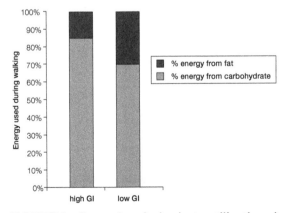

FIGURE 8: Fat and carbohydrate utilisation during walking exercise following a high GI or low GI breakfast.

Low GI foods: when and how much?

Let's start with when. Generally, low GI foods are best eaten 2 to 4 hours before you exercise so that the meal will have left your stomach but remains in your small intestine, slowly releasing glucose energy for hours afterwards.

The slow rate of carbohydrate digestion that is a characteristic of low GI foods helps to ensure there is a steady release of glucose into your bloodstream. Most importantly, during prolonged exercise, this steady release of glucose provides an essential energy source when muscle glycogen stores start to become depleted. This is how low GI pre-exercise foods can improve endurance performance.

However, you may need to experiment with different timings – eating 2, 3 or 4 hours before exercising – to see what works best for you. It can be difficult to get the right balance between not feeling too full and not feeling hungry before you start your exercise session.

It is also important to experiment with food choices to find ones that suit you and your digestive system best. Some low GI foods – particularly those with a high fibre content – can cause discomfort like stomach cramps and/or flatulence. Luckily there are many low GI, low fibre foods to choose from, including pasta (not wholemeal), noodles, rice such as basmati, or Doongara Clever Rice, and the new low GI white breads (look for the GI Symbol).

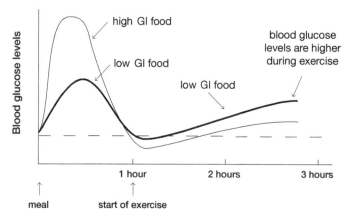

FIGURE 9. Comparison of the effect of low and high GI foods on blood glucose levels during prolonged strenuous exercise.

And how much? What we know from research is that athletes can substantially improve endurance performance when they consume 200–300 grams of carbohydrate 2 to 4 hours before exercise (that's equivalent to around seven to ten slices of bread).

However, if you are essentially exercising for your health and fitness or for weight loss, or if you are not training on a daily basis, your overall carbohydrate requirements before exercise will be much, much less. In the study of recreational exercisers outlined above, the women ate a breakfast that contained 1 gram of carbohydrate per kilogram of their body mass – i.e. 70 grams if they weighed 70 kilograms.

What about carbs during exercise?

You only need to consume carbs while you are exercising for events lasting 90 minutes or more. Many people – both athletes and weekend warriors – make the mistake of gulping down sports drinks which contain large amounts of glucose during exercise so they end up consuming just as much energy as they are expending!

If you do need to consume carbs during exercise, then this is when the high GI ones come in handy. High GI foods are digested in a flash and their glucose is released into the bloodstream very quickly. This means the glucose is available to your muscles almost immediately.

Although we don't actually know the ideal amount of carbohydrate intake during exercise, it is generally recommended that athletes consume 30–60 grams an hour. This is when sports drinks come into their own as they are an ideal way of providing fuel to the working muscle as well as helping with that vital rehydration.

What other options are there? Well, several sports bars and gels are available; jelly beans or other jelly sweets will also provide a rapid source of glucose.

The highs and lows of GI and recovery

Post-exercise recovery is a critical challenge for athletes and recreational exercisers, and one that's all too often overlooked. Good nutrition between training sessions is vital for rapid and effective recovery. This is the time when you need to top up your muscle and liver glycogen stores. And if you are an athlete who trains or competes twice a day, you really need to replenish your glycogen stores fast.

How? Well, you can achieve this by increasing both insulin and glucose concentrations in the blood stream rapidly during the immediate post-exercise period. During the first 30–60 minutes after exercise, your muscles are particularly sensitive to increases in insulin and there is increased activity of a glycogen-storing

If your recovery period is longer than a few hours or restoring muscle glycogen after exercise is not your goal, then you don't need to eat large amounts of high GI carbs after exercise.

enzyme called glycogen synthase. This means that when you eat or drink something, the glucose virtually 'speeds' into the muscle cells and is converted to glycogen. Consuming high GI carbs as soon as possible means you can really make the most of this window of opportunity.

What does this mean in practical terms? It means having 50–75 grams of carbs within the first 30 minutes after exercise and then a further 50–70 grams every two hours until you have consumed a total of 500 grams, or until you have eaten a high carb meal.

When it comes to the GI of your diet, exercise and recovery, it's very much what suits the individual. The type of exercise for example, whether the session is intense or intermittent, can make a difference.

Where do you get 50 grams of carbs?

Cereals	Breads and cakes
4 Weet-Bix	3 slices of raisin toast
10 tablespoons cornflakes	2 muffins
14 tablespoons Bran Flakes	3 crumpets
2 average servings of porridge	4 slices white bread

Fruit	Biscuits and sweets
2 large bananas	4 fruit 'pillows'
410 g can fruit	2 Milky Way bars
4 medium apples	8 boiled sweets
125 g dried apricots	1 Mars Bar
8 tablespoons sultanas	3 cereal bars

Drinks	Grains
850 ml 6 per cent carbohydrate sports drink	75 g rice (uncooked)
1 litre diluted orange cordial	70 g pasta (uncooked)
475 ml Coca-Cola	425 g canned spaghetti

Dr Stevenson and her colleagues from Loughborough University ran a trial in which they asked athletes to run on a treadmill for 90 minutes at 70 per cent of their maximum capacity (to reduce their muscle glycogen stores). Then over the following 24-hour period, they gave the athletes a high GI or low GI diet consisting of 8 grams of carbohydrate per kilogram of body mass in mixed meals that would typically form part of an athlete's diet. Back at the lab the following morning, they asked the athletes to run to exhaustion on a treadmill at 70 per cent of their maximum capacity.

What they found was that the athletes' endurance capacity was significantly improved after a low GI recovery diet compared with a high GI diet. In the low GI trial, the athletes used more fat as a fuel source which meant they 'spared' their muscle glycogen stores for later in the exercise session.

But when they repeated this trial with intermittent exercise (typical of soccer, hockey, netball and rugby) rather than an intense exercise session, they found no differences in recovery of endurance capacity between high GI and low GI diets.

However, if you are exercising primarily for your health and fitness or for weight loss, a low GI post-exercise meal may help your body maintain a higher rate of fat burning (oxidation). Your body's fat oxidation will be elevated post-exercise but will be rapidly suppressed if you eat high GI carbohydrates. This is because your body's higher insulin response to the blood glucose spike after a high GI meal or snack suppresses enzymes that oxidise fat. This basically means you burn less fat and more carbohydrate.

Your body's lesser insulin response after a low GI carb meal or snack suppresses fat oxidation to a lesser extent. What's the benefit? It means your body continues using fat as an energy source long after you have finished exercising. Because weight gain tends to creep up on most of us, every little bit counts!

> If you are exercising primarily for your health and fitness or for weight loss, a low GI post-exercise meal may help your body maintain a higher rate of fat-burning.

Is your diet fit for peak performance?

Take the diet fitness quiz below and see how well you score. It's a good idea to use this quiz regularly to pick up on areas where you may need to improve your diet.

1. CIRCLE YOUR ANSWER.

- I eat at least 3 meals a day with no longer than 5 hours in between.   Yes/No

EATING PATTERNS

Carbohydrate checker

- I eat at least 4 slices of bread each day
  (1 roll = 2 slices of bread).   Yes/No
- I eat at least 1 cup of breakfast cereal each day or an extra slice of bread.   Yes/No
- I usually eat 2 or more pieces of fruit each day.   Yes/No
- I eat at least 3 different vegetables or have a salad most days.   Yes/No
- I include carbohydrate such as pasta, rice and potatoes in my diet each day.   Yes/No

Protein checker

- I eat at least 1 and usually 2 servings of meat or meat alternatives (poultry, seafood, eggs, dried peas/beans, or nuts) each day.   Yes/No

Fat checker

- I spread butter or margarine thinly on bread or use none at all.   Yes/No
- I eat fried food no more than once per week.   Yes/No
- I use polyunsaturated or monounsaturated oil (canola or olive) for cooking (circle yes if you never fry in oil or fat).   Yes/No
- I avoid oil-based dressings on salads.   Yes/No

- I use reduced-fat or low-fat dairy products.   Yes/No
- I cut the fat off meat and take the skin off chicken.   Yes/No
- I eat fatty snacks such as chocolate, chips, cookies, or rich desserts/cakes, etc. no more than twice a week.   Yes/No
- I eat fast or takeaway food no more than once per week.   Yes/No

Iron checker

- I eat lean red meat at least 3 times per week or 2 servings of white meat daily or, for vegetarians, include at least 1–2 cups of dried peas and beans (e.g. lentils, soybeans, chickpeas) daily.   Yes/No
- I include a vitamin C source with meals based on bread, cereals, fruits and vegetables to assist the iron absorption in these 'plant' sources of iron.   Yes/No

Calcium checker

- I eat at least 3 servings of dairy food or soy milk alternative each day (1 serving = 250 ml milk or fortified soy milk; 1 slice (40 g) hard cheese; 200 g yoghurt).   Yes/No

Fluids

- I drink fluids regularly before, during and after exercise.   Yes/No

Alcohol

- When I drink alcohol, I would mostly drink no more than is recommended for the safe driving blood alcohol limit (circle yes if you don't drink alcohol).   Yes/No

2. SCORE 1 POINT FOR EVERY 'YES' ANSWER

Scoring scale

18–20 Excellent	15–17 Room for improvement
12–14 Just made it	0–12 Poor

Note: Very active people will need to eat more breads, cereals and fruit than on this quiz, but to stay healthy no one should be eating less.

Common questions

How relevant is the GI for athletes?

The GI can be useful to help athletes select the right type of carb to eat before and after exercise. Studies have consistently reported that a low GI pre-exercise meal results in a better maintenance of blood glucose during exercise and a higher rate of fat oxidation. This is likely to mean reduced muscle glycogen utilisation during prolonged exercise and possibly improve endurance. High GI meals before exercise may result in plasma glucose concentrations peaking before the exercise, then hypoglycaemia within the first 30 minutes of the exercise. There is little data available on the effect of the GI of carb eaten before intermittent, power- or strength-related sports.

During recovery from exercise, muscle glycogen resynthesis is of high metabolic priority. Eating high GI carbs after exercise increases plasma glucose and insulin concentrations, leading to muscle glycogen resynthesis. If, however, you are exercising for weight-loss or involved in weight-restricted sports, low GI carbs after exercise may be more beneficial as the lower glucose and insulin will not suppress fat.

Low GI basics

Carbohydrate quality makes all the difference to exercise – from intense athletic training to exercise for health and fitness or to lose weight. Low GI eating can be for your specific exercise needs and to more efficiently burn your carbohydrate and fat stores to get the most out of workout.

Tips for managing GI and exercise

- It is best to eat low GI foods 2 to 4 hours before exercise so that your meal will have left your stomach but remains in the small intestine, releasing much-needed glucose energy for a long period of time.
- Experiment with different timing for eating to see what works for you and the type of exercise you are doing. Likewise with low GI food choices and what types of food you enjoy.
- Only reach for sports drinks or gels, high energy bars and high GI foods when you are exercising intensely for 90 minutes or more.

Part 3

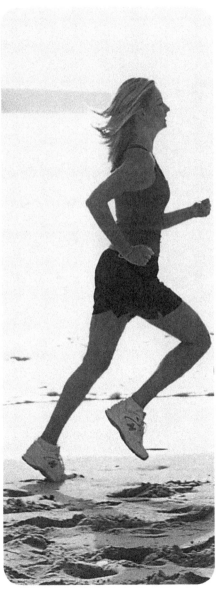

Your guide to a low GI diet for life

- Getting started
- Low GI menus
- Ready, set, go — move it & lose it!

With low GI eating:

- you won't go hungry
- you'll feel better
- you'll look better, and
- you'll have more energy.

Chapter 13

Getting started

Eating a low GI diet is easy. The crux of it is to be smart with your carbohydrate choices. Replace highly refined carbohydrates such as white bread, sugary treats and crispy puffed cereals with less processed carbohydrates such as grainy bread, pasta, legumes, fruit and vegetables. While this sounds simple, it also has science on its side. There's no measuring, no numbers, just eating the foods your body is designed for.

One of our most frequently received requests is 'Just tell me what to eat!' So, in this section, we focus on food and give you some simple guidelines about making the switch to everyday low GI eating, in 10 steps in 10 days. There's no specific order in which you have to do things and no strict week-by-week list of diet 'dos' and 'don'ts'.

Exactly how you incorporate low GI eating into your life is up to you. Some people want to eat low GI foods all the time, others some of the time. That's OK. There's room for both approaches – and, in reality, that's how most of us eat, anyway.

This for that: substitute low GI for high GI

The fact that everyday low GI eating is easy may surprise you if you've struggled to follow other nutrition programs. Simply substituting high GI foods with low GI alternatives will give your overall diet a lower GI and deliver all the benefits of low GI eating. This could mean eating muesli for breakfast instead of cornflakes, wholegrain bread instead of white, or fruit in place of biscuits, for example. Whatever your usual diet, use the table overleaf to help you identify the low GI choices.

This for that: substituting low GI for high GI foods

High GI food	Low GI alternative
Biscuits	A slice of wholegrain low GI bread with jam, fruit spread or nut spread or a slice of fruit bread.
Breads such as soft white or wholemeal	Dense breads with whole grains, stone-ground flour, sourdough and commercial breads with the GI symbol.
Breakfast cereals – most commercial processed cereals	Traditional rolled oats, muesli and commercial low GI brands; look for the GI symbol.
Cakes and pastries	Raisin toast, fruit loaf and fruit buns, particularly the wholegrain varieties.
Chips and packet snacks e.g. Twisties®, pretzels	Grab a handful of fresh grapes or cherry tomatoes, dried fruit or nuts.
Doughnuts and croissants	Try a skim milk cappuccino or smoothie instead.
French fries	Leave them out! Have salad or extra vegetables instead. Corn on the cob or bean salad are better takeaway options.
Lollies	Chocolate is lower GI but high in fat. Healthier options are nuts, sultanas, dried apricots and other dried fruits.
Muesli bars	Make a homemade version or try dried fruit and nuts instead; look for low GI labelling.
Potato	Baby chat potatoes, Carisma potatoes, Nicola potatoes, sweet potato, sweet corn, taro, yam and chestnuts.
Rice	Longer grain varieties such as basmati, SunRice Doongara CleverRice™ or try Asian rice noodles.
Soft drinks	Use a 'diet' or low joule variety if these are a regular part of your diet. Juice has a lower GI but isn't lower in kilojoules. Water is best.
Sugar	Moderate the quantity; consider pure floral honey, fructose (Sweetaddin® or Fruisana®) as alternative sweeteners.

1, 2, 3 . . . Putting it on the plate

Main meals for most Australians and New Zealanders consist of some sort of meat (or chicken or fish) with vegetables and potato (or rice or pasta). This is a good start and a little fine-tuning will ensure a healthy, balanced meal. All you need to do is adjust your proportions to match our 'plate'. Here are the three simple steps to put together a balanced low GI meal.

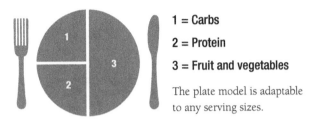

1 = Carbs

2 = Protein

3 = Fruit and vegetables

The plate model is adaptable to any serving sizes.

- As long you keep food to the proportions shown here, the meal will be balanced.
- As long as the types of food you choose fit within the guidelines for healthy eating, then you should have a healthy diet overall.

1 is for carb

It's an essential, although sometimes forgotten, part of a balanced meal. What do you feel like? A grain like rice, barley or cracked wheat? Bread, pasta, noodles or bean vermicelli? Or perhaps a starchy vegetable like sweetcorn, potato, sweet potato, chickpeas, lentils or dried beans? These foods supply energy-rich carbohydrates plus B-group vitamins, minerals and fibre. Include at least one low GI carb per meal.

2 is for protein

Including some protein at each meal lowers the glycemic load by replacing *some* of the carbohydrate — not all! It also helps satisfy the appetite. Meat, poultry, fish and seafood, eggs, tofu, nuts, chese and legumes all fit the bill here.

3 is for fruit and vegetables

This part of a meal, which is often skipped, should have the highest priority, but a meal based solely on fruit and low carb vegetables won't be sustaining for long.

Sometimes, fruit may form part of the carbohydrate in a meal and root vegetables such as carrot, parsnip and beetroot will also contribute some carbohydrate. However, relying on these sources of carbohydrate alone will mean your diet is very low in this nutrient. Fruit and vegetables are essential for vitamins B, C and folate, minerals such as potassium and magnesium and a host of anti-oxidants.

10 steps to a healthy low GI diet

The best way for any of us to eat is to choose from a wide variety of fresh foods that we enjoy and which satisfy us. Of course we need to have sufficient protein and moderate amounts of carbohydrate and fats and a whole host of vitamins and minerals as well. So how can you be sure you'll meet all your nutritional needs? As well as incorporating your low GI carbohydrate choices, the following 10 steps will give you a blueprint for eating a healthy and low GI diet for life. More information on specific low GI foods can be found in The top 100 low GI food finder in Part 4.

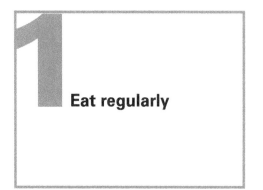

Eat regularly

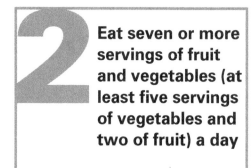

Eat seven or more servings of fruit and vegetables (at least five servings of vegetables and two of fruit) a day

3 Eat low GI forms of breads and cereals

4 Eat more legumes – beans, peas and lentils

5 Use low-fat dairy and calcium-enriched soy milk

6 Include fish, seafood or an alternative source of omega-3

7 Eat unsalted nuts regularly

8 Choose lean red meats, skinless chicken and eggs or plant proteins such as tofu

9 Minimise your salt intake

10 If you drink alcohol, drink in moderation

STEP 1

Eat regularly

Remember the basics: three meals a day is a must, but eating as often as three-hourly is regular eating for some. It depends on your level of hunger. The main thing is that you don't skip meals. Going a long time between meals (more than about 5 hours) can trick your body into starvation mode. This gives the signal that food is in short supply and your body responds by slowing down its metabolic rate (the rate at which it burns energy). In this state, when you do eat, your food will be metabolised differently – it will be directed to storage to enhance survival. What's more, when the next meal time arrives you could be absolutely famished and tend to gorge.

Eating regularly appears to have a connection with body weight. Studies have found that people who eat on four to six occasions in a day have healthier body weights than those who eat only two to three meals, even if the total amount of food is similar. Even three meals a day is better than one or two when it comes to blood fat levels, too. Eating regularly tends to give structure to your eating habits, allowing you to become more aware of what you eat. This makes it easier to establish good habits and identify problem eating.

Eat a good breakfast. Fire up your engine with low GI carbs. A good breakfast recharges your brain and speeds up your metabolism after an overnight fast. Choosing a low GI cereal is one of the most important things you can do to start your day – a bowl of traditional porridge in winter or muesli in the summer will sustain you through the morning.

Give priority to eating. Think about where you'll be at your next meal or snack time. Be prepared to let eating take precedence over some other activities. Carry a snack with you (for example, a piece of fruit, a nut bar, a small pack of dried fruit and/or nuts). Make meals a time to relax and enjoy eating – you are more likely to feel satisfied if you do.

Refuel at lunchtime to maintain energy levels right through the afternoon.
Hold back on the high GI carbs to minimise that post-lunch energy dip. And take
time over one main meal every day to make sure you aren't missing out on the vital
vegetables you need.

Eat small: think of the size of your fist. The bigger the portion in front of
you, the more you'll end up eating, so serve small and eat more often if you need
to. Don't let fast food chains upsize your serving for a little extra money. If it's
not in front of you, you won't eat it.

Plan meals ahead. Cook and freeze for when you come home tired. Take some
time on the weekend to think about meals for the week ahead. Write a shopping
list. Take food with you when you will be away from home for a meal. Avoid
grabbing food on the run.

Listen to your stomach. Stop eating when you are comfortably full, not stuffed.
And if you're unsure whether you've eaten enough, stop anyway and wait. It takes
20 minutes for your stomach to signal fullness to your brain, so give it a chance
for the message to get through. If you don't feel hungry when mealtimes come
around just eat a very small portion.

**Eat a little of whatever you
really feel like.** Be mindful
when you eat it. Take the time
to enjoy it fully, free of other
distractions. Denying yourself
can create cravings and lead
to binge eating.

**Studies have shown
that people who weigh
themselves nearly every
day gain less weight over
time than people who weigh
themselves less often.**

STEP

2

Eat seven or more servings of fruit and vegetables (at least five servings of vegetables and two of fruit) per day

Fruit and vegetables are a pivotal part of a healthy low GI diet. Nutrient rich and low in kilojoules, they are the sort of foods you can't really overdo. A high fruit and vegetable intake has consistently been linked with protection from cancer, obesity, heart disease, macular degeneration and other age-related diseases. Unique combinations of vitamins and anti-oxidants in fruit and vegetables keep your skin and eyes healthy and function like personal bodyguards, protecting cells throughout the body from the damage that occurs as a natural part of ageing and from pollutants in the environment. For more information on the benefits of fruit and vegetables plus extra serving suggestions see The top 100 low GI food finder in Part 4.

Easy ways to eat more vegetables

- Add extra vegetables (frozen are easy) to stir-fried meat.
- Chop up leftover vegetables, heat and serve as topping for toast.
- Try stuffed vegetables for something different.
- Include salad ingredients in a sandwich or bread roll.
- Throw some vegies onto the BBQ with the meat. Try zucchini, corn, capsicum, mushrooms, eggplant or thick slices of par-boiled sweet potato.
- Drink vegetable juices occasionally.
- Try a vegetarian main meal dish at least once a week.
- Add grated carrot and onion to rissoles.
- Choose take-away meals that include vegetables such as:
  - a regular hamburger with salad
  - doner kebabs with less meat, more salad
  - Asian dishes with stir-fried vegies
  - salad sandwiches or rolls
  - pasta with a Mediterranean sauce
  - vegetable pizza
  - jacket potato with beans, salsa and cheese
  - a side order of salad, not fries!
- Keep strips of celery, capsicum and carrot and florets of broccoli or cauliflower to munch on with a dip or in a lunch box for a snack.
- Try a vegetarian lasagne.
- Try a new type of vegetable.

Easy ways to eat more fruit

- Carry a piece of fruit with you for an on-the-run snack.
- Take fruit to work every day.
- Make a fruit smoothie or milkshake.
- Put a plate of sliced apple beside you to nibble on while you work, read or watch TV.
- Slice fresh fruit over your breakfast cereal or add diced fruit to low-fat yoghurt snacks.
- Prepare a fruit platter for all to share after a meal.
- Make sure you buy the best quality fruit you can afford and treat yourself with an exotic fruit rather than chocolate or cake.
- Keep diced melon in a clear container in the fridge for easy consumption.
- Add sliced apple, pear, pineapple or banana to sandwich fillings or salads.
- Serve slices of pan-fried apple or pear with pork.
- Toast thick cut slices of Tres Bon™ continental fruit loaf. Spread with light cream cheese that has been sweetened with a spoonful of caster sugar and a few drops of vanilla essence. Top with fresh fruit – sliced banana, peach, or strawberries, or whole fresh blueberries or raspberries. Dust with icing sugar to serve for a decorative touch.
- Bake whole peaches or nectarines in a moderate oven in a small amount of poaching liquid (see below) and baste with warmed honey regularly during baking (about 30 minutes). Serve with natural yoghurt.
- Grill fresh whole figs by cutting a cross across the top of them and filling with finely chopped macadamia nuts and brown sugar. Place under a hot grill for 5 minutes until the sugar is melted. Serve with fresh ricotta cheese sweetened with a little honey.
- Poach pears, plums, nectarines or peaches by first peeling and removing seeds or stones. Combine 1 cup of water with ½ cup of sugar, flavour with a cinnamon stick, vanilla pod, cardamom pods or a liqueur, bring to the boil and simmer 10 minutes to create a thin syrup. Place your fruit in this and simmer 5 to 15 minutes until the fruit is tender. Serve with light vanilla Fruche.
- Chop up a mango, strawberries and an orange. Mix with fresh passionfruit pulp and serve with frozen yoghurt.

STEP 3 Eat low GI breads and cereals

Cereal grains including rice, wheat, oats, barley, rye and their products (bread, pasta, breakfast cereal, flour) are the most concentrated sources of carbohydrate in our diet. Because of this the form in which we eat these foods has a major impact on the GI of our diet. To eat breads and cereals with a low GI use:

- Densely grained breads, traditional sourdough or commercially made low GI breads
- Barley – for example pearl barley in soup, casseroles, salads or a barley risotto
- Wholewheat or cracked wheat such as bulgur in tabbouli
- Low GI rice such as basmati, Doongara and Moolgiri
- Traditional rolled oats for breakfast as porridge or in muesli, and
- Pasta and noodles.

If you have to eat a gluten-free diet, then wheat, rye, barley, oats and triticale and foods made from these grains are off the menu.

The good news is that there are now low GI gluten-free breads and breakfast cereals on the supermarket shelves (see the tables in Part 5). And you can also make the most of other low GI cereal grains and products, including:

- Sweetcorn, a great standby on its own or added to soups, salads and casseroles
- Quinoa, to make porridges or tabbouli or serve as an accompaniment
- Buckwheat, can be added to soups and casseroles or used to make a tabbouli
- Rice noodles and vermicelli, can be added to Thai salads, rice paper rolls or Asian soups, and
- Buckwheat and bean thread noodles (check they are completely gluten free) can be used in place of rice.

STEP

4

Eat more pulses – beans, peas and lentils

Pulses, including lentils, chickpeas, soybeans and kidney beans, are an important part of a low GI diet. It is recommended that you eat them at least twice a week. The average Australian's intake of these foods is low, being less than 5 grams a day versus the 30 or more grams per day eaten by Asian and Mediterranean populations. Easy ways to eat pulses include using them in soups, salads and sauces. Pulses are easy on the budget, versatile, filling and packed with nutrients, providing a valuable source of protein, carbohydrate, B vitamins, folate, iron, zinc, magnesium and fibre. They are also low in kilojoules, free of saturated fat and cholesterol and a pulse-based meal staves off the hunger pangs for a lot longer.

A bean meal doesn't always have to be vegetarian – try using beans in place of grains or potatoes. You could serve a bean salsa with fish, or cannellini bean purée with grilled meat. Butter beans can also make a delicious potato substitute.

Because they are high in protein, legumes are an ideal substitute for meat. Introduce them to your family gradually by incorporating them in meals with meat – as chilli con carne or a filling for tacos or burritos, for example. You could also try:

- Three-bean mix with a salad
- Canned kidney beans in a bolognaise sauce
- Hommous dip or spread
- Make some dhal (lentils or split peas cooked with spices) as an accompaniment to curry
- Pea and ham soup
- Potato bake with onions, beans and lean bacon, or
- Firm tofu cubed, marinated and added to stir-fries.

Of all foods eaten by populations around the world, legumes are associated with the longest lifespan.

Use low-fat dairy and calcium-enriched soy products

Dairy products provide energy, protein, carbohydrate, vitamins A, B and D, calcium, phosphorus and magnesium. Virtually all dairy foods have low GI values – largely thanks to lactose, the sugar found naturally in milk, which has a low GI of 46. By choosing low-fat varieties of milk, yoghurt, ice-cream and custard, you will enjoy a food that provides you with sustained energy, boosting your calcium intake but not your saturated fat intake. Low-fat milk supplies as much (and usually more) calcium than full-cream milk:

- 1 cup (250 ml) of low-fat milk contains about 415 mg calcium and only 0.5 g fat;
- 1 cup (250 ml) of regular milk contains about 295 mg calcium and 9.7 g fat.

Calcium is the most abundant mineral in our bodies. It builds our bones and teeth and is involved in muscle contraction and relaxation, blood clotting, nerve function and regulation of blood pressure. Research shows that calcium-rich low-fat dairy products:

- Can help lower high blood pressure
- May protect against cancer, particularly cancer of the bladder, bowel and colon, and possibly against breast, ovarian, pancreas and skin cancers
- Can favourably influence blood fat levels and reduce the risk of stroke
- Can reduce the risk of kidney stones, and
- Can assist in weight regulation.

If you eat only plant foods or want to avoid dairy products, soy products such as soy drinks, yoghurts and desserts are the answer. Oat milk and rice milk are both high GI, although nut milks such as almond milk could be expected to be low GI. Alternative milk products are not naturally high in calcium, so look for calcium-fortified products if you are relying on them as a source of calcium. Sesame seeds, dried apricots and figs, Asian greens and the edible bones of fish also contain calcium.

To meet our calcium requirements, it is recommended that adults eat two to three servings of dairy products every day. Good low-fat dairy choices include skim, no fat or low-fat milk and no fat or low-fat yoghurts. A serving is: 1 cup (250 ml) milk, 40 grams cheese or 200 grams yoghurt.

It only takes 21 days to start building a new health habit. Here are some simple ways to get started and make sure you get at least two serves of dairy foods each day.

- Start your day with a fruit smoothie.
- Top your breakfast cereal with yoghurt.
- Relax with a caffè latte mid-morning.
- Add a slice of cheese or a dollop of ricotta to your sandwich.
- Reach for a glass of cool milk for a refreshing snack.
- Follow your main meal with a dairy dessert.
- End the day with warm milk and honey to ensure a good night's sleep.

It only takes 21 days to start building a new health habit.

6

Include fish, seafood or an alternative source of omega-3

Eating fish regularly is associated with a reduced risk of heart disease, improvements in mood and lower rates of depression, better blood fat levels and enhanced immunity. It is likely that the protective components are omega-3 fatty acids. Exactly how they work is a topic of much research. They can reduce inflammation in the body, iron out irregularity in heart beat, reduce blood fat levels and might play a valuable role in treating depression and Alzheimer's disease. Modern Western diets almost certainly do not provide enough of the polyunsaturated omega-3 fats. Our bodies only make small amounts of these unique fatty acids, so we rely on dietary sources, especially fish and seafood, for them.

While the very long chain omega-3 fats are also found in some other animal foods, seafood contains 10–100 times more than in other food groups. For this reason, we suggest you aim to have at least one to two fish meals per week.

Which fish?

Oily fish, which tend to have darker coloured flesh and a stronger fish flavour, are the richest source of omega-3 fats.

- Fresh fish with higher levels of omega-3s are: Atlantic salmon; smoked salmon; Atlantic, Pacific and Spanish mackerel; sea mullet; southern bluefin tuna; and swordfish. Eastern and Pacific oysters and squid (calamari) are also rich sources.
- Canned pink and red salmon (including the bones), sardines, mackerel and, to a lesser extent, tuna, are all rich sources of omega-3s; look for canned fish packed in water, canola oil, olive oil, tomato sauce or brine, and drain well.
- Fish fingers have a measurable GI (GI 38) because of their breadcrumb coating. Although low GI, they may be high in saturated fat, depending on the oil used in their manufacture. Check the food label carefully. Oven baking or grilling are the healthiest ways to cook them and, of course, serve them with plenty of vegetables or salad.

Alternative sources of omega-3 fats

If you don't eat seafood omega-3 fats can also be found in:

- Lean red meat, kidney and liver
- Regular and fish-oil-enriched eggs, and
- Some manufactured products also have encapsulated tuna oil added to them as a source of omega-3, for example high omega-3 bread.

Plant sources of omega-3

A shorter chain form of omega-3, alpha-linoleic acid (ALA), is also found in plants. Our bodies can convert this to a longer chain form but to support conversion it is important you avoid eating too much of the omega-6 class of fats (found especially in sunflower, safflower, soybean and corn oils). Good sources of ALA are:

Linseed/flaxseed oil This is the richest plant source of ALA. However, it is extremely prone to turning rancid with heat and time and (ironically) develops a fishy odour and taste. Purchase it in very small quantities and store carefully. It is best used in salad dressings. Alternatively, linseeds can be freshly ground and sprinkled on cereal or added to cakes and muffins.

Canola oil and mustard seed oil Both these oils are high in monounsaturated fat but also contain significant amounts of ALA. Mustard seed oil has the lowest saturated fat content of any Australian oil. Margarines are available based on canola oil and these are also a source of ALA.

Walnuts and pecans.

Soybeans and soy beverages enriched with omega-3 Soybean oil is also a source of omega-3 but its high omega-6 content makes it less desirable as a source of ALA.

Green leafy vegetables Particularly broccoli, cabbage, spinach and silverbeet, kale and parsley.

Note: Olive oil is not a rich source of omega-3 but is considered 'omega-neutral' in that the fatty acids it contains do not oppose the action of omega-3s.

STEP 7
Eat nuts regularly

People who eat nuts once a week have lower levels of heart disease than those who don't eat any nuts. There are probably several reasons for this. Nuts contain lots of protein and a variety of anti-oxidants which keep blood vessels healthy; arginine, an amino acid that helps keep blood flowing smoothly; and folate and fibre, both of which can lower cholesterol levels. Nuts have even been shown to help blood glucose control in people with diabetes.

Although nuts are high in fat (averaging around 50 per cent), it is largely unsaturated, so they make a healthy substitute for foods such as biscuits, cakes, pastries, potato chips and chocolate. Because they are so nutrient and energy dense, a little goes a long way – we suggest you have about 30 grams most days (or the equivalent). They also contain relatively little carbohydrate, so most do not have a GI value.

- Nuts are perfect for staving off hunger as a between-meal snack. Enjoy a small handful on their own or with a little dried fruit.
- Use nuts in food preparation. For example, use toasted cashews in a chicken stir-fry, sprinkle walnuts or pine nuts over a salad; top fruity desserts with almonds, or add chopped nuts to muesli.
- Use hazelnut spread on bread or try peanut, almond or cashew butter rather than butter or margarine.
- Sprinkle a mixture of ground nuts and linseeds over cereal or salads, or add to baked goods such as muffins.

For more nut suggestions see The top 100 low GI food finder in Part 4.

STEP 8

Choose lean red meats, skinless chicken or tofu/plant-based protein and eggs

Reducing your intake of saturated fat doesn't mean you need to avoid meat. Red meat is the best dietary source of iron, the nutrient used in carrying oxygen in your blood, and the main source of zinc, which is a part of over 100 enzymes active in the body. Good iron and zinc status can improve energy levels and exercise tolerance. A chronic shortage of iron leads to anaemia, with symptoms including pale skin, excessive tiredness, breathlessness and decreased attention span. Even mild iron deficiency can cause unexplained fatigue.

Although chicken contains about one-third the iron of red meat, it is readily absorbed, as it is from red meat, and provides a versatile, nutrient-rich alternative.

If you enjoy meat, we suggest eating lean red meat two to three times a week, accompanying it with salad and vegetables. Trim all visible fat from meat and remove the skin (and the fat just below it) from chicken. Game meat such as kangaroo, rabbit and venison are not only lean but are also good sources of omega-3 fatty acids. So are organ meats such as liver and kidney. Leaner deli meat products are pastrami, silverside, roast beef, leg ham and rolled turkey breast.

Eggs also contain valuable amounts of the nutrients found in meat, although the iron is not as well absorbed. It used to be thought that eggs should be limited because of their high cholesterol content, but it has been found recently that our bodies compensate for an increased cholesterol intake by reducing the liver's cholesterol production. This means that most people (adults and children) can eat an egg a day, for example, without harming their heart. However, a small percentage of people have an inherited condition called familial hypercholesterolaemia, which impairs this self-regulation. To enhance your intake of omega-3 fats, you may like to use omega-3-enriched eggs. These are produced by feeding hens a diet (including canola and linseeds) that is naturally rich in omega-3s.

STEP 9

Minimise your salt intake

An estimated 75 per cent of the salt we eat is from salt already existing in foods, not salt we voluntarily add. Bread and butter/margarine, for example, contributes much of the salt in our diets. Low salt breads take some time to adjust the tastebuds to, but low salt margarines are easy to find on the supermarket shelves and are not noticeably different in taste.

Salt causes the body to hold onto fluid, which then increases blood pressure. High blood pressure, or hypertension, is a serious health problem, particularly for those with heart disease or diabetes. Even children eating a high salt diet are at risk of an increase in blood pressure. Lowering salt intake lowers blood pressure, although some people will respond more than others. A high salt intake has other consequences:

- The more salt we eat the more calcium we excrete, so a high salt intake is a risk for osteoporosis (where calcium is leached from our bones).
- Bronchial reactivity (the chance of our bronchial tubes going into spasm) is linked to sodium balance, so there is some evidence that the severity of asthma is related to salt intake.
- For Ménière's disease (causing vertigo, tinnitus, and intermittent hearing loss), although the cause is uncertain, a low salt diet is advised as part of treatment.
- Risk of stroke, gastric cancer and kidney stones is also increased according to some studies.

We recommend that you minimise the frequency with which you eat salty foods. Once your tastebuds adapt to a lower salt intake – over three to four weeks – you will find it easier to eat less salt and harder to eat salty foods.

Foods high in salt include:

- canned, bottled and packet soups, sauces and gravy bases and stock cubes
- sausages, ham, bacon and other cured meats
- pizza, meat pies, sausage rolls, fried chicken and other takeaway foods
- pickles, chutneys, olives, and
- snack foods such as potato chips.

Check food labels for salt content of foods (listed as 'sodium'). A low salt food contains less than 120 mg sodium per 100 grams. Aim for less than 450 mg per 100 grams with convenience and ready-to-eat foods. Don't routinely add salt to your food at the table or when cooking and ensure that any salt that you do use in the home is iodised (as an additional dietary source of iodine).

Salt causes the body to hold onto fluid, which then increases blood pressure.

STEP 10

If you drink alcohol, drink in moderation

Of everything we drink, alcohol could be considered the most fattening, not simply because of its kilojoule content, but because it has priority as a fuel over other nutrients: as long as there's alcohol in your system, anything else is surplus until the alcohol is burned up – and surplus kilojoules are stored largely as body fat. Looking at it another way, just one can of beer replaces all the kilojoules burnt by 20 minutes of brisk walking.

There is no doubt that large quantities of alcohol should be avoided, but several studies have suggested that a moderate alcohol intake can exert a protective effect against heart disease in some people. People who drink one or two standard drinks per day, but not necessarily every day, show a reduced risk of heart disease, with the effect being greatest among those with other risk factors for heart disease. It is important to note the finding that having three or more drinks per day actually increases the risk of death!

Who shouldn't drink alcohol?

If you have a fatty liver, high triglycerides, pancreatitis, advanced neuropathy or any form of liver disease you should not drink any alcohol.

Also, if you are pregnant, planning to have a baby, or breastfeeding, we recommend you do not drink any alcohol.

Tips for drinking less

If you think you are drinking too much, try some of the following ideas to help reduce your alcohol intake:

- Drink some water or a diet soft drink before you drink any alcohol, so you are not thirsty when you start
- Order a glass of wine and a glass of water at the same time
- Sip your alcoholic drink slowly, and
- Drink a non–alcoholic drink after every alcoholic drink (e.g. water or a diet soft drink).

Taking control

The current guidelines for a low risk to health from drinking alcohol from the National Health and Medical Research Council are that men and women consume two standard drinks or less in any one day. A standard drink is:

- 100 ml wine
- 285 ml beer
- 30 ml (a nip) spirits, and
- 60 ml fortified wine such as sherry.

For information, counselling or other assistance to help moderate your alcohol intake, contact the drug and alcohol service in your area.

What is the GI of alcoholic beverages (beer, wine and spirits)?

Alcoholic beverages contain very little carbohydrate. In fact, most wines and spirits contain virtually none, although beer contains some (3 or 4 grams per 100 ml). A middy of beer (10 ounces) contains about 10 grams of carbohydrate compared with 36 grams in the same volume of soft drink. For this reason, a beer will raise glucose levels slightly. If you drink beer in large volumes (not a great idea) then you could expect it to have a more significant effect on blood glucose. As for enjoying an occasional drink, researchers from the University of Sydney found that a pre-dinner drink tends to produce a 'priming' effect, flicking the switch from internal to external sources of fuel and keeping blood glucose levels low.

10
days to switch to a low GI diet

Let's show you how easy it is to eat the low GI way with some simple guidelines. There's no specific order in which you have to do things, no strict week-by-week list of diet do's and don'ts, no counting, calculating or measuring. However, there are some basics – daily and weekly eating and activity habits essential to good health. After all, this is not a magic pill. It's an eating plan that will help you nourish your body, feel better and promote optimum health. Following is a quiz to make it easier to see how your daily diet rates and what changes you might be able to make to help you make the switch to a low GI diet.

1
Day 1
Scrutinise your
current food intake

2
Day 2
Stock up!

Day 3
Adjust your food
environment

Day 4
Check your
portion sizes

Day 5
Give your
fibre intake
a boost

Day 6
Improve what
you choose
when...

Day 7
Tackle the snacks

Day 8
Put protein in
perspective

Day 9
Give legumes
a go

Day 10
Eat yourself to
health

How does your daily diet rate?

Try our quick quiz.

1. I mostly eat reduced fat or low-fat dairy foods. ❑ YES ❑ NO

2. I include at least one cup of milk or yoghurt or calcium-enriched soy alternative every day. ❑ YES ❑ NO

3. When I drink alcohol, I would mostly drink no more than two standard drinks per day. (Tick YES if you don't drink alcohol.) ❑ YES ❑ NO

4. I generally don't eat takeaway/fast food more than once a week. ❑ YES ❑ NO

5. I eat regular meals. ❑ YES ❑ NO

6. I eat skinless chicken. ❑ YES ❑ NO

7. I avoid adding salt to my food. ❑ YES ❑ NO

8. I include fish or some other seafood at least once a week. ❑ YES ❑ NO

9. I rarely eat packaged snacks such as potato chips. ❑ YES ❑ NO

10. I would usually eat five or more different vegetables in a day. ❑ YES ❑ NO

11. I use an unsaturated margarine spread rather than butter. (Tick YES if you use neither.) ❑ YES ❑ NO

12. I use unsaturated oils such as olive, canola, sunflower, sesame, macadamia and mustard seed for cooking and food preparation. ❑ YES ❑ NO

13. I eat at least one piece of fruit every day. ❑ YES ❑ NO

14. I limit fatty meats such as sausages, devon, cabanossi, hamburger mince, lamb chops to less than once a week. ❑ YES ❑ NO

Score 1 point for each YES

What your score means.

12–14	Excellent. It looks like you have the balance right and your basic dietary habits are sound. Read on to make sure what you are eating is low GI.
9–11	It sounds like your dietary habits aren't bad but you have work to do in achieving the right balance and lowering the GI of your diet.
Less than 9	Oops! Room for a lot of improvement here – just to boost the basic nutritional quality of your diet. So, back to the basics and good luck.

Making the switch to a low GI diet – the basics

Every day you need to:

- Eat at least three meals – don't skip meals. Eat snacks too if you are hungry.
- Eat fruit at least twice – fresh, cooked, dried or juice.
- Eat vegetables at least twice – cooked, raw, salads, soups, juices and snacks.
- Eat a cereal at least once – such as bread, breakfast cereal, pasta, noodles, rice and other grains in a wholegrain or low GI form.
- Accumulate 60 minutes of physical activity (including incidental activity and planned exercise).

Every week you need to:

- Eat beans, peas and/or lentils – at least twice. This includes baked beans, chickpeas, red kidney beans, butter beans, split peas and foods made from them such as hommous and dhal.
- Eat fish and seafood at least once, preferably twice – fresh, smoked, frozen or canned.
- Eat nuts regularly – just a tiny handful.

Start with something simple

Nothing inspires like success so attack the easiest changes first, such as eating one piece of fruit every day.

Do it gradually

Choose one aspect of your diet that you want to work on, for example, eating more vegetables, and make that your focus for at least six weeks. It can take at least this long for a new behaviour to become habit.

Don't expect 100 per cent success

A lapse in your eating habits is not failure. It's a natural part of developing new habits. Falling over is easy, but getting up and keeping going can take real effort. Believe in yourself. You can do it!

DAY 1
Scrutinise your current food intake

Today the aim is to take a closer look at what you are already eating and hunt down the high GI parts of your diet.

Take a pen and paper and begin by recalling the meals of your day, starting with breakfast. Write down the different foods you eat for each meal. Have a look in your pantry and fridge to help jog your memory. And remember to include snacks.

Look back over your day and circle the foods which are high GI choices. Key culprits are most biscuits and crackers, most breads and breakfast cereals, potato, bread rolls, crumpets, doughnuts, scones. These are the targets to change and today's job is basically to identify them and start looking up some alternatives and preparing a shopping list.

You can approach the change in a few different ways. One is to replace high GI foods with their low GI counterpart (the table This for that in Chapter 13 could help here). Another is to choose smaller portions of high GI foods, for example eat smaller portions of mashed potato. If one of the high GI foods is something you particularly like, another option is to choose it less often. You might love oven-fresh crusty white bread for example so you might allow yourself to buy a loaf once a month. Even better, you can combine your high GI food with a low GI option to moderate the glycemic impact.

Take your first step

Take a 20-minute walk today. Any time, any place, 10 minutes out and 10 minutes back. Move at a pace that gets you slightly out of breath, but keep moving. Listen to music, take a friend, take the dog, but do it today. Take an umbrella if you need to!

Our Menu

Breakfast

A bowl of All-Bran topped with sliced pear and low fat milk OR wholegrain toast spread with ricotta cheese and sliced banana

Snack

2-3 Fruit slice biscuits OR a piece of fruit

Lunch

100g tuna on whole rye crackers with sliced tomato and Lebanese cucumber followed by low fat yoghurt OR roast beef, pork, turkey or chicken on a wholegrain sandwich with salad

Snack

Fresh fruit OR a handful of toasted almonds

Dinner

Grilled white fish fillets with tomato, onion, parsley and lemon on top of green beans and baby potatoes OR chicken, sweetcorn and vermicelli noodle soup with steamed Asian greens

Snack

Few squares of dark chocolate OR fruit and low-fat yoghurt

DAY 2 Stock up!

To help yourself start eating differently you need to make sure the right foods are available, so referring to yesterday's research, finalise your shopping list and let's stock the larder!

Prepare your shopping list under headings like we've used in Low GI smart shopping in Part 5 of this book. The key sections where you are likely to be trying something new are:

Bread & Bakery – you'll need an everyday low GI loaf and possibly a fruit or seeded snack option.

Chilled Foods – ensure you have a range of low fat dairy options, including yoghurts, dairy desserts or reduced-fat cheese for snacks.

General Groceries – look for a low GI breakfast cereal, e.g. a tasty muesli, as well as pasta, noodles, some Basmati rice and legumes.

Going up

You will easily walk for at least 30 minutes today when you are shopping but to give your energy expenditure an extra boost add the task of using the stairs (and not a lift or escalator) wherever possible. This is really going to test your aerobic fitness, especially if you are overweight and may not be suitable if you have knee and joint problems. If you have convenient access to a set of stairs it is a great way of gradually working on building your fitness as you increase the number of sets you can do.

Our Menu

Breakfast

Raisin toast and a low fat milk drink OR Bircher muesli soaked in apple juice overnight then served with low-fat Greek style yoghurt and chopped fresh fruit

Snack

Fresh fruit OR a handful of fruit and nuts

Lunch

Baked beans on toast OR tuna, celery, mayonnaise and lettuce on a wholegrain roll

Snack

Handful of corn chips with avocado or tomato salsa OR fruit

Dinner

Saté chicken or beef skewers with savoury rice and vegetables or salad and peanut sauce OR pan-fried pork with apple and onion served with mashed sweet potato and steamed greens

Snack

Lemon sorbet OR fruit crumble with low fat ice-cream

DAY 3 Adjust your food environment

Talking to people about what they eat often makes us realise how easily we fall victim to our environment. If there is a bowl of lollies in front of you aren't you likely to eat one? If someone offers you a chocolate, wouldn't it be unusual to refuse? Isn't it easier to take that little packaged snack with us to watch TV, instead of preparing a plate of fruit? Perhaps you don't relate to all these scenarios but they illustrate the point that what many of us eat really depends on what is in front of us. So today's task involves a bit of housekeeping:

- Get rid of temptations: Clear out the pantry, removing unhealthy foods, or putting your indulgence foods in high cupboards or out of sight.
- Keep the shopping list you prepared yesterday to fine tune as you try things but stick to it when you are shopping. Do not buy crisps, chocolate biscuits and cakes even if they are on sale.
- Start collecting favourite recipes or record easy meal ideas and keep them in a folder, handy in the kitchen.
- Prepared some of the fresh fruit you've bought by mixing up a fruit salad or laying out a fruit platter – ready to pull out of the fridge whenever you are hungry.
- Use small snap-lock bags or containers to package up dried fruit and nuts, ready to use for snacks on the go.

Keep moving

Another walk is all that's needed. If you did it on Day 1 you can do it again today. Remember it's just 10 minutes out and 10 minutes back, but feel free to stretch it if you can. If you've got some stairs handy, add them into your exercise routine. Plan on doing it in the morning – it's the time when things tend to get done.

Our Menu

Breakfast

A couple of slices of wholegrain toast with your favourite spread and a small OJ OR vegetable omelette with wholegrain toast

Snack

Fresh fruit OR a nut bar

Lunch

Felafel Roll made on Lebanese bread with hommous, tabbouli and salad OR a toasted sandwich on wholegrain bread

Snack

Wholegrain crispbread with your favourite spread OR fruit and yoghurt

Dinner

Zucchini and salmon slice with salad and sourdough bread OR steamed ginger fish with Asian greens and Doongara rice

Snack

Fruit and low-fat custard OR toasted fruit muffin

DAY 4

Check your portion sizes

It's not uncommon for us to come across clients who are very unsure about how much they ought to be eating. The 'serving size' on packaged foods cannot be relied on as a guide, nor can the amount served in restaurants. A simplified, ever-ready guide to portion sizes exists in the palm of your hand, so compare your portion sizes with the following guide at your next meal. Unless someone else is serving for us we tend to fall into usual habits of eating a certain amount but it is an easy way to end up overeating! You can easily check your portion size using your hand:

- meat or protein serves fit the palm of your hand
- starchy carb serves match the size of your clenched fist
- and use 2 cupped hands for your vegetable/salad serve.

Circuit training

To build some more exercise into your day look at where you could do a little circuit training. Your circuit could be 1 minute of jogging on the spot, 5 flights of stairs (at the train station, in an office block, or in your own home), a few laps of the shopping centre or the infamous 20 times round the Hill's Hoist. If you can find a circuit that suits you it could be just the motivation you need to help keep exercise going.

Our Menu

Breakfast

Banana smoothie made with low fat milk, ripe banana, low fat yoghurt and honey OR fruit salad topped with yoghurt and a sprinkle of crunchy toasted muesli

Snack

Dried fruit and nut mix OR fresh fruit

Lunch

Wholegrain sandwich made with chicken, avocado, grated carrot, beetroot, lettuce and mayonnaise OR wholegrain toast topped with melted cheese and baked beans

Snack

Yoghurt and fruit OR a slice of low GI bread and jam

Dinner

Minced beef, chilli and kidney bean burritos with diced tomato, lettuce and grated reduced-fat cheese OR homemade chicken and mushroom casserole served alongside basmati rice and steamed vegetables

Snack

Skim hot chocolate OR low-fat ice-cream and strawberries

DAY 5

Give your fibre intake a boost

If you've never tried it you'll be surprised at how well an adequate fibre intake can make you feel. The main sources of fibre in our diet are cereal grains, fruits and vegetables. Nuts and seeds make a significant contribution too. You might be surprised to know that you could be making low GI choices but not eating a particularly high fibre diet. Wholemeal, brown foodstuffs like wholemeal bread, pasta and brown rice are high in fibre but not any lower GI than their white counterpart. To give your low GI diet a high fibre boost try incorporating one of these foods daily:

- A high fibre breakfast cereal, e.g. All–Bran®, Guardian which have a low GI
- Psyllium husk, a soluble fibre, e.g. sprinkled on cereal or mixed in juice
- Dried fruit like prunes, dried apricots and sultanas
- Legumes, e.g. brown lentils in a salad, kidney beans with beef in chilli, chickpeas in a curry or hommous

Bend & stretch

Gentle stretching is recommended as part of your warm-up prior to exercise and it targets another aspect of fitness that is often overlooked – flexibility. It declines significantly as we age unless we do something to stop it, so do make sure that prior to your walk today you explore the range of movement you have in your muscles with stretching exercises.

Our Menu

Breakfast

Wholegrain toast spread with peanut butter, sliced banana and a drizzle of honey OR boiled egg, wholegrain toast and a small fresh orange juice

Snack

Fruit OR low-fat yoghurt with a sprinkle of trail mix

Lunch

Minestrone soup topped with shaved Parmesan and a rye sourdough roll OR marinated chicken and Caesar salad with sourdough bread on the side

Snack

Hommous dip with vegetable crudités, olives and pita chips OR fruit

Dinner

BBQ lamb with tomato, brown lentil and mint salad OR steak with sweet potato wedges, corn on the cob and garden salad

Snack

Small handful of nuts OR fresh fruit salad

DAY 6

Improve what you choose when…

If you started the switch to a low GI diet on a Monday, then today is the first weekend day for you. Different challenges arise as a result of a change to routine and so today we want you to work on improving what you choose when …

- you meet a friend for coffee
- you eat out in a restaurant
- you're on the go all day and don't want to stop to eat

It might seem impossible to stick to low GI choices but most menus will have an option if you look hard enough. Take a look at the following pages for hints.

Enjoyable exercise

You know the saying; Exercise – you don't have to take it seriously, just regularly. Whether it's an active pastime, a job that needs to be done or a sport you like to play – lots of things you like to do can be counted as exercise. If we use a benchmark of 7500 steps as a daily target, here are some things you might like to try to put towards your total:

Activity equivalent	Steps
Grocery shopping with a trolley for 30 minutes	2800
Playing table tennis for 15 minutes	1600
Window shopping for an hour	2000
Vigorous sexual activity for 15 minutes	750
Washing the car by hand	3700
10-pin bowling for 15 minutes	1200
Mowing the lawn for 30 minutes	4700

Our Menu

Breakfast

Bowl of natural muesli with milk and yoghurt, topped with fresh or canned fruit OR poached eggs on wholegrain toast with grilled tomato or sautéed mushrooms

Snack

Wholegrain crackers with your favourite topping OR fruit

Lunch

Smoked salmon, light cream cheese and dill on rye sourdough bread OR sweet potato, marinated mushroom, semi-dried tomato, baby spinach, cheese and seeded mustard on a tortilla wrap

Snack

Trail mix OR low-fat milk drink

Dinner

Your favourite pasta with semi-dried tomato or basil pesto and shaved Parmesan and a fresh green salad and vinaigrette OR tandoori chicken with basmati rice and steamed vegetables

Snack

Fruit and a small chunk of cheese OR fruit with low-fat ice-cream

DAY 7
Tackle the snacks

Poor snack choices can be the downfall of your diet if you aren't careful. For most people it's the late night or mid-afternoon snacks that muck them up. Making what you recognise as a poor choice can have a negative impact on your thinking for the rest of the day so that one small indulgence ends up creating an avalanche of poor food choices. It's far better to see an indulgence as exactly what it is and not let it lead your entire diet astray.

One of the strategies that can help you control snack foods is to deliberately plan snacks into your diet. If there is something you really enjoy as indulgence schedule it into your day. In this case it's important you don't miss the snack because that can leave you over-hungry when meal-time comes around.

Rest or relaxation

Your choice today. Perhaps you can get one of those enjoyable or necessary exercise activities into the day.

Our Menu

Breakfast

Scrambled eggs made with low-fat milk and unsaturated margarine, served with grilled tomato and wholegrain toast OR 9-Grain muffin, toasted and topped with margarine and a drizzle of honey and a low-fat milk drink

Snack

Muesli bar OR bakery fruit bun

Lunch

Roast vegetable frittata with green salad and vinaigrette OR lunch-box salad made with 4-bean mix, tuna in vinaigrette, diced capsicum, celery and shallot

Snack

Toast with peanut butter OR a piece of fresh fruit

Dinner

Spicy pork stir-fry with Asian vegetables and Hokkein noodles OR beef or vegetarian lasagne with tossed green salad and vinaigrette

Snack

Fresh fruit OR a few squares chocolate

DAY 8

Put protein in perspective

If you still feel hungry after meals you could benefit from including a little more protein. Next to carbohydrate, protein is the most satiating nutrient: it can make your meals more satisfying and give you extra staying power. It's the reason why we suggest combinations like fruit and cheese or nuts and dried fruit for a snack. Why not try it out for yourself today by adding a protein-rich food to your snacks, e.g.: a matchbox-sized piece of cheese, a small can of tuna, a dollop of cottage cheese, a tablespoon of nuts, or an egg.

Protein foods are excellent sources of micronutrients such as iron, calcium, zinc, vitamin B12 and omega-3 fats. Lean red meat is the best source of iron you can get. Fish and seafood are important sources of omega-3 fats. Dairy foods supply the highest amounts of calcium. Eggs are great sources of several essential vitamins and minerals including vitamins A, D and E and B-group vitamins, in addition to iron, phosphorus and zinc. Legumes are nutritional powerpacks – high in fibre, a valuable source of carbs, B vitamins and minerals and potent phytochemicals. Nuts are one of the richest sources of 'good fats' and the anti-oxidants vitamin E and selenium.

Put up some resistance*

You know weight training doesn't have to necessitate a set of dumbbells. You can work your biggest muscle groups simply by standing. Begin some strength training today with the simple exercise of sit-to-stand. Sit up straight in a dining room (armless) chair, then stand and sit, stand and sit, repeatedly, aiming for a total of 16 times. Build up to a couple of sets with a rest in between and incorporate into your exercise routine 2 or 3 times a week.

*This exercise may not be suitable for those with limiting injuries or arthritis. If you feel pain you should stop the exercise. Consult a qualified personal trainer for an individualised exercise program.

Our Menu

Breakfast

Wholegrain toast topped with avocado and sliced tomato or baked beans OR traditional rolled-oat porridge cooked with milk and water and a tablespoon of sultanas, topped with a drizzle of honey

Snack

An apple with a small chunk of cheese OR skim milk drink e.g., latte

Lunch

Sushi, followed by fresh fruit if you are still hungry OR chicken, vegetable and pasta salad

Snack

Small handful of almonds and a sparkling apple juice OR dried fruit and nuts

Dinner

Vegetarian pizza OR Thai beef salad

Snack

Low-fat yoghurt OR a piece of toast with nut spread

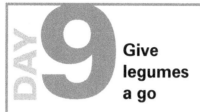

**Give
legumes
a go**

If you're serious about a low GI diet then legumes really should be taken at least twice a week. Aside from baked beans, if you grew up in a Western household, they probably haven't featured much in your diet up till now. Being one of Nature's superfoods means it is time you got acquainted. A good way to get started is to try dishes that incorporate legumes from restaurant menus. This way you are likely to be tasting them prepared at their best. A little questioning in the restaurant and some research with recipes at home can have you preparing your own delicious legume dishes.

Today's task is to include legumes in one of your meals and find a recipe including legumes that you would like to try.

Hydrate yourself

How much water do you usually drink in a day? More than 3 glasses? Then skip this section. If you cannot recall drinking water on at least 2 routine occasions in your day, then how about giving it a go today? Its too late once you're thirsty because dehydration precedes this. It might also save you mistaking thirst for hunger and help cut down your food intake. A good way to start is with a routine glass of water in the morning and another in the evening. During the day, carry a water bottle with you.

Our Menu

Breakfast

A mug of hot chocolate made with skim milk and raisin toast OR a wholegrain muffin, toasted and topped with creamed corn, mushroom and melted cheese or your favourite topping

Snack

Fruit OR a muesli slice

Lunch

Ham and tomato omelette with sourdough bread, green salad and vinaigrette OR combine salmon with diced tomato, red onion, chickpeas and French dressing to make a salad

Snack

Vegetable sticks with hommous OR fresh fruit

Dinner

Lean roast lamb with dry-roast sweet potato, pumpkin and parsnip and steamed greens OR baked fish in sun-dried tomato marinade served with steamed Doongara rice and baby green beans

Snack

2 squares dark chocolate OR 1 scoop of your favourite ice-cream

DAY 10

Eat yourself to health

Eating a low GI diet isn't only about choosing the right carbs. By working through these days you will now be eating a whole range of healthier foods and you should be feeling the benefit of it. As one final check today, we'll finish as we began – by scrutinising the foods you eat today. This time we'll make it a little easier for you. Using our example below, draw up your own checklist and tick off foods as you eat them. Ticks in all the bolded boxes reflects a balanced intake.

Your daily food intake checklist

BREAD & CEREALS	VEGETABLES	FRUIT	DAIRY	MEAT & ALTERNATIVES
☐ ☐ ☐	☐ ☐ ☐		☐	
☐ ☐ ☐	☐ ☐ ☐	☐ ☐	☐	☐
☐ ☐	☐ ☐	☐ ☐	☐	☐

Remember you can easily check your portion size using your hand:

- meat or protein serves fit the palm of your hand
- starchy carb serves match the size of your clenched fist
- and use 2 cupped hands for your vegetable/salad serve.

Our Menu

Breakfast

Traditional rolled-oat porridge served with berries and a dollop of low fat Greek style yoghurt OR a slice or two of wholegrain toast spread with your favourite topping, followed by a piece of fruit and a low-fat milk drink such as a latte or hot chocolate

Snack

Fruit OR wholegrain crackers topped with a generous spread of cottage cheese, sliced ripe tomato and ground black pepper

Lunch

Sardines with fresh lemon juice on wholegrain toast and a green side salad with vinaigrette OR chunky soup, based on vegetables with barley, lentils or pasta and some crunchy wholegrain crackers to munch on the side

Snack

Wholegrain fruit loaf spread with ricotta cheese and a sprinkle of cinnamon OR fresh fruit

Dinner

Your favourite pasta with a Bolognese sauce, sprinkle of parmesan and salad and vinaigrette alongside OR grilled steak or fish with sweet potato mash, sautéed mushroom and steamed greens

Snack

2 squares dark chocolate OR frozen fruit and yoghurt

Low GI basics
Simple steps to developing good eating habits

Listen to your appetite

Eat when you are hungry and put your knife and fork down when you are full (not stuffed). If you have a tendency to overeat, serve food in the kitchen and bring it to the table to remove the temptation of helping yourself to seconds and thirds at the table. Also, be aware that we all have 'hungry days', so it's quite normal to eat more on some days and less on others.

Watch for signs of non-hungry eating

It's also normal to reach for food when you are tired, bored or stressed. We call this 'non-hungry eating'. It isn't wrong, but it tends to contribute to overeating. If you are aware of it, you can do something about it – such as drink a glass of water or make yourself busy.

Think about what to eat, rather than what not to eat

Be positive. Try something new. Look through recipe books or use our food finder in Part 4 for your meals and simple preparation techniques that make healthy foods into satisfying meals.

Eat regularly

Remember the basics: three meals a day is a must. It's probably easier to stick to regular meal and snack times to start with, too. So make meals a time to relax and enjoy food whether you are on your own or with family or friends – you are more likely to feel satisfied if you do.

If it's healthy, keep it handy

Stock your cupboards and fridge with healthy low GI foods and snacks. Increase your chances of eating them by keeping them handy!

Keep occasional foods out of sight

Make overeating as hard as possible by putting occasional and treat foods well out of sight, preferably out of easy reach.

Chapter 14	Low GI menus

Putting it on the plate

Needing more ideas of what to actually eat? To show you how the many different aspects of nutrition can fit together to create a new low GI way of living, we've designed some typical healthy menus based on putting our three simple meal-planning steps into action. By using our 1, 2, 3 steps (see page 143) you will get the right balance of low GI carbs, protein and fruit and vegetables on your plate – every meal and every day. It will also make it easier for you to adapt your usual meals to the low GI guidelines. You'll find all recipes and menus in this chapter have an emphasis on including low GI carbohydrates, plenty of fruit and vegetables, lean meats and seafood and healthy oil in your diet.

Different body types, different lives

The body types menus from pages 208 to 217 have been given slight modifications to cater for four different body types. We have deliberately left quantities off most of the menus because it is not our intention to prescribe an amount of food to you (particularly considering we don't even know you!). We all have different energy needs and appetites – needs that vary from day to day – and consequently the amount of food we eat usually varies from day to day. This is normal and beneficial, particularly if our food choices reflect a similar variety. If you would like more specific guidance with your diet we suggest you see an Accredited Practising Dietitian.

7 everyday low GI breakfasts

You know it's a good idea to eat breakfast if you want to keep healthy, but did you realise that your food choices may also be a critical factor? Eating breakfast can improve: speed in short-term memory tests; alertness, which may help with memory and learning; and mood, calmness and reduce feelings of stress. Firing up your engine with high GI crispy flakes or soft, light toast provides a short-lived fuel supply that will send you in search of a top-up within a few hours. If you want something to nourish your body and sustain you right through the morning, follow our breakfast basics.

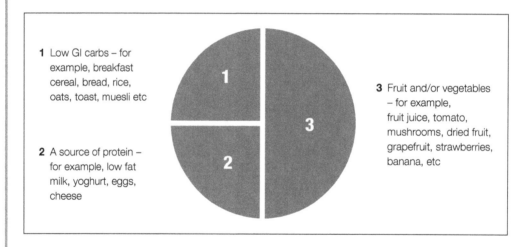

1 Low GI carbs – for example, breakfast cereal, bread, rice, oats, toast, muesli etc

2 A source of protein – for example, low fat milk, yoghurt, eggs, cheese

3 Fruit and/or vegetables – for example, fruit juice, tomato, mushrooms, dried fruit, grapefruit, strawberries, banana, etc

Breakfast basics

Choose foods from each group – carbohydrate, protein and fruit and vegetables.
1. **Carbohydrate** – breakfast cereal, bread, baked beans
2. **Protein** – low-fat milk, calcium-enriched soy milk, low-fat yoghurt, eggs, tofu, lean ham or bacon, sardines or a little cheese
3. **Fruit and vegetables** – the choice is yours, fresh, frozen or canned fruit and vegetables, dried fruit, fruit or vegetable juice

Kaye's Favourite Breakfast

1. **Carbohydrate:** natural muesli
2. **Protein:** skim milk, low-fat natural yoghurt
3. **Fruit:** strawberries

Add a little skim milk to a big bowl of natural muesli to moisten, plus a generous dollop of low-fat natural yoghurt. Top with a handful of chopped strawberries (or any other fruit).

Creamy Porridge

1. **Carbohydrate:** rolled oats
2. **Protein:** skim milk
3. **Fruit:** raisins, honey

Cook traditional rolled oats according to the packet instructions in skim milk to make a creamier porridge. Serve topped with a scattering of raisins and a drizzle of honey.

Fruit Toast with Ricotta and Pear

1. **Carbohydrate:** dense fruit and nut bread
2. **Protein:** reduced-fat ricotta cheese
3. **Fruit:** pear

Spread thick slices of a dense fruit and nut bread with reduced fat ricotta cheese and top with sliced fresh pear (peeled if you prefer). Sprinkle with cinnamon sugar to serve.

Eggs with Mushrooms and Parsley

1. **Carbohydrate:** soy and linseed bread
2. **Protein:** eggs
3. **Vegetables:** mushrooms, parsley

Slice a generous handful of button mushrooms and cook in a little olive oil. When softened, add some fresh chopped parsley and season with salt and pepper if desired. Serve on toasted soy and linseed bread with poached or scrambled eggs. A grilled tomato alongside makes this breakfast extra tasty.

everyday low GI breakfasts

Oats with Apple, Raisins and Almonds

1. **Carbohydrate**: rolled oats
2. **Protein**: skim milk
3. **Fruit and nuts**: apple, raisins, almonds

Soak traditional rolled oats in skim milk in the refrigerator overnight. Next morning add 1 grated Granny Smith apple, a small handful of raisins and a sprinkle of slivered almonds, stir and serve.

Smoothie On the Go

1. **Carbohydrate**: processed bran cereal
2. **Protein**: low-fat milk, low-fat yoghurt
3. **Fruit**: banana, honey

Combine 1 banana, 1 tablespoon of bran cereal, 1 cup of low-fat milk, 2 teaspoons of honey and 100 grams of low-fat yoghurt in a blender. Blend until smooth and thick.

Lazy Weekend French Toast

1. **Carbohydrate**: sourdough bread
2. **Protein**: eggs, skim milk
3. **Fruit**: pear or apple

Beat together 2 eggs, ¼ cup of skim milk and 1 teaspoon of pure vanilla extract. Dip 4 thick slices of sourdough bread in the egg mixture, then cook over medium heat in a lightly greased non-stick frypan for 2–3 minutes on each side until golden. Serve topped with pan-fried pear or apple slices and a sprinkling of cinnamon.

7 everyday low GI lunches

It is important to take a break and refuel properly at lunchtime. A healthy low GI lunch will help maintain energy levels and concentration throughout the afternoon and reduce the temptation to snack on something indulgent later in the day. It does not need to be a big meal. In fact, if you find yourself feeling sleepy in the afternoon, cut back on the carbs and boost the protein and light vegetables at lunchtime. (Of course a cup of coffee may help too!) Try these light meal suggestions for lunch – or for dinner if you prefer to eat your main meal at lunchtime.

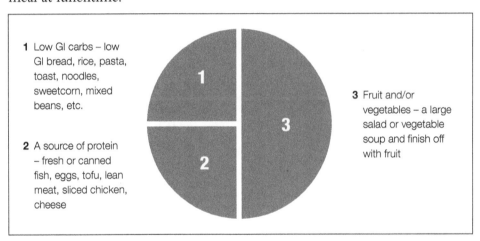

1 Low GI carbs – low GI bread, rice, pasta, toast, noodles, sweetcorn, mixed beans, etc.

2 A source of protein – fresh or canned fish, eggs, tofu, lean meat, sliced chicken, cheese

3 Fruit and/or vegetables – a large salad or vegetable soup and finish off with fruit

Lunch and light meal basics

Choose a food or foods from each group – carbs, protein and fruit and vegetables.

1. **Start** with a low GI carb such as wholegrain or sourdough bread, pasta, noodles, sweet corn or canned mixed beans.
2. **Add** some protein such as fresh or canned salmon or tuna, lean meat, sliced chicken, reduced-fat cheese or egg.
3. **Plus** vegetables or salad to help fill you up. A large salad made with a variety of vegetables would be ideal. Round off the meal with fruit.

7 everyday low GI lunches

Minestrone and Toast

1. **Carbohydrate**: beans, pasta, sweet potato, barley, rice, low GI bread
2. **Protein**: Parmesan, beans
3. **Vegetables**: tomato, carrots, onion, celery and other soup vegetables

When making minestrone yourself or buying it ready-made, choose a filling combination that includes legumes and plenty of chopped vegetables. Serve topped with some freshly shaved Parmesan and enjoy with low GI toast or a crusty grainy roll.

Snack Bar Sandwich

1. **Carbohydrate**: mixed grain, soy and linseed or seeded bread
2. **Protein**: canned salmon, tuna or hardboiled egg
3. **Vegetables**: tomato, sprouts, grated carrot, finely sliced onion rings, mixed salad greens

Try a smear of mayonnaise on the bread instead of margarine.

Lebanese Roll-ups

1. **Carbohydrate**: wholemeal flatbread, hommous
2. **Protein**: reduced-fat cheese, hommous
3. **Vegetables**: tabbouli, shredded lettuce

Spread flatbread with hommous, roll up around a filling of tabbouli and shredded lettuce sprinkled with grated cheese and warm through in a sandwich press.

Mexican Bean Tortilla

1. **Carbohydrate**: Mexican beans, corn tortilla
2. **Protein**: reduced-fat cheese, red kidney beans
3. **Vegetables**: avocado, lettuce, tomato

Warm ½ cup of beans (red kidney beans in a tomato and mild chilli sauce) and serve in a corn tortilla with 2–3 avocado slices, lots of shredded lettuce, tomato slices and grated reduced-fat cheese.

Simple Long Soup

1. **Carbohydrate:** vermicelli noodles, creamed sweetcorn
2. **Protein:** chicken stock, chicken, egg
3. **Vegetables:** carrot, shallots

Bring 2 cups of chicken stock to the boil, add a handful of dry vermicelli noodles and 1 finely diced carrot. Cook the noodles and carrot for 3–4 minutes then stir in ½ cup of creamed corn, strips of cooked chicken (a great way to use leftovers) and chopped shallots. Heat through. Beat 1 egg and slowly pour it into the boiling soup in a thin stream, stirring quickly.

Frittata

1. **Carbohydrate:** sweet potato, sweet corn kernels
2. **Protein:** egg, skim milk, lean ham, reduced fat-cheese
3. **Vegetables:** zucchini, red and green capsicum, tomato, onion, mushroom, shallots and parsley

Stir-fry about 1 cup of chopped vegetables with 2 slices of chopped ham in a little oil until soft. Beat 2 eggs with ½ cup of skim milk and season with freshly ground black pepper and 1 tablespoon of chopped parsley. Pour the egg mixture over the vegetables and cook over a low heat (preferably covered) until set. Sprinkle a little grated cheese over the top and brown under a hot grill.

Salmon Salad with Chilli Dressing

1. **Carbohydrate:** sourdough or wholegrain bread
2. **Protein:** red salmon
3. **Vegetables:** cherry tomatoes, red onion, red and yellow capsicum, mixed salad and baby spinach leaves

Combine 1 small can of red salmon (drained and flaked) with ½ punnet of cherry tomatoes, slices of red onion, red and yellow capsicum strips and mixed salad and baby spinach leaves. Toss in a chilli dressing made from olive oil, lemon juice and minced chilli and serve with bread or a crusty roll.

7

everyday low GI main meals

What to make for dinner is the perennial question. Most people know that eating well is important, but it can be hard to get motivated to cook at the end of a long day. You don't have to spend hours preparing. If your cupboards and refrigerator are stocked with the right foods, you should be able to put a meal together in under 30 minutes.

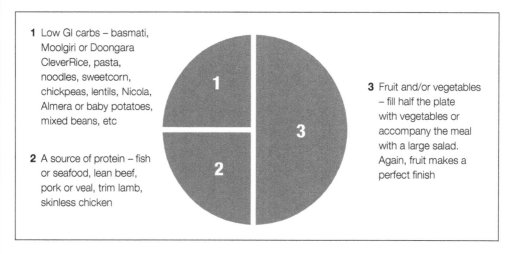

1 Low GI carbs – basmati, Moolgiri or Doongara CleverRice, pasta, noodles, sweetcorn, chickpeas, lentils, Nicola, Almera or baby potatoes, mixed beans, etc

2 A source of protein – fish or seafood, lean beef, pork or veal, trim lamb, skinless chicken

3 Fruit and/or vegetables – fill half the plate with vegetables or accompany the meal with a large salad. Again, fruit makes a perfect finish

Main meal basics

Choose a food or foods from each group – carbs, protein and fruit and vegetables.

1. **Start** with a low GI carb such as sweet potato, pasta, noodles, sweet corn, legumes.
2. **Add** some protein such as lean meat or chicken, fish or seafood, eggs and legumes.
3. **Plus** plenty of vegetables and salad to help fill you up – remember our plate model at the start of this chapter. A large salad made with a variety of vegetables would be ideal. Round off the meal with fruit.

Peppered Steak with Sweet Potato Mash

1. **Carbohydrate**: sweet potato
2. **Protein**: fillet, rump or topside steak
3. **Vegetables**: mushrooms, green beans, salad vegetables including tomato

Sprinkle steak (allow 120 grams per person) with pepper seasoning and barbecue or pan-fry. Serve with steamed sweet potato (allow 150 grams per person) mashed with low-fat milk, sliced mushrooms cooked in a little olive oil, steamed green beans and a crisp salad tossed in a vinaigrette dressing.

Lamb and Vegies

1. **Carbohydrate**: canned or baby new potatoes (allow 2–3 per person), sweetcorn on the cob (allow 1 small cob per person)
2. **Protein**: trimmed lamb loin chops or cutlets (allow 200 grams per person) or lean lamb fillet (allow 150 grams per person)
3. **Vegetables**: carrot, broccoli (allow ½ cup per person)

For extra flavour, coat the meat with a spice blend such as chermoula or garlic and rosemary and allow to 'dry marinate' for about 20 minutes. Barbecue or grill lamb (trim off the fat if you are cooking chops). Serve with steamed vegetables – baby new potatoes, corn cob, sliced carrots and broccoli florets – and your favourite condiments.

Thai-style Kebabs

1. **Carbohydrate**: Basmati rice
2. **Protein**: chicken, beef, firm white-fleshed fish, or tofu (allow 500 grams for 4 kebabs)
3. **Vegetables**: zucchini, onion, mushrooms (add extra vegetables such as red capsicum if you like)

Prepare a marinade using the following ingredients: juice and grated rind of 2 limes, 1 teaspoon of crushed garlic, 1 tablespoon of grated ginger, 2 teaspoons of chopped chilli, 1 tablespoon of chopped lemongrass and 1 tablespoon of chopped coriander.

Marinate 500 grams of diced chicken, beef, firm fish or tofu, 2 zucchinis sliced into rounds, 1 onion quartered and layers separated and 8 mushrooms, halved, or quartered if they are large, for at least 20 minutes, longer if you have the time. Thread the different ingredients alternately on skewers, brush with a little oil and barbecue or grill under a preheated grill for about 10 minutes, turning regularly and basting with the marinade. Serve with Basmati rice and lime wedges.

Honey and Mustard Pork

1. **Carbohydrate**: baby new potatoes (allow 2–3 per person), or sweet potato (allow 120 grams per person)
2. **Protein**: pork cutlets (allow 200 grams per person)
3. **Vegetables**: red capsicum, broccoli

Prepare a marinade with the following: 1 tablespoon of olive oil, 1 tablespoon of seeded mustard, 2 teaspoons of honey,

everyday low GI main meals

2 tablespoons of lemon juice and freshly ground black pepper. Trim the fat off the pork cutlets, marinate for an hour then pan-fry for about 5 minutes on each side. Cut the capsicum into strips lengthwise and stir-fry in the remaining marinade. Serve with steamed broccoli florets and potato or sweet potato, spooning the juices over the meat. Serve with additional mustard or apple sauce.

Spaghetti with Tomato Salsa and Feta

1. **Carbohydrate**: spaghetti (or your favourite pasta shapes)
2. **Protein**: feta cheese
3. **Vegetables**: tomato, onion, basil, olives, salad vegetables

To make about 2 cups of salsa (enough for 4 people), chop 4 tomatoes, ½ red onion, a bunch of basil leaves and 80 grams of pitted kalamata olives and combine in a bowl. Toss cooked spaghetti in a little olive oil and top with the tomato salsa and 150 grams of crumbled feta. Serve with a crispy green salad.

Spicy Fish with Rice and Vegetables

1. **Carbohydrate**: Basmati rice
2. **Protein**: firm white fish fillets (allow 150 grams per person)
3. **Vegetables**: frozen vegetable combination (peas, carrots, beans, sweet corn, etc.)

Brush firm white fish fillets with your favourite curry paste blended with some lemon juice. Pan-fry and serve with Basmati rice and steamed vegetables.

Red Lentil and Vegetable Curry

1. **Carbohydrate**: split red lentils, Basmati rice
2. **Protein**: lentils, yoghurt
3. **Vegetables**: onion, pumpkin, carrots, vegetable stock, English spinach, coriander

Cook 1 finely chopped onion in a little oil in a large frypan until soft and golden. Add 2 tablespoons of curry paste, 400 grams of diced pumpkin, 2 diced carrots and ½ cup of split red lentils. Stir in 2 cups of vegetable stock and simmer, uncovered, until just cooked. Stir in the leaves from a bunch of English spinach and simmer gently just until they wilt. Serve over steamed Basmati rice with natural yoghurt, topped with finely chopped fresh coriander. Serves 4 people.

Involve everybody
at mealtimes

When you can, involve everybody in the household in choosing
and preparing meals. Even if you love cooking, it's fun having
an offsider – someone to spin the lettuce, turn the meat, set the
table, or simply chat to while you chop or stir, etc. It's also a
great opportunity to find out about what's happening in other
family members' lives! Lots of our readers say they hate cooking,
but preparing and cooking meals is an integral part of healthy
eating. Easy meals for family and friends can revolve around
platters of foods on the table from which everyone can serve
themselves. This avoids any complaints about being served foods
they don't like.

If you live alone . . .

If you live alone why not prepare food for two and put a meal away
for another night? To avoid overeating on the night you cook, divide
up all the food before you sit down to eat. Make use of partially
prepared convenience foods such as chopped salads, filled pastas
and frozen mixed vegetables to make meal preparation a little
easier.

   If you like using frozen meals, choose a low fat type and add your
own cooked vegetables to bulk it out. Make a point of taking time
over your meal and enjoy what you're eating. Don't gulp it down
without thinking in front of the television – you can end up eating
more than you should. The experts have even given this habit a
name: 'mindless eating'.

7 everyday low GI desserts

The idea of dessert puts a smile on everyone's face but so often we keep sweet treats for special occasions. Well, you don't need to worry with these recipe ideas – they are easy, everyday fare made with just a few ingredients in a matter of minutes. Finishing your meal with something sweet can help signal satiety/satisfaction to the brain's appetite centre, and stop you hunting around the kitchen afterwards. They're also a great source of fruit and calcium- and protein-rich dairy foods.

Does filo pastry have a low GI?

Pastry by itself hasn't been GI tested. It's not something you normally eat as a meal. But the real problem with most shortcrust and flaky pastry products is that they tend to be very high in fat, particularly saturated fat (remember the ingredients for making pastry are essentially flour and butter with a little water plus sugar for a sweet pastry). The reason we occasionally recommend recipes with filo pastry is that you can get that lovely crisp in the mouth pastry feel with a lot less fatty pastry. Just two or three sheets of filo lightly sprayed with olive oil (not melted butter), or even orange juice for a dessert, will do the job. So a strudel using a few sheets of filo can provide a delicious after-dinner treat.

Caramelised Apples

Cut 4 apples into quarters, remove the core and seeds and slice thinly. Cook in 1 tablespoon margarine for 4–5 minutes, or until golden. Reduce the heat and add 2 tablespoons brown sugar, stirring until it dissolves. Increase the heat and add 150 ml light evaporated milk and stir to combine and heat through. Serve the apples with the sauce and a dollop of low-fat natural yoghurt.

Honey Banana Cups

Slice a large banana and halve 2 fresh passionfruit. Divide half a 200 g tub of low-fat honey-flavoured yoghurt between 2 small cups or glasses. Top with half the banana and one of the passionfruit. Top with the rest of the yoghurt and remaining banana, finishing with the passionfruit. Serve with a coconut macaroon alongside.

Strawberries with Honey Yoghurt

Toss 2 punnets of washed, hulled strawberries with 2 tablespoons of caster sugar in a frying pan for 5 minutes. Serve with low-fat natural yoghurt combined with 1–2 tablespoons of honey, to taste.

Peaches with Cinnamon Ricotta

Beat 300 g of low-fat ricotta cheese with 2 tablespoons of icing sugar, ½ teaspoon of cinnamon and ½ teaspoon of vanilla essence. Divide dollops of the mixture between 4 side plates and add a halved fresh peach (or any other fruit) and 2 almond wafers.

Banana Split

Cut 4 bananas in half lengthways and place in dessert bowls. Add 2 scoops of low-fat ice-cream and top with the pulp of ½ passionfruit.

Summer Fruit Salsa

Dice a large mango, a handful of strawberries and a peeled orange into 1 cm pieces. Mix with fresh passionfruit pulp and serve with low-fat ice-cream or frozen yoghurt.

Fruit Toast

Toast thick slices of continental fruit loaf and spread with light cream cheese or ricotta sweetened with a teaspoonful of caster sugar and a few drops of vanilla essence. Top with fresh fruit: sliced banana, peach or strawberries, or whole fresh blueberries or raspberries. Sprinkle with icing sugar to serve.

7 everyday low GI snack ideas

Most people feel like eating every 3 to 4 hours. Eating frequently can help you avoid becoming too hungry and lessen the chance of overeating when meal times come around. Depending on what you choose, snacks can also make a valuable contribution to your vitamin and mineral intake.

Quick snacks you can make in minutes

- fresh fruit salad
- ice-blocks made with fruit juice
- a handful of fresh or frozen grapes
- sticks of celery, cucumber, carrots, red capsicum and zucchini with hommous or yoghurt-based dip
- low-fat natural yoghurt with fresh fruit
- a smoothie made with fruit and low-fat milk and yoghurt
- 1 scoop of low-fat ice-cream
- hommous with pita bread
- a bowl of cereal with low-fat milk
- a slice of fruit or raisin toast
- an apple muffin
- 2 oat biscuits with a slice of cheese and an apple
- wholewheat breakfast biscuits with milk (Note: eating sweetened cereals dry is hazardous for teeth – always add milk.)

Portable pack-and-go snacks

- a juicy orange
- a small banana
- a large peach or pear
- single-serve pear or peach snack pack in natural juice
- a handful of dried fruit and nut mix
- a handful of dried apricots, apple rings, sultanas or raisins
- a tub of low-fat yoghurt or a dairy dessert
- a Weiss bar
- low-fat cheese or cheese sticks
- popcorn
- 4 squares (25–30 g) of chocolate (very occasionally for a treat)

Hot snacks for cold days

- corn on the cob
- a mug of vegetable soup with toast or crackers
- toasted sandwich on low GI bread
- small can of baked beans
- small serving of instant noodles with vegetables
- toasted fruit loaf lightly spread with margarine or low-fat ricotta
- low GI toast fingers lightly spread with Nutella®, peanut butter, honey, fruit spread or Vegemite®

Nibbles

- a small handful of unsalted, roasted nuts
- a small handful of dried fruit and nut mix
- carrot, celery and other vegetable sticks
- fruit platter – berries, orange segments, dried fruit, nuts, etc.
- marinated vegetable platter (use paper towel to soak up some of the oil before arranging the platter) with pita bread

Snacks make a valuable contribution to your vitamin and mineral intake.

7 everyday low GI drinks

Water

It's kilojoule-free and cheap – surely two good reasons for drinking water. However, it isn't necessary to drink eight glasses a day. Food contributes at least one-third of our daily fluid requirement, so we need five to seven cups of fluid to make up the remainder. Aim to make at least two or three of these water.

Fruit juice

It's widely considered a healthy drink, but if your diet includes fruit and vegetables, fruit juice really isn't necessary. If you like to include it, one glass a day is enough, and think of it as a (low fibre) serving of fruit.

Tea

Drinking a cup of tea often provides the opportunity to take time out and relax – there is a benefit in this. Tea has also been recognised recently as a valuable source of anti-oxidants which may protect against several forms of cancer, cardiovascular disease, kidney stones, bacterial infection and dental cavities. A maximum of two to three cups of tea a day is recommended.

Coffee

Did you know that 80 per cent of the world's population consumes caffeine daily? For most people two cups of coffee a day is recommended, but if you are pregnant, caffeine sensitive or have high blood pressure it is probably best to cut down to one cup per day. Both tea and coffee are a major source of anti-oxidants in the diet, simply because they are so widely and frequently consumed.

Milk

Milk is a valuable source of nutrients for adults and children but, being a liquid, it is easily overconsumed. Think of it as food in a liquid form. Recommended intakes vary for different ages, but for normal, healthy, non-pregnant adults, around 300–450 ml of low-fat milk a day is suitable.

Drinks

- a small glass of fruit juice (200 ml)
- low-fat milk or calcium-enriched soy milk
- low-fat flavoured milk
- warm flavoured milk drink (Milo etc.)
- a low-fat smoothie
- caffé latte or cappuccino with low-fat milk

What's the GI of a caffé latte and a cappuccino?

Most milky drinks will have a low GI and won't add too many kilojoules either, so long as you don't sweeten them with more than a teaspoon or so of sugar and you say no to those flavoured syrups lined up on the counter. In fact a caffé latte, cappuccino, café au lait or flat white can be the perfect mid-morning snack and an easy way to help you get your two to three serves of dairy foods a day. Regular or skim, milk has a low GI (27–34) – a combination of the moderate glycemic effect of its sugar (lactose) plus milk protein, which forms a soft curd in the stomach and slows down stomach emptying. Regular whole milk is high in saturated fat, but these days there's a wide range of reduced fat milks including low fat and skim types. If you prefer soy milk (GI 36–45 reduced fat) make sure you opt for calcium fortified and of course, reduced fat. Note that rice milk is not a suitable substitute; it has a high GI (79). How much milk are you getting with your coffee? Well, to some extent it depends on the barista and where you buy it. But here are some standard definitions.

- A caffé latte is a single shot of espresso with steamed milk – approximately a 3:1 ratio of milk to coffee.
- A cafe au lait is similar except it is generally made with brewed coffee instead of espresso in a ratio of 1:1 milk to coffee.
- Cappuccino is traditionally equal parts espresso, steamed milk and frothed milk.
- Flat white is similar to a cappuccino, but with latte proportions of foam.

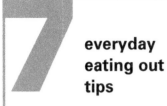

everyday eating out tips

Controlling what you eat and how you eat is easy at home or work as you can cook your own food or pack your own lunch to take away. There are times and circumstances where this is difficult and you will find yourself grabbing lunch from a takeaway restaurant or sandwich bar or you are out at meetings or functions. Being focused on a low GI way of eating shouldn't stop you from eating out at your favourite restaurant from time to time either. Here are some suggestions to help you make the food choices that suit you and your low GI everyday eating.

Fast-food outlets

Burgers and French fries are a bad idea – quickly eaten, high in saturated fat and rapidly absorbed high GI carbs that fill you with kilojoules that don't last long. Some fast-food chains are introducing healthier choices but read the fine print. Look out for lean protein, low GI carbs, good fats and lots of vegetables.

You can choose:
- marinated and barbecued chicken, rather than fried
- salads such as coleslaw or garden salad; eat the salad first
- corn on the cob as a healthy side order
- individual menu items rather than meal deals, and never upsize

Lunch bars

Steer clear of places displaying lots of deep-fried fare and head towards fresh food bars offering fruit and vegetables. Tubs of garden or Greek salad finished with fruit and yoghurt make a healthy, low GI choice.

With sandwiches and melts, choose the fillings carefully. Including cheese can make the fat exceed 20 grams per sandwich (that's as much as chips!).

Make sure you include some vegetables or salad in or alongside the sandwich.

You can choose:
- mixed grain bread rather than white
- salad fillings for sandwiches or as a side order instead of fries
- pasta dishes with both vegetables and meat
- Lebanese kebabs with tabbouli and hommous
- grilled fish rather than fried
- vegetarian pizza
- gourmet wraps

In cafés

Whether it's a quick snack or a main meal, catching up with a friend for coffee doesn't have to tip your diet off balance. Pass on breads, but if you really must, something like a dense Italian bread is better than a garlic or herb bread.

Whatever you order, specify: 'no French fries – extra salad instead' so temptation does not confront you. If you want something sweet try a skim iced chocolate or a single little biscuit or slice.

You can choose:
- skim milk coffee rather than full-cream milk
- sourdough or wholegrain bread instead of white or wholemeal
- bruschetta with tomatoes, onions, olive oil and basil on a dense Italian bread rather than buttery herb or garlic bread
- salad as a main or side order, with the dressing served separately so you control the amount
- char-grilled steak or chicken breast rather than fried or crumbed
- vegetable-topped pizza – such as capsicum, onion, mushroom, artichoke, eggplant
- lean meat pizza – such as ham, fresh seafood or sliced chicken breast
- pasta with sauces such as marinara; Bolognese; Napolitana; arrabiata (tomato with olives, roasted capsicum and chilli); and piccolo (eggplant, roasted capsicum and artichoke)
- seafood such as marinated calamari, grilled with chilli and lemon or steamed mussels with a tomato sauce
- water, mineral water or freshly squeezed fruit and vegetable juices rather than soft drinks

7 everyday eating out tips

Asian meals

Asian meals including Chinese, Thai, Indian and Japanese offer a great variety of foods, making it possible to select a healthy meal with some careful choices.

Keeping in line with the 1, 2, 3 steps to a balanced meal, seek out a low GI carb such as Basmati rice, dhal, sushi or noodles. Chinese and Thai rice will traditionally be jasmine and although high GI, a small serve of steamed rice is better for you than fried rice or noodles.

Next add some protein – marinated tofu, stir-fried seafood, Tandoori chicken, fish tikka or a braised dish with vegetables. Be cautious with pork and duck, for which fattier cuts are often used; and avoid Thai curries and dishes made with coconut milk because it's high in saturated fat.

And don't forget, the third dish to order is stir-fried vegetables!

You can choose:
- steamed dumplings, dim sims or fresh spring rolls rather than fried entreés
- clear soups to fill you up, rather than high-fat laksa
- noodles in soups rather than fried in dishes such as pad Thai
- noodle and vegetable stir-fries – if you ask for extra vegetables you may find that the one dish feeds two
- seafood braised in a sauce with vegetables
- tofu, chicken, beef, lamb or pork fillet braised with nuts, vegetables, black bean or other sauces
- salads such as Thai salads
- smaller serves of rice
- vegetable dishes such as stir-fried vegetables, vegetable curry, dhal, channa (a delicious chickpea curry) and side orders such as pickles, cucumber and yoghurt, tomato and onion
- Japanese dishes such as sushi, teriyaki, sashimi, salmon steak or tuna, teppanyaki (which is char-grilled) in preference to tempura, which is deep-fried

Airlines and airports

Airports are notoriously bad places to eat. Fast-food chains, a limited range, pre-made sandwiches, sad-looking cakes, a lack of fresh fruit and vegetables, and expensive!

In airline lounges you will do better, although, again, the range is limited. Fresh fruit is always on offer and usually some sort of vegetables either as salad or soup. The bread is usually the super-high GI white French type and with crackers as the only other option, you would do better to rely on fruit, fruit juices, yoghurt or a skim milk coffee for your carbs.

In-flight, unless you have the privilege of a sky chef, meals are fairly standard fare, including a salad and fruit if you're lucky. Many airlines offer special diets with advance bookings and although there's no guarantee it meets your nutritional criteria, it may give you healthier choices compared to what everyone else is having.

Travelling domestic economy these days, it's probably best to eat before you leave, take your own snacks with you and decline the in-flight snack (you really will be better off without that mini chocolate bar, biscuit, cake or muffin, and on some airlines you have to pay for it).

You can choose:
- fresh fruit, soup and salad items in airline lounges rather than white bread, cheese, cakes and salami
- small meals in-flight, rather than eating everything put in front of you
- water to drink, wherever you are
- dried fruit, nut bars, bananas or apples that you have taken along yourself

body-type low GI diet menus

1 for everybody

These menus are designed for the average adult. They are also suitable for people with type 1 diabetes, with the inclusion of snacks.

2 for bigger bodies

These menus have been modified for people trying to lose weight, including those with type 2 diabetes. The emphasis is on a moderate carbohydrate intake, to satisfy appetite, with a small amount of fat to save on kilojoules. If appetite is not a problem you may choose to use the menus for EveryBody, which are slightly higher in fat, but to lose weight you will need to moderate the serve size or the kilojoule intake could be excessive.

3 for kids' bodies

These menus have been modified for children. Children are best fed a nourishing mix of carbohydrates and fats. The children's menus include variations on the dishes in the adult menus, with the inclusion of healthy snacks. Many of the snack foods children eat are high in fat and quickly digested, high GI carbohydrate, which may increase their risk of obesity. We suggest some healthier alternatives.

GETTING YOUR KIDS TO EAT SOMETHING DIFFERENT

Children are born with a liking for sweet tastes but they also prefer what they are familiar with. Initial rejection of a new food can eventually turn to acceptance if children are given lots of opportunities to sample the new food in a favourable environment. A small taste is all it takes, but changes in taste do occur gradually so 8 to 10 small tastes may be required.

DRINKS FOR CHILDREN

Offer children water to drink with their meals and limit the amount of cordial and soft drink they have. Around 200 ml of fruit juice and 400 ml of milk a day is sufficient for school-age children.

4 for busy bodies

These menus have been modified for very active people. Active people need a high carbohydrate intake to fuel their muscles, but this needn't all be low GI. So in these menus you'll find large quantities of carbohydrate of different types. We've indicated the GI ranking of the carbohydrate in these menus and offer the following tips on when to use high and low GI carbohydrates for best performance.

USING THE GI TO BOOST YOUR SPORTS PERFORMANCE

Scientific research has so far identified three key applications of the GI to enhance sports performance:

1 Use high GI foods after exercise, in the recovery phase to enhance glycogen replenishment.

2 Use high GI foods or fluids during exercise to maintain food glucose levels.

3 A low GI pre-event meal may enhance endurance in prolonged exercise.

low GI diet menu ideas for everybody

monday

BREAKFAST
- Bürgen toast with avocado, sliced tomato and black pepper
- Fresh citrus fruit or juice

LUNCH
- Minestrone soup with a crusty bread roll
- Low-fat yoghurt and berries

DINNER
- Deep sea bream fillets with semi-dried tomato marinade
- Doongara rice, green bean, rocket and baby tomato salad

tuesday

BREAKFAST
- Swiss natural muesli topped with low-fat yoghurt and sliced banana or berries
- Apple juice

LUNCH
- A mixed Mediterranean salad of lettuce, tomato, cucumber, capsicum, olives and sprouts with balsamic dressing served with chunky oven-baked sweet potato wedges and guacamole
- A bunch of grapes

DINNER
- Grilled fish fillet or basted chicken breast served with sweet potato, potato and garlic mash, spinach and snow peas

wednesday

BREAKFAST
- Semolina and low-fat milk flavoured with honey and vanilla
- Plate of fresh melon slices: rockmelon, watermelon, honeydew
- Low-fat hot chocolate

LUNCH
- Sardines on toast with low GI bread served with lettuce, sliced cucumber, shredded carrot and beetroot, and sprouts

DINNER
- Vegetable and noodle stir-fry
- Rhubarb with honey and strawberries topped with natural yoghurt and a sprinkle of toasted walnuts

thursday

BREAKFAST
- Poached egg with slow roasted tomatoes and wholegrain toast
- Fresh grapefruit or juice

LUNCH
- Toasted Turkish bread with hommous and tabbouli
- Sliced kiwi fruit and banana

DINNER
- Pork fillet with roasted pears and Basmati rice served with steamed carrot and zucchini or other fresh vegetables

friday

BREAKFAST
- Sautéed mushrooms, shallots and parsley served on wholegrain toast
- Tomato juice

LUNCH
- Sourdough rye with lean roast beef and horseradish or smoked salmon and light cream cheese and capers
- Fresh fruit or juice

DINNER
- Vegetarian lasagne with a green salad
- Peaches and low-fat ice-cream

saturday

BREAKFAST
- Wholegrain toast with peanut butter or Vegemite
- Orange juice

LUNCH
- Salmon omelette with wholegrain bread and salad greens

DINNER
- Pilaf with butter bean, capsicum and prawns
- Diced nectarine and banana topped with low-fat fruit yoghurt and a sprinkle of toasted almonds

sunday

BREAKFAST
- All Bran™ with low-fat milk or yoghurt and fresh or canned fruit

LUNCH
- Chargrilled vegetables and beans with pasta and a mixed green salad with olive oil vinaigrette
- Fresh fruit

DINNER
- Lean lamb roast brushed with oil, rosemary and dried mint, baked over water, served with char-grilled garlic potatoes and sweet potato and fresh steamed greens
- Apple and ginger crumble

low GI diet menu ideas for bigger bodies

monday

BREAKFAST
- 2 slices wholegrain toast spread with ½ an avocado and topped with sliced tomato and black pepper
- Grapefruit or tomato juice

LUNCH
- A hearty winter vegetable soup with a wholegrain roll and a small apple

DINNER
- Deep sea bream fillets with semi-dried tomato marinade served with ½ cup of Doongara rice, and green bean, rocket and baby tomato salad

tuesday

BREAKFAST
- Natural muesli (about ½ cup) with low-fat yoghurt and fresh strawberries

LUNCH
- A mixed salad of cherry tomatoes, chopped cucumber and celery, baby beets, marinated mushrooms and mesclun lettuce with a cornmeal, capsicum and chive muffin

DINNER
- Grilled fish fillet or basted chicken breast (120 g) served with sweet potato, potato and garlic mash, spinach and snow peas

wednesday

BREAKFAST
- ⅓ cup of raw rolled oats and a tablespoon of raisins with low-fat milk
- Fresh grapefruit

LUNCH
- Open sandwich with ricotta, avocado and sprouts
- Sliced rockmelon

DINNER
- Vegetable and noodle stir-fry
- Rhubarb with honey and strawberries topped with a dollop of low-fat natural yoghurt

thursday

BREAKFAST
- Multigrain toast with a smear of canola margarine, Vegemite and a boiled egg
- Tomato or orange juice

LUNCH
- Toasted Turkish bread with hommous and tabbouli
- Sliced kiwi fruit

DINNER
- Pork fillet with roasted pears and ½ cup of Basmati rice served with steamed carrot and zucchini or other fresh vegetables

friday

BREAKFAST
- Sautéed mushrooms with chopped parsley and shallots, seasoned with soy sauce, served with 2 slices mixed grain toast
- Skim milk cappuccino

LUNCH
- A sandwich of low GI bread filled with salmon and lemon juice, lettuce and tomato
- Fresh fruit

DINNER
- Vegetable lasagne with green salad
- Peaches and a scoop of low-fat ice-cream

saturday

BREAKFAST
- 2 slices of wholegrain toast spread with canola margarine and Vegemite or marmalade
- Small glass of orange juice

LUNCH
- Combine leftover pasta with a can of tuna, chopped tomato, celery, cucumber and parsley; dress with balsamic vinaigrette or a dessertspoon of canola mayonnaise

DINNER
- Pilaf with butter beans, capsicum and prawns
- Diced nectarine with a dollop of low-fat vanilla yoghurt and a slice of crisp almond bread

sunday

BREAKFAST
- ½ cup of All Bran with low-fat milk or yoghurt topped with ½ cup fresh or canned peach slices or berries

LUNCH
- Chickpea, tomato and eggplant with toasted bread and a mixed green salad with olive oil vinaigrette

DINNER
- Lean lamb roast brushed with oil, rosemary and dried mint and baked over water, served with chargrilled garlic potatoes and sweet potato and fresh steamed greens
- Fresh fruit plate

low GI diet menu ideas for kids' bodies

monday

BREAKFAST
- Banana smoothie with vanilla yoghurt, honey and wheatgerm

SNACK
- Raisin toast with canola margarine

LUNCH
- Ham sandwich with cherry tomatoes
- Small apple and mini yoghurt

SNACK
- Frozen orange quarters

DINNER
- Barbecued chicken with corn cobs and salad
- Low-fat custard served over canned pear halves

tuesday

BREAKFAST
- An apricot and muesli muffin and a bowl of fruit salad with yoghurt

SNACK
- A bag of home-popped popcorn

LUNCH
- Wholemeal lavosh bread topped with hommous, shredded lettuce, cheese, tuna and carrot
- Sliced fresh apple

SNACK
- Toast with Vegemite

DINNER
- Oven-fried fish with chunky chips. Choose products cooked in canola oil. Offer fresh raw vegetable sticks alongside
- Stewed apples with low-fat vanilla yoghurt

wednesday

BREAKFAST
- Low GI toast with peanut butter, honey and sliced banana

SNACK
- Milk and Milo

LUNCH
- Low GI toast topped with creamed corn, mushroom and melted cheese

SNACK
- Crumpet and honey

DINNER
- 'Home-made' chicken and noodle soup: add slivers of chicken and pasta to salt-reduced packet mix. Boil 10 minutes. Add mixed frozen vegies and chopped shallots near the end of cooking
- Top canned fruit with muesli and bake in moderate oven for 10 minutes. Serve with low-fat vanilla yoghurt

thursday

BREAKFAST
- Nutri-Grain with low-fat milk and sliced banana

SNACK
- Snack pack of peaches

LUNCH
- Jacket potato topped with beans and cheese

SNACK
- Chopped strawberries, banana, grapes and peach with fruit yoghurt

DINNER
- Fish and vegetable kebabs with pineapple pieces, button mushrooms and cherry tomatoes. Grill, basting with a mix of oil, soy sauce and warmed honey. Serve with noodles or rice

friday

BREAKFAST
- Baked beans on toast
- Fresh fruit

SNACK
- A slice of cheese and wholemeal crackers

LUNCH
- Salmon and lettuce on Performax low GI bread

SNACK
- Fruit yoghurt
- Choc chip cookies

DINNER
- Vegetarian lasagne
- Fresh strawberries with a scoop of low-fat ice-cream

saturday

BREAKFAST
- Porridge with low-fat milk, sultanas and juice

SNACK
- 2 oatmeal biscuits and a glass of low-fat milk

LUNCH
- Tuna, chopped celery and mayonnaise roll
- Fruit juice

SNACK
- Vegetable strips with corn relish and cottage cheese dip

DINNER
- Vegetable and noodle stir-fry
- Low-fat ice-cream with sliced banana, nuts and chocolate syrup

sunday

BREAKFAST
- Shredded wheat with low-fat milk
- A slice of raisin toast
- Hot chocolate

SNACK
- Paddle-Pop

LUNCH
- Spaghetti or pasta shapes with basic tomato sauce
- A bowl of small chunks of fresh fruit offered with toothpicks and yoghurt to dip.

SNACK
- Cheese and fruit plate with water crackers

DINNER
- Lean lamb roast with potato and sweet potato chunks, peas and mint sauce

low GI diet menu ideas for busy bodies

We have indicated the GI rating of the carbohydrate foods in the following meals and snacks to help you choose the right type of food for your circumstances.

Δ = High GI carbohydrate   ‡ = Low GI carbohydrate

monday

BREAKFAST
- 4 slices wholegrain fruit and nut loaf‡, toasted and topped with light cream cheese, slices of apple‡, and cinnamon
- A glass of low-fat milk‡

LUNCH
- 2 sandwiches on mixed grain bread‡ with tuna, tomato, onion, cucumber
- A banana and fruit juice‡

DINNER
- Garlic prawns, capsicum and coriander pasta‡, green salad and bread roll
- Fresh fruit‡

tuesday

BREAKFAST
- Large serve of chunky fresh fruit salad‡ topped with low-fat yoghurt‡ and low-fat toasted muesli‡
- Apricot and muesli muffin

LUNCH
- Lavosh bread with lettuce, tomato, grated cheese and canned Mexican beans‡
- An apple‡
- Low-fat flavoured milk‡

DINNER
- Roasted sweet potato, garlic and rosemary pilaf‡
- Summer pudding‡

wednesday

BREAKFAST
- Rolled oats‡ cooked with mixed dried fruit‡, topped with pecans or walnuts
- Toast with honey
- Low-fat milk or juice‡

LUNCH
- 3 sandwiches with lean roast meat and salad
- Juice‡

DINNER
- Antipasto (vegetarian) with sourdough bread
- Vegetarian pizza
- GelatoΔ

thursday

BREAKFAST
- Banana and honey jaffles made with low GI bread‡. (Use a light spread of canola margarine.)
- Skim milk cappuccino‡

LUNCH
- Beef and lentil burgers‡ on a toasted wholemeal roll∆, served with mixed lettuce, sliced tomato and chilli sauce
- Flavoured mineral water∆

DINNER
- Warm lamb salad with 2 bread rolls
- Poached pears‡ with low-fat vanilla yoghurt‡ and toasted flaked almonds

friday

BREAKFAST
- Baked bean and light cheese melts on low GI bread‡
- Canned peach slices‡

LUNCH
- Vegetable and rice noodle‡ Vietnamese soup
- Fruit salad‡

DINNER
- Vegetable bake with a bread roll∆
- Fresh rockmelon∆ with low-fat ice-cream‡

saturday

BREAKFAST
- 4 slices low GI toast‡ with peanut butter and honey
- Orange juice‡

LUNCH
- Marinated BBQ chicken noodle salad‡
- Canned fruit‡

DINNER
- Thai green chicken curry with Doongara rice‡
- Mango lassi‡

sunday

BREAKFAST
- Just Right™ topped with a sliced banana, low-fat milk
- A couple of slices of wholegrain toast‡ with jam
- An apple and fruit juice‡

LUNCH
- Spaghetti‡ with basic tomato sauce
- Bread roll∆ and fruit juice‡

DINNER
- Seared tuna steaks with red capsicum sauce, Doongara rice‡
- Fresh fruit platter‡

snacks

- Dried fruit and nut mix‡
- Raisin toast‡
- Fresh fruit‡
- Low-fat milk with chocolate flavouring‡
- Low-fat yoghurt‡

- A fruit smoothie‡
- Muffins
- Snack packs of canned fruit‡
- Scones and jam∆
- Banana sandwich∆

- Creamed rice
- Sustagen™ ‡
- Pancakes∆
- Pikelets∆
- Toast and honey∆
- Bowl of Nutri-Grain

Chapter 15

Ready, set, go – move it & lose it!

When we explained the basics of everyday low GI eating at the beginning of this section, we mentioned that one of the golden rules is to accumulate 60 minutes of physical activity every day, including incidental activity and planned exercise. This will help you control your weight and provide a host of other benefits. To make a real difference to your health and energy levels, exercise has to be regular and some of it needs to be aerobic. But every little bit counts – and, best of all, any extra exercise you do is a step in the right direction.

Though some people can make a serious commitment to 30-plus minutes of planned exercise three or four times a week, most of us have a long list of excuses. But there's good news. Research tells us that the kilojoules we burn in our everyday activities are important too, and that any amount of movement is better than none at all.

Changing the habits of a lifetime isn't easy. We know how hard it can be to find time to fit everything into a day, especially if you are working and have a family. That's why we suggest you move it *and* lose it with our '1, 2, 3 one step at a time, in your own time' approach.

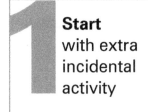

Start
with extra
incidental
activity

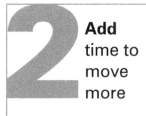

Add
time to
move
more

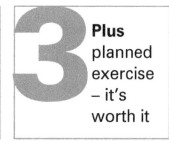

Plus
planned
exercise
– it's
worth it

Start
with extra
incidental
activity

Incidental activity is the exercise we accumulate each day as part of our normal routines – putting out the garbage, making the bed, doing chores, walking to the bus stop, popping out for a coffee and walking up a flight of stairs. If you make a conscious effort to increase the amount of this kind of activity in your day, it will eventually become second nature.

With just a little extra effort, you can build more incidental physical activity into your life. You've probably heard these ideas before, so read this list as a timely reminder. It would be great if you could use just one of these ideas regularly.

- Use the stairs instead of taking the lift. Walk up them as quickly as you can. Try taking them two at a time – to strengthen your legs.
- Don't stand still on the escalator – walk up and down.
- Take the long way around whenever you can – popping down to the corner shop, getting a drink from the office water cooler, going to the bathroom.

If you do regular exercise you:

- will tend to have lower blood pressure
- will feel more energetic
- are less likely to have a heart attack or develop diabetes
- will reduce your insulin requirements if you have diabetes
- will find it easier to stop smoking
- will be better able to control your weight
- can increase levels of 'good' HDL cholesterol
- will sleep better

- Make the time to walk your children to or from school.
- Catch up with a friend by meeting for a walk, rather than talking on the phone or over coffee.
- Get off your chair and talk to your colleagues rather than sending endless emails.
- Walk the dog instead of hitting tennis balls for him or her to chase and retrieve.
- Get rid of the leaf blower and rake the leaves or sweep the courtyard the old-fashioned way.
- Park the car at the opposite end of the carpark and walk to the ATM, post office or dry cleaners.
- Walk to a restaurant (or park a good distance from it) to force yourself to take a walk after dinner.

Think of extra incidental activity as an opportunity not an inconvenience. The following table shows how 'spending' 5 minutes here and there every day can add up to potential fat 'savings' in the long term.

Take 5 minutes every day to:	Potential savings in kilos of fat*	
	in 1 year	in 5 years
Take the stairs instead of the lift	3.7	18.5
Vacuum the living room	0.7	3.5
Walk 150 m from the car to the office	0.7	3.5
Carry the groceries 150 m to the car	0.9	4.5

* Figures based on a 70 kg (11 stone) person

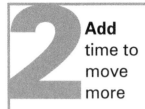

Add
time to
move
more

Exercise is more likely to be achieved when scheduled into your day, just like any other appointment. So think about your day, make a note in your diary and prioritise exercise. To reap the benefits, exercise doesn't have to be intense: exercise of moderate duration and intensity – including walking – is associated with reduced risk of disease. While brisk walking is best, even slow walkers benefit!

For most of us, walking fits the bill perfectly. It keeps us fit, it's cheap and convenient, it gets us out and about, and it becomes even more important as we grow older. You can walk alone, or with friends. In fact, talking while you walk can have important emotional benefits: Not only do our bodies produce calming hormones while we walk, but the talk itself can be great therapy – and good for relationships in general. But don't hesitate to walk alone if you prefer, or with your dog – your pet will love you all the more for it. And you'll be able to take some time to think and relax.

How often? Try to walk every day. Ideally you should accumulate 30 minutes or more on most days of the week. The good news is, you can do it in two 15-minute sessions or six 5-minute sessions. It doesn't matter.

How hard? You should be able to talk comfortably while you walk. Find a level that suits you. If you feel sore at first, don't worry; your body will adapt and the soreness will decrease. Stretching for 2 minutes before and after your walk will help minimise aches and pains.

Getting started Before beginning a walking (or any exercise) program, see your doctor if you have:

• been inactive for some time
• a history of heart disease or chest pains
• diabetes
• high blood pressure

Or if you:
• smoke
• weigh more than you should

How many steps will make a difference?

Go out and buy a cheap pedometer (step counter). Research has shown that every day we need to take about:

- ❑ 7500 steps to maintain weight
- ❑ 10 000 steps to lose weight
- ❑ 12 500 steps to prevent weight regain

For most of us this means taking a walk on top of our incidental activity. In the normal course of a day – just living and working – it is virtually impossible (unless you deliver the mail or walk other people's dogs for a living!) to achieve that 10 000 steps a day.

The following table gives you an idea of how many steps are equivalent to 15 minutes of certain activities.

15 minutes of activity	Equivalent number of steps
Moderate sexual activity	500
Watering the garden	600
Vigorous sexual activity	750
Clearing and washing the dishes	900
Standing cooking at the barbecue	950
Standing while playing with kids	1100
Carpentry – general workshop	1200
Playing golf at the driving range	1200
Food shopping with a trolley	1400
General house cleaning	1400
Sweeping and raking	1600
Digging the garden	2000
Mowing the lawn with a hand mower	2350
Moving furniture	2350
Carrying bricks or using heavy tools	3150

To achieve:

- 4000 steps you need about 30 minutes of moderately paced walking
- 7500 steps you need about 45 minutes of moderately paced walking
- 10 000 steps you need about 60 minutes of briskly paced walking

3

Plus planned exercise – it's worth it

Exercise and activity speed up your metabolic rate (increasing the amount of energy you use) which helps you to balance your food intake and control your weight. Exercise and activity also make your muscles more sensitive to insulin and increase the amount of fat you burn.

A healthy low GI diet has the same effect. Low GI foods reduce the amount of insulin you need, which makes fat easier to burn and harder to store. Since body fat is what you want to get rid of when you lose weight, exercise or activity in combination with a low GI diet makes a lot of sense.

Best of all, the effect of exercise doesn't end when you stop moving. People who exercise have higher metabolic rates and their bodies burn more kilojoules per minute even when they are asleep!

If you are ready to improve your fitness, making a commitment to a planned exercise program including aerobic, resistance and flexibility/stretching exercises will give you the best results. Variety is also important.

Planned exercise doesn't mean having to sweat it out in a gym. The key is to find some activities you enjoy – and do them regularly. Just 30 minutes of moderate exercise each day can improve your health, reducing your risk of heart disease and type 2 diabetes. If you prefer you can break this into two 15-minute sessions or three 10-minutes sessions. You'll still see the benefits. Remember, every little bit counts.

What about personal trainers?

Working with a personal trainer can be a great way to improve your health and fitness and work towards your goals. A good trainer will design an exercise program tailored to your needs and fitness level as well as providing motivation and support. Many personal trainers now provide services for a reasonable rate and you can choose to use a health club or train at home or outdoors. If cost is an issue, you could train with a small group of three or four others with similar fitness levels, or you could just have a few sessions initially. If you can, try to budget for at least 10 sessions. This will help you achieve your goals and increase your confidence with the new exercises.

How to find a good personal trainer

Many trainers are attached to health clubs, but if you don't belong to one or you would prefer to train at home or outdoors, look in your local newspaper or search online for someone in your area. Ask to see their qualifications – they should have a Certificate IV in personal training. A good trainer should offer you at least one complimentary session to 'try before you buy'.

What to expect when you see a personal trainer

In your first session, a good personal trainer will ask you about your current lifestyle, your goals and expectations and any health or medical problems. He or she will then work out a program to help you reach your goals and work closely with you to implement the plan, supervising each of your exercise sessions to make sure you are performing the exercises correctly and pushing you to the next level. He or she will also help to motivate you when the going gets tough.

Here are some ideas to get you started

- aerobics
- aquarobics
- cycling
- dancing
- exercise balls
- exercise bikes
- exercise classes
- exercise DVDs and videos
- golf
- health clubs and gyms
- paddling, rowing and kayaking
- Pilates
- spin classes
- surfing and bodysurfing
- swimming
- table tennis
- tai chi
- team sports
- tennis, squash and other racket sports
- treadmills
- weight training
- yoga

Part 4

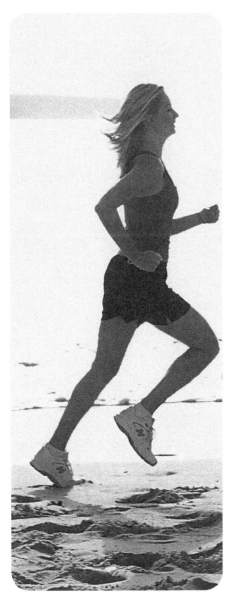

The top 100 low GI diet food finder

- Fruit & vegetables
- Bread, breakfast cereals & grains
- Noodles
- Pasta & couscous
- Rice
- Wholemeal cereal grains
- Legumes
- Nuts
- Fish & seafood
- Lean meat & chicken, eggs & plant protein alternatives
- Dairy foods
- Dairy alternatives

Chapter 16	# Low GI diet food finder

To pick the top 100 low GI foods and to give you plenty of choice, we pushed our shopping trolley up and down the supermarket aisles. We have listed the foods in this section A to Z within their food category to make meal planning and shopping easier.

We are often asked about foods such as lean red meat, chicken, eggs, fish and seafood – foods that don't have a GI because they don't contain carbs. As a result we have also included brief sections on these protein-rich foods because they are an important part of a healthy diet.

Which brand?

Low GI eating often means making a move back to staple foods – legumes, whole cereal grains, vegetables and fruit – which naturally have a low GI, so it doesn't matter what brand you buy. Brands are important, however, when it comes to choosing carb-rich processed foods such as breads and breakfast cereals whose GI values can range from low to high.

To find the GI of your favourite brands you can:

- Look for the certified GI Symbol on foods.
- Check the nutritional label – some manufacturers include the GI.
- Visit www.glycemicindex.com to search a reliable database of GI values.
- Check the GI tables in Part 5.

LOW GI

Fruit & Vegetables

Fruit and vegetables play a central role in a low GI diet. While we all remember being told to eat our greens, we now know that it's important to eat seven or more serves of fruit and vegetables every day for long-term health and well-being. The greater the variety, the better.

When it comes to fruit and vegetables think colour, think variety, think protective anti-oxidants, and give these foods a starring role in your meals and snacks.

Green

- artichokes, Asian greens, asparagus, avocados, green beans, bok choy, broccoli, broccolini, Brussels sprouts, cabbage and Chinese cabbage, green capsicum, celery, chard, chicory, choko, choy sum, cress, cucumber, endive, green onions, leafy greens, leeks, lettuce, mesclun, okra, peas (including snowpeas and sugar snap peas), rocket, silverbeet, spinach, spring onions, sprouts, squash, watercress, witlof, zucchini
- green apples, feijoas, figs, green grapes, honeydew melons, kiwi fruit, limes, green pears

Red/pink

- red capsicum, radishes, red onions, tomatoes, yams
- red apples, blood oranges, cherries, cranberries, red grapes, pink/red grapefruit, guavas, plums, pomegranates, raspberries, rhubarb, strawberries, tamarillo, watermelon

White/cream

- bamboo shoots, cauliflower, celeriac, daikon, fennel, garlic, Jerusalem artichoke, kohlrabi, mushrooms, onions, parsnips, potatoes (white-fleshed), shallots, swedes, taro, turnips, white corn
- bananas, lychees, nectarines, white peaches, brown pears

Orange/yellow

- butternut squash, carrots, yellow/orange capsicum, pumpkin, squash, sweetcorn, sweet potato, winter squash, yellow beets, yellow tomatoes
- yellow apples, apricots, custard apple, gooseberries, grapefruit, lemons, mandarins, mangoes, nectarines, oranges, papaya, paw paw, peaches, persimmons, pineapple, rockmelon, tangerines

Blue/purple

- beetroot, eggplant, purple asparagus, radicchio lettuce, red cabbage
- blackberries, blackcurrants, blueberries, boysenberries, purple figs, purple grapes, plums, raisins

Why are fruit and vegetables so important?

A high fruit and vegetable intake has been consistently linked with better health. It could be because they are packed with anti-oxidants – nature's personal bodyguards – which protect body cells from damage caused by pollutants and the natural ageing process.

Some key anti-oxidants

Beta-carotene – the plant form of vitamin A, used to maintain healthy skin and eyes. A diet rich in beta-carotene may even reduce damage caused by UV rays. Apricots, peaches, mangoes, carrots, broccoli and sweet potato are particularly rich in beta-carotene.

Vitamin C – nature's water-soluble anti-oxidant found in virtually all fruits and vegetables. Some of the richest sources are guavas, capsicum, oranges, kiwi fruit and rockmelon. Vitamin C is used to make collagen, the protein that gives our skin strength and elasticity.

Anthocyanins – the purple and red pigments in blackberries, blueberries, capsicum, and eggplant also function as anti-oxidants, minimising the damage to cell membranes that occurs with ageing.

LOW GI Fruit

Naturally sweet and filling, fruit is widely available, inexpensive, portable and easy to eat – just like other snack foods, but without the added fat and sugar. So, buy the best you can and enjoy a lifetime of benefits.

The sugars in fruits and berries have provided energy in the human diet for millions of years. It shouldn't come as too much of a surprise, therefore, to learn that these sugars have low GI values. Fructose, in particular – a sugar that occurs naturally in all fruits and in floral honey – has the lowest GI of all. Fruit is also a good source of soluble and insoluble fibres which can slow digestion and provide a low GI. And as a general rule, the more acidic a fruit is, the lower its GI value.

Temperate climate fruits – apples, pears, citrus (oranges, grapefruit) and stone fruits (peaches, plums, apricots) – all have low GI values.

Tropical fruits – pineapple, paw paw, papaya, banana, rockmelon and watermelon tend to have higher GI values, but their glycemic load (GL) is low because they are low in carbohydrate. So keep them in the fruit bowl and enjoy them every day if you wish as they are excellent sources of anti-oxidants.

Eating fruit regularly is a great way to keep hydrated: some fruits such as watermelon contain up to 90 per cent water. If you're not well hydrated, all your body functions, from joint lubrication and muscle contraction through to digestion and mental performance can be compromised.

Fruit juice

It's all too easy to overdo the kilojoules when drinking juice. For example, if you buy a 'large' orange juice in a café or fast food outlet that offers value-for-money portions, you may find you are consuming the equivalent of ten oranges (3000 kJ)! Remember, one serve is 125 ml (½ cup).

When buying juice look for labels that say: '100 per cent pure fruit juice' or 'unsweetened'.

FOOD	QUICK RECIPE IDEAS

APPLES

Just one fresh apple will give you about one-third of your vitamin C needs for the day and by stimulating saliva it can also help prevent dental decay. Apples are a good source of dietary fibre, particularly pectin, which promotes a healthy balance of bacteria in the intestine. On top of this, apples, particularly the skins, are packed with anti-oxidants. Cooking apples is likely to raise the GI slightly.

- Add coarsely grated apple to your muesli or favourite low GI breakfast cereal, or to muffin mixes when baking.
- Bake or microwave whole apples for a warm and filling dessert, or core and stuff with dried fruit, a little honey and a sprinkle of cinnamon, then bake.
- Add apple slices to sandwiches and salads or serve apple slices with fruit and cheese platters.
- Slice into segments and use to make stewed apple with cloves, open apple tarts or apple crumbles with a crunchy toasted muesli topping.

APPLE RINGS, DRIED

A rich source of fibre, dried apple rings are great for lunch boxes, and a tasty ingredient to chop and add to muesli and other breakfast cereals, fruit and nut mixes, health bars and fruit slices and desserts. Drying concentrates the kilojoules, so count about 4 rings as a serve.

- Make a compote by microwaving or simmering dried apple with other dried fruits and a cinnamon quill in just enough water to cover.
- Soak dried apple in boiling water for about 30 minutes and use in desserts or baking or to make an apple sauce for serving with meat.

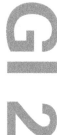

FOOD	QUICK RECIPE IDEAS

GI 40

APPLE JUICE
(unsweetened)
Apple juice is a good source of vitamin C and potassium. The fibre, however, is lost during processing, along with many of the other nutrients in apple skin. When buying juice, look for unsweetened, 100 per cent juice.

- Sip on a long apple spritzer made with ½ cup of juice plus plenty of crushed ice, soda water and fresh mint leaves.
- Make apple juice ice-blocks to cool down on hot days.
- Start the day with muesli moistened with apple juice rather than low-fat milk.
- Use apple juice to sweeten breakfast cereal and other foods.
- To make your own, quarter and core two apples and cut into pieces that will fit into the food tube of your juicer, process and enjoy a small glass of juice (125 ml) as a snack or to finish a meal. Add sticks of celery, carrot or a little fresh ginger for variety.

Are you eating enough fibre?

Many low GI foods are good sources of dietary fibre, which is a terrific bonus since we need about 30 grams of fibre a day for bowel health and to keep regular. Filling, high fibre foods can also help you maintain a healthy weight by reducing hunger pangs.

Dietary fibre comes from plant foods – it is found in the outer bran layers of grains (corn, oats, wheat and rice and in foods containing these grains), fruit and vegetables and nuts and legumes (dried beans, peas and lentils). There are two types – soluble and insoluble – and there is a difference.

- *Soluble fibres* are the gel, gum and often jellylike components of apples, oats and legumes. By slowing down the time it takes for food to pass through the stomach and small intestine, soluble fibre can lower the glycemic response to food.
- *Insoluble fibres* are dry and branlike and commonly thought of as roughage. All cereal grains and products made from them that retain the outer coat of the grain are sources of insoluble fibre, e.g. wholemeal bread and All-Bran, but not all foods containing insoluble fibre are low GI. Insoluble fibres will only lower the GI of a food when they exist in their original intact form, for example in whole grains of wheat. Here they act as a physical barrier, delaying access of digestive enzymes and water to the starch within the cereal grain.

FOOD	QUICK RECIPE IDEAS

APRICOTS

For fragrance and flavour, fresh apricots are almost irresistible. This sweet low GI fruit is delicious as a snack or to finish a meal. Like all orange–yellow fruits and vegetables, they are rich in beta-carotene and a good source of vitamin C, fibre and potassium. To eat your fill of apricots year round, choose canned apricots in natural juice (GI 51) or dried apricots (GI 30).

- Cooking apricots brings out their flavour, so they are delicious stewed.
- If they are not quite ready for eating when you buy them, they should ripen in a day or two at room temperature in your fruit bowl (or in a paper bag away from heat and light).
- Grill apricot halves (stones removed) and serve with low-fat custard, ice-cream or yoghurt.
- Halve fresh apricots, remove the stones, stuff with a teaspoon of ricotta and top with chopped nuts.
- Gently poach whole or halved apricots in fruit juice with cloves or a cinnamon quill.

GI 34

APRICOTS, DRIED

Dried apricots can be so more-ish it's often hard to stick to just a handful – five or six halves is the equivalent of a serve. However, if you do overindulge, remind yourself of their health benefits: they are high in fibre, a rich source of beta-carotene and provide reasonable amounts of calcium, iron and potassium. Dried apricots are a delicious snack food whether you are on the run or desk bound.

- Simmer dried apricots in a little water, white wine or fruit juice to soften and plump up and serve on their own or with a dollop of low-fat yoghurt or ice-cream.
- Add chopped apricots and other dried fruits to homemade muesli.
- Dice and add dried apricots to the mix when baking fruit slices and cookies.
- Make a Moroccan-flavoured casserole with diced lamb or chicken, onions, dried apricots and spices such as paprika and cumin.

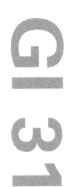

GI 31

FOOD	QUICK RECIPE IDEAS

GI 52

BANANAS

Eat this versatile fruit raw or cooked; whole, sliced or mashed; or as a snack or part of a dessert, fruit salad or meal. They are also a nutritional goldmine: high in fibre, folate and vitamin C and rich in potassium, which is why sportspeople consume them in great numbers after intense exercise to replace nutrients and help maintain peak performance.

- If the bananas in your fruit bowl are looking over-ripe, freeze them in their skins, then peel and add to the blender. They make the most delicious ice-cream alternative for creamy thickshakes and smoothies.
- Enjoy banana custard or ice-cream made with low-fat milk or soy drink.
- Add mashed banana to the mixing bowl for muffins and fruit breads.
- Gently fry banana slices in a little margarine and brown sugar and serve with pancakes or a dollop of low-fat yoghurt – or both.
- Bake or steam green bananas (about 30 minutes) and serve with barbecued meats.

GI 53

BLUEBERRIES

Blueberries, like most berries, don't contain much carbohydrate. As one of today's superfoods, they are bursting with nutrition and flavour while being very low in kilojoules and of course they are packed with anti-oxidants. The blueberries in the shops locally are cultivated 'highbush' blueberries (*Vaccinium corymbosum L*). In the US, you can also buy frozen wild blueberries (*V. angustifolium*). They are smaller and have a more intense flavour.

- Combine blueberries with a little caster sugar and a tablespoon or two of balsamic vinegar or a little white wine or orange juice. Let the flavours develop for 30 minutes then serve.
- Make blueberry smoothies with low-fat milk, soy milk or yoghurt for breakfast or a meal in a glass when you are on the run. If you use frozen fruit you don't need ice cubes.
- Add ½ cup berries to your morning cereal or yoghurt.
- Toss berries into pancake batter or muffin mix.
- Sprinkle berries on green and fruit salads.

FOOD	QUICK RECIPE IDEAS

BERRIES

Apart from strawberries (GI 40), most berries have so little carbohydrate it's difficult to test their GI. Their low carbohydrate content means their glycemic load (GL) will be low, so enjoy them by the bowlful. A good source of vitamin C and fibre, some berries also supply small amounts of folate and essential minerals such as potassium, iron, calcium, magnesium and phosphorus.

- Top gelato, low-fat ice-cream or yoghurt with a spoon or two of berries for a snack or dessert.
- Purée berries for coulis, salsas, sauces, sorbets and ice-creams.
- Serve berries for breakfast with muesli or your favourite low GI cereal and a dollop of low fat vanilla or honey yoghurt.

GI 40

CANNED FRUIT, IN NATURAL JUICE

Canned fruit in natural juice is a great way to help you get to your two serves of fruit every day. Keep an eye out for bottled sour pitted cherries (GI 41). Canned fruit in syrup (even 'light' syrup) has a higher GI – and more kilojoules per serving.

- Served canned fruit with muesli or your favourite low GI breakfast cereal.
- Top canned fruit with a dollop of yoghurt and enjoy for dessert (or breakfast).
- Combine your favourite low GI canned fruits to make a fruit salad.
- Along with traditional favourites such as apricot or pear halves or peach slices you can find interesting combinations such as peaches and grapes (GI 46), pineapple and papaya (GI 53) and orange and grapefruit segments (GI 53).

GI 25–54

	FOOD	QUICK RECIPE IDEAS

GI 52

CRANBERRY JUICE COCKTAIL

(unsweetened)
Cranberries have earned a reputation for promoting urinary tract health and research is now confirming that there maybe something in this. Whole cranberries are an excellent source of iron, vitamin C and fibre and are packed with anti-oxidant power. Like all juices, enjoy it in moderation as drinking a large glass can mean you are taking on board more energy (kilojoules) than you intended – or need.

- As an alternative, try a cranberry spritzer with ice and soda. You can also get an artificially sweetened light version.
- Create a **tangy cranberry cooler** by combining 1 cup of cranberry juice with ½ banana, a tub of low-fat yoghurt, ½ cup fresh or frozen raspberries and 1 cup of crushed ice
- Whip up a **creamy cranberry-banana flip** for two. Blend 1 small banana with ½ tub of vanilla low-fat yoghurt, 1 cup of cranberry juice and ½ cup skim milk. Add more yoghurt if you like it when the straw stands up straight!

GI 54

CUSTARD APPLES

Creamy custard apples taste like a tropical fruit salad and are virtually a complete low GI food source on their own. They also provide some protein, carbohydrate and fibre along with many essential vitamins and minerals, including vitamin C, potassium and magnesium. Cooking alters the flavour, so stir segments into savoury dishes or curries just before serving to heat through.

- Add fresh custard apple segments or purée to desserts such as cheesecake, sorbets, parfait and ice-cream.
- Power your day with an energy breakfast of muesli moistened with fresh orange juice and topped with custard apple segments.
- For a meal on the run, sip a custard apple smoothie made with low-fat yoghurt and milk and honey to sweeten.
- Fold custard apple purée into low-fat yoghurt for a quick and creamy dessert.
- Serve segments of custard apple with fruit and cheese platters – remembering to lightly brush them with a little lemon juice first to prevent discolouring.
- Sleep soundly after a custard apple egg nog made with low-fat milk and honey to taste.

FOOD	QUICK RECIPE IDEAS
DATES, DRIED Dates are one of the oldest cultivated fruits and a staple food throughout the Middle East. Rich in carbohydrate, they are a good source of fibre, minerals such as iron, potassium and magnesium and vitamins B6, niacin and folate. Like all dried fruits, a little goes a long way because they are a concentrated source of carbohydrate. Think of a serving as 4 or 5 regular size dates.	• They make a delicious snack when you are on the run – especially pitted dates! • Add chopped dates to stuffings, pilafs, muffins and winter warming desserts.

GI 39–45

FOOD	QUICK RECIPE IDEAS
GRAPEFRUIT Half a grapefruit contains about 35 mg of vitamin C, which is almost your recommended daily intake. This is one of the lowest GI fruits and provides some fibre too. Choose fruit that feels 'heavy' for its size – this tends to indicate a thinner skin and plenty of juice. Store in your fruit bowl as they are juicier eaten at room temperature.	• Start your day with zest with juicy grapefruit's refreshing tang. Halve a grapefruit, loosen the segments and eat as is, or sweeten with a little sugar or a drizzle of floral honey. • Toss segments in salads with smoked salmon and avocado; prawn and avocado; or witlof, radicchio, beetroot and avocado; or simply add to Asian greens and a citrus dressing. • Combine with chopped capsicum, finely chopped onion and a little chilli for a tangy salsa to accompany barbecued meats. • Enjoy as part of a winter fruit salad with sweeter ingredients such as oranges and raisins and a drizzle of honey.

GI 25

FOOD	QUICK RECIPE IDEAS

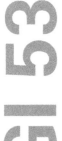

GI 48

GRAPEFRUIT JUICE
(commercial)
Cool and refreshing as a snack or after a workout, one small glass of grapefruit juice is rich in vitamin C. The grapefruit juice you buy in the supermarket has a much higher GI than the whole fruit, possibly because manufacturers reduce its acidity to produce a juice with wide consumer appeal. If you squeeze your own grapefruit for juice, however, the GI should be similar to that of whole fruit.

- Combine with soda or mineral water for a cool spritzer.
- Add juice to desserts such as sorbets and mousses.

GI 53

GRAPES
Grapes are a perfect low GI finger food fruit – grab a small bunch and enjoy as a no-mess, no-fuss snack or with a fruit or cheese platter to finish a meal. They are a good source of vitamin C, provide some fibre and red-skinned grapes contain protective anti-oxidants called anthocyanins. Choose bunches with plump, undamaged fruit (avoid split, sticky or withered grapes) and don't be shy about asking if you can taste-test for flavour.

- Top cereal with low-fat vanilla yoghurt and a handful of fresh grapes to start the day.
- Put a bowl of grapes on the table after dinner.
- Add red and green grapes to fruit salads and side salads.
- Cool off with frozen fruit skewers – grapes, strawberries, banana slices and melon or pineapple chunks make a colourful combination.

FOOD	QUICK RECIPE IDEAS

KIWI FRUIT

The furry kiwi fruit provides plenty of vitamin C – just one will meet your daily requirements. They are also rich in fibre, a good source of both vitamin E and potassium and a moderate source of iron. They are renowned as a meat tenderiser thanks to the enzyme actinidin – simply rub cut or mashed fruit over the meat and leave for about 30–40 minutes before barbecuing or grilling. Shop for kiwis with care. Choose plump, firm fruit with just a little give – if it feels soft to touch the flesh will be mushy.

- The best way to eat them is simply to cut them in half and scoop out the flesh. Alternatively peel and slice or dice and add to fruit and green salads, and fruit and cheese platters, or purée and serve with low-fat yoghurt, ice-cream, gelato and sorbets.
- Toss kiwi fruit slices with watercress and avocado chunks in a light citrus dressing.
- Add slices of kiwi fruit to chunks of pineapple, paw paw and mango, strawberry halves, passionfruit and a dash of lime juice to make a colourful tropical fruit salad.
- Bring colour and variety to a cheese platter with slices of kiwi fruit, small bunches of purple–red grapes, dried apricot halves and walnuts.

GI 53

MANGOES

Mangoes are one of the few tropical fruits that squeeze into the low GI range. They are also a rich source of vitamin C (one provides your recommended daily intake) and beta-carotene, and a useful source of fibre and potassium.
This versatile fruit is delicious fresh, sliced and puréed in desserts, or combined with fish, meat, poultry along with flavours such as lime juice, chilli and coriander for main meals.

- Stir-fry strips of duck or chicken breast and make a warm salad tossed with golden mango slices, bean sprouts, chopped onion, chilli, fresh mint leaves and a tangy Thai dressing.
- Combine diced mango with chopped red onion, tomatoes, red capsicum and coriander and a dash of lime juice to serve as a salsa with seafood.
- Try chopped fresh mango with a scoop of low fat chocolate ice-cream and an almond wafer for a delicious and easy dessert.

GI 51

FOOD	**QUICK RECIPE IDEAS**

GI 42

ORANGES

One orange is something of a personal protection powerhouse, providing you with your whole day's vitamin C requirement. Oranges are rich in anti-oxidants and are good sources of folate and potassium.

- Peel and enjoy the juicy segments with breakfast cereal, as a snack, or as an after-dinner palate cleanser.
- Chop into fruit salads, toss into salads, add to soups or casseroles or to couscous.
- Slice and add to fruit punch.
- Carrot and orange make a great couple – enjoy this perfect partnership in soup, salad or juice.
- Oranges (and mandarins) make delicious desserts – jellies, sorbets, soufflés, crepes, ice-cream.
- Try a citrus salad with orange and grapefruit segments, a can of chickpeas, cherry tomatoes and peppery rocket tossed in an oil and lemon juice dressing.

GI 50

ORANGE JUICE

**(unsweetened)
Freshly squeezed juice has most of the health benefits of a whole orange, but lacks the fibre unless you throw in the pulp. If you are buying oranges specifically for juicing, choose ones that are firm and heavy for their size. When shopping look for unsweetened, 100 per cent juice.**

- Use orange juice to moisten breakfast cereal as a change from milk, or add to meat dishes, couscous or spinach salads to help increase iron absorption. And remember, it's all too easy to overdo your juice intake – a serve is just 125 ml (½ cup).
- Add juice to fruit punches, fruit salad, milk shakes and egg nog.
- Use orange juice's zesty flavour in marinades, sauces and dressings.
- Freeze juice to make summer treats such as ice-blocks and icy poles.

FOOD	QUICK RECIPE IDEAS

PAWPAW

Pawpaws (and papayas) are from the same juicy family and, like other yellow-range fruit, are rich in beta-carotene. It's nice to know that as the mango season ends, the pawpaws will be arriving in the greengrocer's. Like many tropical fruits, we think that they are just about unbeatable eaten fresh. You can use them as a meat tenderiser too, as they contain papain. Just purée and rub a little over the meat, leave for 20 minutes then cook.

- Serve pawpaw or papaya slices for breakfast sprinkled with lemon or lime juice for a fresh tasting start to the day or dice papaya and add to tropical fruit salads with mangoes, kiwi fruit, passionfruit and berries.
- Purée and use as a sauce or topping or to flavour sorbets and ice creams (but not jellies – fresh papaya will not set in gelatine desserts).
- Serve seafood or chicken with a coriander and pawpaw/papaya salsa.

GI 56

PEACHES & NECTARINES

It's nice to know that something as juicy and delicious as a ripe, fresh peach (GI 42) or nectarine (GI 43) is so healthy. Peaches and nectarines are good sources of vitamin C, potassium and fibre. Canned peaches in natural juice (GI 43) have many of the nutritional benefits of fresh fruit (with a little less vitamin C) along with a low GI and the convenience of being available year round.

- Top grainy toast with ricotta and thinly sliced fresh peaches or nectarines for an easy breakfast or a tasty snack.
- Halve, stone and poach peaches or nectarines in champagne, white wine or fruit juice with or without the skin and serve with low-fat yoghurt or ice-cream.
- Sip on a fruity whip of puréed peaches or nectarines blended with ice and orange juice.
- Sprinkle fresh peach or nectarines halves with a little cinnamon and lightly grill.
- Try single serving cans or tubs as a snack.
- Dried peach (GI 35) also makes a handy snack.

GI 42–43

FOOD	QUICK RECIPE IDEAS

GI 38

PEARS

Juicy, sweet pears are one of the world's most loved fruits. They are renowned as a non-allergenic food, thus a favourite when introducing babies to solid foods. An excellent source of fibre and rich in vitamin C and potassium, fresh pears have a low GI because most of their sugar is fructose. Canned pears in 'natural juice' also have a low GI (43).

- Dip pear slices in lemon juice and serve with cheese and walnuts.
- Toss in salads – try pear, avocado, rocket or radicchio and walnuts.
- Poach or bake pears in a light citrus syrup or red wine with a touch of cardamom.
- Try topping a bowl of porridge with grilled pear slices and a drizzle of honey or some brown sugar.
- Dried pears (GI 43) are delicious added to compotes.
- Pack a pear for lunch or to snack on during the day – there's no need to peel as the skin is a good source of fibre.

GI 43

PINEAPPLE, CANNED IN JUICE

When you get to the canned fruit section of the supermarket, it seems to be dominated by pineapple. So it's amazing to think that before the canning industry got going, pineapples were a real status symbol and very few people could afford them! People love canned pineapple because the flavour is so consistent. It can be trickier buying them fresh (GI 59) as they don't ripen or get any sweeter once they have been picked. Unsweetened pineapple juice also has a low GI (46).

- Canned pineapple, with its sweet tangy flavour, is a great complement to all types of dishes including appetisers, mains, salads, sides, beverages and desserts.
- Grill pineapple rings (fresh or canned) with chicken or lean beef, lamb or pork burgers.
- Add a few chunks of pineapple to fruit or green salads.
- Serve pineapple rings or chunks with a scoop of low-fat frozen yoghurt or your favourite dairy dessert.
- Add pineapple to banana smoothies for extra tang
- Mix a little crushed pineapple into cottage cheese for dips with crunchy crudités like carrot or celery sticks or capsicum strips.

FOOD	QUICK RECIPE IDEAS

PLUMS

Plum pudding, plum jam, Chinese plum sauce – this fruit is popular the world over. It's also a good source of fibre and provides small quantities of vitamins and minerals.

Choose plump, undamaged fruit (no splits, bruises or signs of decay) with a slight whitish bloom and enjoy fresh as a snack or to finish a meal.

- Halve, remove stone and add to fruit salads and compotes or serve with cheese or fruit platters.
- Purée for making sauces and delicious sorbets and ice-cream – or plum soup.
- Top stewed plums with a sprinkle of toasted muesli and a dollop of yoghurt for a breakfast with a difference.
- Poach plums in red or white wine with a stick of cinnamon and serve hot or cold.

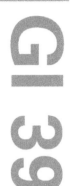

PRUNES

Prunes have a reputation for keeping us regular (as does prune juice), but there's more to this tasty dried fruit than that. They are a concentrated source of many nutrients including beta-carotene, B vitamins, potassium and phosphorus. Prunes are also a useful source of iron for vegetarians.

You can buy prunes with stones or pitted – but check for the occasional stone as the processing is not always perfect.

- Combine prunes with an equal amount of water in a small pan and gently simmer for about 5–10 minutes. Add a slice of lemon or some spices for extra flavour.
- To soften in the microwave, pour fruit juice or water over prunes, cover and cook.
- To soften overnight, place prunes in a heatproof bowl and just cover with boiling water. When cool, cover and store in the refrigerator.
- A great low GI food for snacks on their own or as part of a fruit and nut mix.
- Soften or 'plump' by simmering or soaking and enjoy in desserts, or add to lamb, pork, chicken and game dishes for a Moroccan flavour.

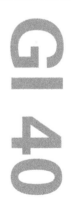

FOOD	QUICK RECIPE IDEAS

GI 40

STRAWBERRIES

It's no wonder deliciously versatile strawberries are popular. You can eat them fresh, add them to fruit salads and frappés, use them in a delicious dessert, decorate cakes with them, or make them into jams, fruit spreads and sauces.
Fresh strawberries are rich in vitamin C, potassium, folate, fibre and protective anti-oxidants. So reap the health benefits as you enjoy them by the bowlful, but hold the cream!

- For a perfect parfait, take a tall glass and arrange layers of sliced strawberries, whole blueberries and dollops of low-fat vanilla yoghurt. Mango slices are delicious with this combination, too
- Blend strawberries for a bright and refreshing coulis to serve with low-fat ice-cream or poached pears. Freeze for fruity ice-blocks.
- Add strawberries to smoothies and shakes with low-fat yoghurt or ice-cream.
- Serve whole with fruit and cheese platters or dip in chocolate for a sweet treat with coffee at the end of a meal.
- Quarter fresh strawberries and soak in balsamic vinegar with a little sugar.
- Add to green salads with baby spinach, bocconcini and a light balsamic dressing.

GI 56

SULTANAS

Sultanas are a good source of fibre and also provide some potassium and vitamin E. They are juicier, softer and sweeter than their cousins the currant and raisin. Keep in mind that the kilojoule content of dried fruit is higher than for fresh fruit.

- Sweeten breakfast cereal and yoghurt with a spoonful of sultanas.
- Simmer sultanas in apple or orange juice with peeled and grated ginger to make a tasty compote for breakfast or dessert.
- Add sultanas to your favourite bread and butter pudding recipe along with chopped dates.
- Make a **fruit compote** with 2 cups of your favourite dried fruits, 1–2 cups fresh orange juice (to cover), a cinnamon stick, and a little sugar or floral honey to taste. Simmer for 10 minutes, cover and set aside to cool. Serve with breakfast cereal or as a dessert.
- Add to all sorts of dishes from casseroles and compotes to couscous, cakes, cookies and crumbles

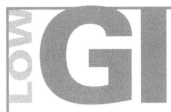

Vegetables

Think of vegetables as 'free' foods – they are full of fibre, essential nutrients and protective anti-oxidants that will fill you up without adding extra kilojoules. And most are so low in carbohydrate that they will have no measurable effect on your blood glucose levels.

Leafy green and salad vegetables, for example, have so little carbohydrate that we can't test their GI. Even in generous serving sizes they will have no effect on your blood glucose levels.

Most varieties of potato tested have a high GI, so if you are a big potato eater, try to replace some with low GI alternatives such as sweetcorn, sweet potato, yam or legumes (but watch your portion sizes). Vegetables such as pumpkin, carrots, peas and beetroot contain some carbohydrate, but a normal serving size contains so little that it won't raise your blood glucose levels significantly.

Storage and cooking tips

Vegetables are best fresh, so shop two or three times a week if you can and use them within two to three days.

To make sure you gain the benefit of all those essential nutrients when cooking:

- Leave the skins on whenever you can, or peel very finely
- Avoid soaking vegetables in water
- Use a steamer or microwave for best results
- Cook vegetables in big chunks rather than coarsely chopped
- Reduce the amount of water you use, cover the pan and cook quickly and as close to serving time as possible; *never* add bicarbonate of soda to the cooking water
- Cook vegetables until they're softened but still firm to bite.

LOW GI Vegetables

Starchy vegetables – 3 things you need to know

When it comes to starchy vegetables like potatoes, sweet potatoes, corn, taro and yams, you need to think of them as the Vegetable Kingdom's equivalent of rice or pasta. Remember, their place is the carb quarter of the dinner plate (and within the inner rim too and not piled up like a pyramid).

1. These starchy vegies are a good source of fibre (when you don't peel them) and micro-nutrients including vitamin A (yellow/orange-fleshed vegies), B vitamins, vitamin C and potassium.

2. They aren't fattening by themselves; it's how you cook them and what you pour over them that adds the kilojoules. They also tend to be 'feel-full' foods. Their high fibre and water contents means that they are bulky, and help to satisfy your appetite.

3. They are great mixers. Combining them in bakes or gratins or pilafs will boost the variety of vitamins, minerals and phyto-nutrients you get and lower the GI if you combine higher GI vegies with low GI ones, e.g. mashed potato with butter beans.

Australia's first and only certified low GI potato

Versatile, compact and full of flavour, Carisma is the only potato in Australia to carry the official low GI symbol from the Glycemic Index Foundation. Available only at Coles supermarkets and harvested all year, the Carisma potato is grown by some of the best potato farmers in Australia in regions such as the Riverland in South Australia, Lockyer Valley in Queensland and various regions in Western Australia. With a GI of 55 (average GI for other Australian potatoes is 77), Carisma is excellent for mashing, roasting, boiling and including in your favourite salads. For more information visit: www.carismapotatoes.com.au

FOOD	QUICK RECIPE IDEAS

CARROTS

Carrots are rich in beta-carotene, a plant form of vitamin A or retinol, which we need to maintain normal vision. A deficiency in vitamin A produces night blindness (an inability to see in dim light). Carrots also provide some vitamin C and fibre, so add them when you're cooking soups, salads, stir-fries, stews, casseroles, cakes and puddings. Carrot juice (GI 43) combines well with other juices for a refreshing drink.

- Grate and add to salads and sandwiches, cut into sticks for dips or snacks, or boil, steam or bake (whole or sliced) and serve with main meals.
- Enjoy a freshly grated carrot salad with a bunch of chopped chives and a dressing of oil and lemon juice.
- For a Middle Eastern flavour toss cooked carrot slices in a little oil and lemon juice with roasted cumin seeds crushed in a mortar and pestle.
- Make a creamy, puréed carrot soup with leeks, a potato, and a good quality chicken stock served with a dollop of low-fat yoghurt.
- Peel and juice a couple of carrots or add other vegetables or fruit such as celery, apple and orange to start your day with a good health glow.

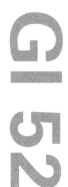

GI 39

PARSNIPS

Parsnips are a good choice because they won't send your blood glucose on a roller coaster ride, so enjoy this sweet, nutty winter vegetable. No need to peel parsnips (a lot of the goodness is just under the skin), just scrub and brush then bake, pan-fry, steam, roast, or boil and mash them like potatoes. Like us, you'll find they make a great substitute for potatoes in many recipes. Don't go for the biggest parsnips in the pile as they may have a woody centre. Choose firm, smooth, creamy white ones and store in the vegetable crisper in your fridge.

- It's hard to go past baked parsnips with a roast dinner.
- Like other starchy vegetables, parsnips are perfect for creamy soups. Curried parsnip soup is a winter favourite.
- Cooked parsnips mashed with a leek (or onion) and a potato or two and flavoured with a little nutmeg makes a delicious side dish.

GI 52

FOOD	QUICK RECIPE IDEAS

GI 51

PEAS, GREEN
Green peas are actually a legume, but we have included them here as most of us think of them as a green vegetable. They are rich in fibre and vitamin C and higher in protein than most vegetables. Although a good source of thiamin, niacin, phosphorus and iron when fresh, cooking will reduce the nutrient levels.

- Boil, steam or microwave peas for about 4–5 minutes (remember, cooking destroys the nutrients) or add to rice dishes such as risottos, pasta dishes, omelettes, soups and stews (at the last minute), or combine with mashed potato or sweet potato.
- Peas with edible pods such as snowpeas and sugar snaps (immature pods) only need the minimum of cooking time, too, and are delicious in stir-fries, or steamed or cooked in the microwave for a side dish.
- Whip up an omelette with onion, a little ham or lean bacon and fresh peas.
- If you feel like comfort food, purée or mash cooked peas with chicken stock.
- Add blanched snowpeas or sugar snaps to salads or serve with vegetable platters and dips.

What about potatoes?

Most people like potatoes – they can be prepared in so many different ways, are nutritious, and taste great whether you bake, steam or mash them. However, we now know that just about any potato in your supermarket or grocery store will have a high GI. But cutting out potatoes is something many people trying to eat a low GI diet to manage their blood glucose levels find really hard to do. So what's the answer?

First of all, there's no need to say 'no' to potatoes altogether just because they may have a high GI. They are fat free (when you don't fry them), nutrient rich and filling. Not every food you eat has to have a low GI. So enjoy them, but just have less and say no thanks to seconds. That means a couple of small spuds on your dinner plate. Alternatively, serve your spuds up in a way that will help you keep your blood glucose levels steady – a potato salad with a vinegary vinaigrette dressing, half a jacket potato topped with baked beans or potato mashed (50/50) with butter or cannellini beans.

Secondly, look for the low or lower GI varieties of potato in the fresh produce aisles; Carisma potatoes carry the GI symbol, too: Carisma (GI 55), Nicola (GI 58), Almera (GI 65).

FOOD	QUICK RECIPE IDEAS

PUMPKIN, BUTTERNUT

Pumpkin only contains a little carbohydrate in a normal serving (that's about a cup) so it won't send your blood glucose up. Pumpkins are high in fibre (especially butternuts roasted or steamed with their skin on) and are a rich source of beta-carotene, which adds up to making them a great alternative to potatoes on your dinner plate.

- Make a **creamy pumpkin soup** with peeled and diced butternut pumpkin, red lentils, chopped onions and vegetable or chicken stock.
- Bake pumpkin chunks with herbs or spices and add to salads or frittatas or serve as a side dish.
- Mashed pumpkin makes a great topping for cottage pie.

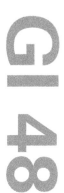

GI 51

SWEETCORN
(on the cob)
Sweetcorn is actually the seed of a type of grass that grew in the Americas for thousands of years before Christopher Columbus arrived on the scene. It is rich in vitamin C and a good source of fibre, folate and beta-carotene. It also has higher amounts of protein and vitamin B than most other vegetables because it's actually a cereal grain. Canned (GI 46) and frozen kernels have a similar GI to corn on the cob.

- Serve piping hot topped with the merest hint of margarine or butter.
- Toss whole baby corn into stir-fries or cut kernels off the cob and add to soups and stews, fritters and frittata, chowders and crepes, salsa and salads.
- Spice up barbecue meats with a tangy corn salsa made from corn kernels, diced tomato, capsicum, onion, chopped chilli (to taste), fresh coriander and a lime dressing.
- Make a sweetcorn frittata with corn kernels, chopped onion, lean bacon, eggs, low-fat milk and parsley and top with a sprinkle of reduced-fat tasty cheese.
- Add the finishing touch to a warm salad of roast sweet potato, red onion, red capsicum, baby eggplant and baby spinach with small corn cob chunks.

GI 48

FOOD	QUICK RECIPE IDEAS

GI 54

TARO

Taro, sometimes called 'elephant ear', is an important food throughout the Pacific Islands. It's a good source of vitamin C and fibre like other traditional staples such as sweet potato and yam. If you haven't tried taro before, look for firm, hairy tubers with no wrinkling of the skin. Wear rubber gloves when peeling as the juices occasionally cause a skin irritation. Taro flesh is similar to sweet potato in flavour and you can use it the same way – steamed, boiled or cut into wedges and baked.

- Try a **taro, chickpea and sweet potato curry** as a side dish (serves 6) or with cooked rice as a main meal (serves 4). Peel and chop 400 grams each of taro and sweet potato into 2 cm chunks and steam for about 10 minutes until half cooked. Remove from the heat and set aside. Heat 2 tablespoons of olive oil in a large pan and lightly sauté 1 tablespoon of freshly grated ginger and 3 cloves of crushed garlic over a medium heat for 2–3 minutes. Add the taro and sweet potato, 2 cups of cooked chickpeas, 1 tablespoon of curry powder and 1 red chilli (peeled, seeded and very finely sliced). Stir gently to coat the vegetables and chickpeas in the curry mix, then cover and cook until the vegetables are tender. Serve topped with 2 or 3 tablespoons of freshly chopped coriander.

GI 38

TOMATO JUICE

Low in kilojoules and so low in carbs it is hard to measure their GI, but they do provide plenty of fibre, vitamins, minerals and lycopene. As you process them, they become more concentrated, which is why tomato juice (GI 38) and tomato soup are a source of carbohydrate for light meals and snacks. Look for salt-reduced brands.

- Oven-roast tomatoes and serve as a side dish with a barbecue or roast or grilled meats.
- Stir a fresh tomato sauce through spaghetti or your favourite pasta shapes.
- Make your own **creamy tomato soup**, Sauté diced onion and potato in a little extra virgin olive oil, add a can of Roma tomatoes and about 3–4 cups of water and simmer until the vegies are tender. Purée, season and serve with a dollop of low-fat yoghurt topped with a scattering of chopped parsley.
- Canned tomato soup (GI 45) is a quick and easy meal with a slice or two of grainy toast and is also great as a base for easy casseroles and sauces.

FOOD	QUICK RECIPE IDEAS
YAM Like sweet potato and taro, yams are high in fibre, nutrient dense and a good source of vitamin C and potassium. They have long been a staple food in Asia, throughout the Pacific Islands and in New Zealand. In Australia the Aborigines ate many varieties of yam. Use yams in your cooking in the same way you would use sweet potatoes, although yams tend to have an 'earthier' flavour.	• Purée yam cooked with leeks and chicken stock to make a creamy soup and flavour with fresh herbs such as dill or chives. • Toss cooked bite-sized chunks of yam with mesclun, onion slices, capsicum and chives in a light oil and vinegar dressing for a satisfying salad. • Steam and mash yam chunks with skim milk and a teaspoon or two of margarine and season with salt and a few twists of freshly ground black pepper to taste. • Bake a gratin at 180°C with overlapping yam slices moistened with chicken stock, sprinkled with a teaspoon of dried sage topped with grated cheddar cheese and freshly grated nutmeg.

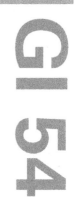

If you have diabetes, should you avoid eating pumpkin?

Definitely not, because, unlike potatoes and cereal products, pumpkin does not contain a lot of carbohydrate. So, despite high GI, (depending on variety) its sometimes glycemic load (GI × carb per serve divided by 100) is medium. These vegetables contain loads of micronutrients and can be consumed as part of a healthy, balanced meal.

LOW GI

Breads, Breakfast Cereals & Grains

Did you know that the type of bread and cereal you eat affects the overall GI of your diet the most? Why? Well, cereal grains such as rice, wheat, oats, barley and rye and products made from them such as bread, pasta and breakfast cereals are the most concentrated sources of carbohydrate in our diet.

These days, supermarket shelves are packed with products based on quickly digested, high GI flours and grains. Breakfast cereals are a good example. Once, a bowl of slowly digested porridge made with traditional rolled oats gave most of us the energy to keep going from breakfast through to lunchtime. Nowadays we are more likely to fill that breakfast bowl with high GI crunchy flakes that will spike our blood glucose and insulin levels and leave us needing a mid-morning snack to keep going.

A simple swap is all it takes to reduce the GI of your diet. To get started, replace some of those high GI breads and breakfast cereals with low GI carbs that will trickle fuel into your engine.

A simple swap is all it takes to reduce the GI of your diet.

LOW GI

Bread

Most breads sold today have a high GI because they are made from quickly digested, highly refined flours – white or wholemeal. Look for the GI Symbol on packaged breads – there's lots to choose from, including low GI white breads. When buying bread from a specialty bakery or hot bread shop, choose the coarse textured, dense grainy varieties, or a traditionally made sourdough, or soy and linseed breads.

Breads, bread rolls and pocket breads are not fattening in themselves. It's what goes on (or in) them that can pile on the kilojoules. A smear of margarine is all you need – or none at all. For a change, try peanut butter, almond or cashew butter, or avocado. Or you can opt for low-fat alternatives like ricotta or cottage cheese or a fresh fruit spread.

What about flour? If I make my own bread (or dumplings, pancakes, muffins etc), which flours, if any, are low GI?

To date there are no GI ratings for refined flour, whether it's made from wheat, soy or other grains. This is because the GI rating of a food must be tested in real people. So far we haven't had volunteers willing to tuck into 50-gram portions of flour on three occasions! What we do know, however, is that bakery products such as scones, cakes, biscuits, donuts and pastries made from highly refined flour – whether white or wholemeal – are quickly digested and absorbed.

What should you do with your own baking? Try to increase the soluble fibre content by partially substituting flour with oat bran, rice bran or rolled oats and increase the bulkiness of the product with dried fruit, nuts, muesli, All-Bran or unprocessed bran. Don't think of it as a challenge; it's an opportunity for some creative cooking.

FOOD	QUICK RECIPE IDEAS

GI 54

FRUIT LOAF

There are several types of fruit loaves or breads which include raisins, sultanas, dried apricots or apple, figs and sometimes nuts and seeds. The dried fruit content means they can be a useful source of iron, protein, fibre, thiamin, niacin, riboflavin and magnesium. Enjoy fresh or toasted for breakfast or as a snack.

- Snack on toasted fruit loaf with a dollop of ricotta.
- Add flavour to a **bread and butter pudding** by making it with slices of fruit loaf – great comfort food or for filling hollow legs. Spread 8 slices of fruit loaf with a tablespoon of margarine. Cut into triangles and place in layers in a round casserole dish. Whisk 3 eggs with 2 cups of low-fat milk or soy milk and 2 tablespoons of sugar or honey and pour over the bread layers. Stand the casserole dish in a baking pan filled with enough water to come halfway up the sides of the dish. Bake in a moderate oven (180°C) for 40 minutes or until browned on top.

GI 50

PUMPERNICKEL

**This traditional rye bread from Germany can be something of an acquired taste. It's a very good source of fibre and thanks to its high proportion of whole cereal grains, has a low GI value. Also known as rye kernel bread, pumpernickel contains 80–90 per cent whole and cracked rye kernels.
It is usually sold thinly sliced and vacuum packed for long shelf life. You can crumble it to use in stuffings and for making desserts, but it is most popular as an appetiser.**

- For an appetiser, top pumpernickel with tangy cheese and apple or pear slivers, spicy sausage and salsa, or smoked salmon, horseradish cream and dill.
- For breakfast, toast pumpernickel, spread lightly with margarine and accompany with a hot chocolate drink made with low-fat milk.

FOOD	QUICK RECIPE IDEAS

SOURDOUGH

Crusty, chewy white sourdough's characteristic flavour (when it is made the traditional way) comes from the slow fermentation process, which produces a build-up of organic acids. It's about the best low GI bread substitute for people who absolutely insist they can only eat white bread. Use for sandwiches and toast (with sweet or savoury spreads and toppings) or serve with main meals, soups and salads. Make bruschetta for a quick and easy light meal or snack.

Simply brush slices of crusty sourdough with a little olive oil then lightly grill or bake on both sides and top with:

- fresh tomato and basil salsa with a dash of balsamic vinegar
- char-grilled red and yellow capsicum with roasted artichoke hearts
- char-grilled eggplant with semi-dried tomatoes
- mushrooms sautéed with garlic, lemon juice and parsley
- tuna, rocket and capers

GI 54–58

SOURDOUGH RYE

Sourdough rye is made with rye instead of wheat flour. Slices of chewy, low GI sourdough rye piled with tasty hot or cold fillings make great sandwiches for workdays, picnics or travel. This bread's compact structure keeps the sandwich with all its fillings intact, while the slightly sour flavour combines well with a wide range of meat, poultry, fish and salad fillings.

Try these sandwich fillings:

- salad (the works) with rare roast beef and horseradish, or smoked ham and grainy mustard
- smoked turkey with cranberry, avocado and sprouts
- egg salad with fresh chopped chives and crispy cos lettuce
- chicken breast with watercress, apple slices and walnuts
- tuna melt – flaked tuna, finely sliced onion rings and a slice of gruyère cheese
- BLT – lean grilled bacon, lettuce and tomato slices

GI 48

	FOOD	QUICK RECIPE IDEAS

GI 52

SOY AND LINSEED BREAD

These moist breads with good keeping qualities are made by adding kibbled soy beans or soy flour and linseeds to bread dough. They are also rich in omega-3 fatty acids (the good essential oils). Unless you are on a very low-fat diet, don't be deterred from enjoying soy and linseed breads as their fat content is unsaturated. They are a good source of fibre.

- Club sandwiches; open-faced sandwiches with cold meats and salad and toasted or grilled sandwiches for light meals and lunches.
- For a satisfying salad in a sandwich, skim two slices of soy and linseed bread with a little avocado and fill with a slice of lean ham, tomato, rocket, grated carrot, beetroot, spring onions and sprouts.
- To make a cheesy melt, spread a slice of soy and linseed bread with wholegrain mustard. Add chopped sun-dried tomatoes, grilled eggplant and a slice of mozzarella cheese. Melt the cheese under the grill, top with salad greens and another slice of soy and linseed, slice diagonally and serve.

GI 39–54

WHOLEGRAIN, MULTIGRAIN OR MIX-GRAIN BREAD

These breads contain lots of 'grainy bits' in the bread (not just on top for decoration). They tend to have a slightly grainy, chewy texture and provide a good source of fibre, vitamins, minerals and phytoestrogens, although this will depend on the flour mix. These are usually made from wholemeal or white flour (or a combination of the two) with kibbled and wholegrains added to the dough.

- Make your own 'submarines' with wholegrain rolls or muffins
- Top a vegetable gratin with grainy breadcrumbs
- Enjoy a beef or chickpea burger on a grainy bun

FOOD	QUICK RECIPE IDEAS

WHITE CORN TORTILLAS

Tortillas are a flat (unleavened) bread traditionally made from corn (maize) flour. Almost any kind of food that is not too liquid – beans, corn or chicken, chilli or salsa – can be placed on or wrapped in the versatile tortilla for a complete meal. Make the most of them with your favourite recipes for burritos, enchiladas, fajitas and quesadillas (but hold the creamy dips) or use as rolls, wraps or scoops.

- To make bean and corn burritos, preheat the oven to 180°C. Combine a 400-gram can of drained corn kernels, drained, a 400-gram can of red kidney beans, rinsed and drained, 2 large ripe tomatoes, chopped, 2 shallots, finely sliced and 75 grams prepared taco sauce in a bowl. Wrap four 15 cm white corn tortillas in foil and warm in the oven for 5 minutes. To assemble, spread shredded lettuce over a warmed tortilla, and top with the bean mixture and a little grated fat-reduced cheese. Fold the bottom of the tortilla over the filling, and roll up to enclose. Serve immediately. Makes 4.
- Corn tortillas are a good alternative to pita and flat bread and make great wraps for salad fillings.

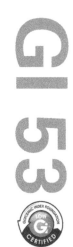

GI 53

Almost any kind of food can be placed on or wrapped in the versatile tortilla for a complete meal.

LOW GI

Breakfast cereals & grains

Whether you like waking up to a crisp, crunchy cereal, a warming bowl of porridge or a chewy, nutty muesli, a good breakfast can set you up for the day. Given the solid evidence that people who eat breakfast are calmer, happier and more sociable, the number of people skipping breakfast is an alarming trend. Studies regularly show that eating breakfast improves mood, mental alertness, concentration and memory. Nutritionists also know that having breakfast helps people lose weight, can lower cholesterol levels and helps stabilise blood glucose levels.

People who eat breakfast are calmer, happier and more sociable.

FOOD	QUICK RECIPE IDEAS
ALL-BRAN **With its malty taste, Kellogg's All-Bran is a good source of B vitamins and excellent source of insoluble fibre. Made from coarsely milled wheat bran, it's among the most fibre-rich of all breakfast cereals on the market. It is also low in sodium and a good source of potassium.**	• Top a bowl of All-Bran with banana slices or canned pear slices, serve with low-fat milk. • Sprinkle a few tablespoons over low-fat yoghurt as a fibre booster. • Blend yourself a honey banana smoothie – a cup of low-fat milk, a small banana, honey to taste and ¼ cup of All-Bran (or more if you like). • Warm up in winter with a fruity blend of canned plums or apricot halves, low-fat milk, honey to taste and ¼ cup of All-Bran; microwave for 30 seconds. • Add ½ cup of All-Bran to muffin mixes, banana and other fruit or vegetable breads, biscuits and slices when baking.
MUESLI, NATURAL **(made with rolled oats, dried fruit, nuts and seeds)** **A good source of thiamin, riboflavin and niacin, its low GI value is the result of the slower digestion of raw oats. Any muesli will fuel your day, but check the information label when buying toasted muesli as it can contain extra fat and sugar.**	• Try our low GI **simple Swiss muesli**: Combine 1 cup of traditional rolled oats, ½ cup of low-fat milk and 2 tablespoons of sultanas in a bowl; cover and refrigerate overnight. Next morning add ½ cup of low-fat vanilla yoghurt, 2 tablespoons of slivered almonds and ½ an apple (grated). Mix well, adjusting the flavour with a little lemon juice if you wish. Serve with your favourite berries – such as strawberries or blueberries. Serves 2.

GI 44

GI 40–55

FOOD	QUICK RECIPE IDEAS

GI 55

OAT BRAN, UNPROCESSED

(unprocessed oat bran, average)
You can buy unprocessed oat bran in the cereal section of supermarkets and in health, natural and organic food stores. Bran is a soft, bland product useful as an addition to breakfast cereals and as a partial substitution for flour in baked goods to help boost fibre and lower the GI. You can also add a tablespoon or two to meatball and burger mixes, use it in making muesli or add to porridge for extra fibre.

- Enjoy low GI **Oat and Apple Muffins** straight from the oven! Preheat the oven to 180°C. Combine ½ cup of All-Bran and ⅔ cup of low-fat milk in a bowl and let stand for 10 minutes. Sift ½ cup of self-raising flour, 2 teaspoons of baking powder and 1 teaspoon of mixed spice into a large bowl. Stir in ½ cup of unprocessed oat bran, ½ cup of raisins and 1 peeled and diced Granny Smith apple. Combine 1 egg, lightly beaten, ¼ cup of honey and ½ teaspoon of vanilla in a bowl. Add the egg and All-Bran mixtures to the dry ingredients and gently stir with a wooden spoon until just combined. Be careful not to overmix. Spoon the mixture into a greased 12-hole muffin pan. Bake for about 15 minutes or until lightly browned and cooked through. Makes 12 muffins.

GI 52–58

PORRIDGE

(made with traditional rolled oats)
A good source of soluble fibre, B vitamins, vitamin E, iron and zinc. Traditional rolled oats are hulled, steamed and flattened. The additional flaking to produce quick cooking or 'instant' oats not only speeds up cooking time, it increases the rate of digestion and the GI. This is why traditional rolled oats are preferred over instant in the low GI diet.

Don't skimp on finishing touches for perfect porridge. Choose toppings such as:

- fresh fruit slices in season
- mixed berries
- unsweetened canned plums
- a teaspoon or two of maple syrup
- a tablespoon or two of dried fruit such as sultanas or chopped apricots
- Follow the instructions on the packet (or use your favourite recipe) to make porridge. A fairly standard rule is one part rolled oats to four parts water. Cooking oats in milk (preferably low-fat or skim) not only produces a creamy dish but supplies you with calcium and reduces the overall GI.

LOW GI

Noodles

Noodles have long been a staple food in China, Japan, Korea and most of South-east Asia. Today, their meals-in-minutes value has made them popular worldwide – they are a great stand-by for quick meals. They are also a good source of carbohydrate, provide some protein, B vitamins and minerals and will help to keep blood glucose levels on an even keel.

Served with fish, chicken, tofu or lean meat and plenty of vegetables, a soup, salad or stir-fry based on noodles gives you a healthy balance of carbs, fats and proteins plus some fibre and essential vitamins and minerals. If they are served crisp, it means that they have been deep-fried.

To cook, follow the instructions on the packet as times vary depending on types and thickness. Some noodles only need swirling under running warm water to separate, or soaking in hot (but not boiling) water to soften before you serve them or add to stir-fries. Others need to be boiled. Like pasta, they are usually best just tender, almost al dente, so keep an eye on the clock.

As it's all too easy to slurp, gulp, twirl and overeat noodles, keep those portion sizes moderate. While they are a low GI choice themselves, eating a huge amount will have a marked effect on your blood glucose. Instead of piling your plate with noodles, serve plenty of vegetables – a cup of noodles combined with lots of mixed vegetables can turn into three cups of a noodle-based meal and fit into any adult's daily diet.

Remember when planning meals that the sauces you serve with noodles and how you cook them can provide a lot more kilojoules than the noodles themselves.

FOOD	QUICK RECIPE IDEAS
GI 46 **BUCKWHEAT (SOBA) NOODLES** Japan's soba noodles are rather like spaghetti in both colour and texture. They are usually made from a combination of buckwheat and wheat flour and are a better source of protein and fibre than rice noodles. You can buy them fresh or dried, but fresh is better if available. Serve soba hot or cold. One of the classic soba recipes is zaru soba, in which boiled soba noodles are eaten cold with a soy dipping sauce.	• Make a **buckwheat noodle salad** by tossing 2 cups of cooked noodles in a dressing made with about 1 tablespoon of light soy sauce, 2 tablespoons of white wine vinegar, 1 teaspoon of sesame oil, 2 teaspoons of mirin, ½ teaspoon of finely chopped ginger, 1 clove of crushed garlic and a pinch of chilli (or to taste). Top with finely chopped spring onions and serve. If you like, add thinly sliced pieces of fresh bean curd, too.
GI 39 **CELLOPHANE NOODLES (MUNG BEANS)** Cellophane noodles, also known as Lungkow bean thread noodles or green bean vermicelli, are fine, translucent threads made from mung bean flour. When soaked they become shiny and slippery and are sometimes called slippery noodles or glass noodles. They are often used in soups, salads and stir-fries. To soften simply soak them in hot (not boiling) water for a couple of minutes before adding them to the dish.	• Make a **spiced seafood salad** using seafood mix from the fish shop (including calamari, crab meat and prawns) with cellophane noodles, chopped Asian greens, snowpeas and a chilli lime dressing. • Use leftover chicken to whip up a salad with noodles, blanched snowpeas, blanched green beans, rocket and a light sesame and hoi sin dressing.

FOOD	QUICK RECIPE IDEAS

INSTANT NOODLES

Dried noodles are very popular as a quick meal or snack. They are a high-carbohydrate convenience food but they also contain a substantial amount of fat – over 35 per cent of their kilojoules in fact. The flavour sachets supplied tend to be based on salt and flavour enhancers. Keep them for occasional use and add fresh or frozen chopped vegetables when preparing. These noodles can also be added to soups and stir-fries.

- For a meal in minutes, make a quick **Thai noodle curry**. Stir-fry sliced onion, red capsicum, baby corn, broccoli florets and snowpeas in a large pan or wok. Add a tablespoon of Thai red curry paste. Prepare instant Asian noodles according to the instructions on the packet. Add to the vegetables with enough stock to make a sauce. Stir in a tablespoon of light coconut milk, heat through and serve.

- Make up a single-serve packet of quick-cook noodles with half the flavour sachet. Add a couple of tablespoons each of frozen peas and corn kernels and then microwave to heat through.

GI 52

RICE NOODLES
(fresh)

Made from ground or pounded rice flour, rice noodles are available fresh and dried. Run hot water through fresh rice noodles to loosen them then drain and combine with other ingredients. Dried rice noodles are rather brittle and need to be soaked for 10 to 15 minutes before adding to soups, salads and stir-fries.

- Enjoy rice noodles in broth served with a little lean meat, chicken or tofu and vegetables including chopped Asian greens, bean sprouts, mint leaves and some finely sliced chilli.

- Make up some **fresh rice paper rolls**: mix together softened chopped rice vermicelli with grated carrot, fresh bean sprouts, chopped roasted peanuts (unsalted), chopped fresh mint and coriander or parsley and a dressing of sesame oil and lime juice with minced garlic, chilli and a pinch of sugar. Roll up spoonfuls of the mixture in softened rice paper rounds and serve alongside sweet chilli sauce for dipping.

GI 40

GI LOW

Pasta & couscous

It's said that pasta (Italian for 'dough') comes in more shapes and sizes than there are days of the year. Whatever the shape, it's perfect for quick meals and scores well nutritionally as a good source of protein, B vitamins and fibre.

Initially we thought that pasta's low GI was due to its main ingredient, semolina (durum or hard wheat flour). Scientists have now shown, however, that even pasta made with plain wheat flour has a low GI and the reason for the slow digestion is the physical entrapment of ungelatinised starch granules in a spongelike network of protein (gluten) molecules in the pasta dough. Pasta and noodles are unique in this regard. Adding egg to the dough lowers the GI further by increasing the protein content.

Al dente ('firm to the bite') is the best way to eat pasta – it's not meant to be soft. It should be slightly firm and offer some resistance when you are chewing it. It's more glucose friendly too – overcooking boosts the GI. Although most manufacturers specify a cooking time on the packet, don't take their word for it. Start testing about 2 – 3 minutes before cooking time is up.

Watch that glucose load. While pasta is a low GI choice, eating too much will have a marked effect on your blood glucose. That's because if you eat too large a portion of even a low GI food the glucose load becomes too large. So, instead of piling your plate with pasta, fill it with vegetables – a cup of cooked pasta combined with plenty of mixed vegetables can turn into three cups of a pasta-based meal and fit easily into any adult's daily diet.

A moderate portion of pasta served with vegetables or tomato sauce or accompaniments such as olive oil, fish and lean meat, plenty of vegetables and small amounts of cheese provides a healthy balance of carbs, fats and proteins.

FOOD	QUICK RECIPE IDEAS

CAPPELLINI

This is the thinnest form of pasta (cappellini literally means 'fine hairs') and is made from semolina. Angel-hair pasta is similar in shape, but its dough is made with eggs. Because cappellini is so thin, it is all too easy to overcook it. For a perfect al dente product, the optimal cooking time is around 4 minutes. Cappellini comes fresh or dried and is best served with light, smooth or spicy sauces such as tomato, marinara or pesto.

- A basic **marinara sauce** is essentially tomatoes and garlic to which seafood (most often these days) is added. To make a basic marinara, cook 2 cloves of crushed garlic and a finely sliced onion in a little olive oil until soft and golden. Add chopped fresh herbs such as parsley and basil (about ½ cup), 2 × 400 gram cans of Italian tomatoes, a splash of white wine, a pinch of sugar and salt and freshly ground black pepper to taste. Simmer uncovered until the sauce is thick, rich and red – about half an hour. Add 250 grams of green prawns (shelled and deveined) towards the end of the cooking time. Cook until the prawns lose their translucency – just a few minutes depending on the size. Makes about 3 cups of sauce.

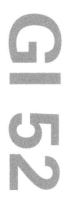

GI 45

COUSCOUS, PEARL

Unlike traditional couscous, pearl couscous, which takes its name from its pearl-like shape and size, is often described as a 'toasted pasta specialty'. Like regular pasta, it is made from hard (durum) wheat and water. But instead of being dried, it is toasted in an open-flame oven. It has a rich, nutty flavour and a chewy texture, with a smooth, almost buttery feel. It makes a perfect side dish to meat, poultry, or fish instead of potatoes, rice, or traditional pastas or couscous. (Blu Gourmet Pearl Couscous is a GI Symbol partner.)

- To make **pearl couscous salad with vegetables** and cashew nuts and a sesame dressing, bring a large pot of water to the boil. Stir in 250 g couscous and cook uncovered for 10 minutes. Drain the couscous, place in cold water to cool, then drain again. In a bowl mix together juice of 1 lemon, 2 tablespoons salt-reduced soy sauce, ½ teaspoon sesame oil, ½ a red chilli sliced, 3 tablespoons olive oil, 80 g roasted unsalted cashew nuts and ½ cup coriander leaves. Add the cold drained couscous and toss gently. Add 300 g cooked green beans and toss together very gently before serving.

GI 52

FOOD	QUICK RECIPE IDEAS

GI 40

FETTUCCINE

This is the familiar flat, long, ribbon-shaped pasta usually about $^1/_2$ cm wide. Fettuccine is the term that Romans use for 'noodles'. It's made from semolina and other ingredients such as spinach, squid ink, tomato paste and even cocoa. Available fresh and dried, it's best with tomato- or cheese-based sauces.

- Toss cooked fettuccine in a tablespoon of pesto with diced tomatoes and top with a little grated Parmesan cheese. Try using a sundried tomato pesto as an alternative and topping with some pitted black olives.
- **Fettuccine** is delicious with seafood. While the pasta is cooking, combine a little finely chopped garlic, chopped red chillies and flat leaf parsley in a bowl (adjust the quantity to suit your tastebuds). Pan-fry about four scallops per person in a little olive oil for 2–3 minutes, then add the garlic mixture and heat through. Stir in the drained pasta and serve topped with more freshly chopped parsley.

GI 47

MACARONI

These short, hollow pasta tubes of 'macaroni cheese' fame combine well with tomato- or other vegetable-based sauces. They are often used in baked dishes, soups and salads.

- To make **macaroni cheese**, preheat the oven to 180°C then cook 400 grams of macaroni following the instructions on the packet. Combine a 250 gram tub of ricotta with 1¼ cups of low-fat milk, 2 beaten eggs, 2 teaspoons of smooth Dijon mustard, 1 teaspoon of Tabasco sauce (or to taste) and freshly ground black pepper in a food processor and blend. Combine the cooked macaroni with 1 cup of shredded low-fat tasty cheddar cheese and 2 cups of baby spinach leaves in a bowl. Stir in the ricotta mixture then spoon into a baking dish. Top with grated Parmesan cheese, grainy breadcrumbs and a little paprika and bake for 20–25 minutes. Serve with a crispy green salad. Serves 4.

FOOD	QUICK RECIPE IDEAS
(STAR) PASTINA Small pasta or 'pastina' comes in many shapes: stars, orzo, acini di pepe, and many more. But just like the larger pasta shapes, pastina is made from durum wheat semolina. It is used in vegetable, chicken and beef soups to provide some bulk and added kilojoules to the soup. Children particularly love the shapes of these smaller pastas.	• Cook 100 grams of star pastina according to the packet instructions and drain. Heat 6 cups of chicken stock and add the cooked pasta plus 2 cups of cooked shredded chicken fillet. Season with salt and freshly ground black pepper and serve with a little grated Parmesan cheese and chopped flat leaf parsley.
RAVIOLI **(meat-filled)** Ravioli are small, square pasta 'pillows' with fillings such as meat, cheese and spinach, mushroom, pumpkin and tofu. Buy them fresh, frozen or vacuum packed and serve with a sauce that brings out the flavour of the fillings.	• A homemade **tomato and basil sauce** with a sprinkle of Parmesan cheese is a classic ravioli dish. What makes it even better is that by adding a large salad and fruit dessert you will have created a low GI meal in less than 20 minutes! • Top a homemade tomato and basil soup with floating ravioli and grated Parmesan cheese.

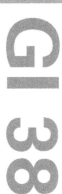

GI 38

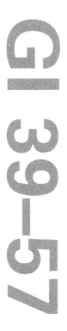

GI 39–57

FOOD	QUICK RECIPE IDEAS

GI 44

SPAGHETTI

Probably the most popular pasta of all, spaghetti's round, long strands are available fresh and dried and in a variety of flavours such as spinach and wholemeal. With its sturdy texture, spaghetti's versatility is endless.

- Serve spaghetti with a low-fat meat sauce made from lean cuts of beef, pork or veal plus chopped tomatoes, carrots, onions, celery and fresh herbs.
- Toss al dente spaghetti with smoked salmon, capers and a little olive oil and finish with a twist of two of lemon juice.
- Make a **spaghetti and tomato salad** – enjoy as a light meal and use leftovers for lunch the next day. Dice 3 medium tomatoes and combine in a bowl with 1 tablespoon of olive oil, 1 tablespoon of capers, 1 crushed garlic clove, the juice of a lemon, a sprinkle of chilli powder (or to taste), a few pitted black olives, freshly ground black pepper to taste and a handful of torn basil leaves. Combine with a cup of cooked spaghetti and serve cold or warm. Serves 2.

GI 42

SPAGHETTI (WHOLEMEAL)

All the low GI virtues of regular spaghetti apply to wholemeal spaghetti and they can be used interchangeably in any recipe with the same sauces and accompaniments. Just keep in mind that you'll be taking in more than double the amount of dietary fibre when you opt for wholemeal spaghetti.

- It blends beautifully with cooked and raw vegetables; any mixture of herbs and spices; meats, poultry, fish and shellfish; sauces containing olive oil, margarine, butter or light cream; and even nuts such as walnuts, pine nuts and sunflower seeds – all of which fit in a healthy, balanced diet.

FOOD	QUICK RECIPE IDEAS

SPIRALI

There are so many dried pasta shapes – from spirals (spirali), shells (conchiglie), bows (farfalle, literally butterflies), quill-shaped tubes (penne and penne rigate), small wheels (rotelle), twists (gemelli, literally twins) to round tubes such as cannelloni which are stuffed then baked. Everyone has their favourites. The great news for pasta lovers is that they all have a relatively low GI. But keep these portions moderate.

- Serve your favourite shapes with lightly steamed cauliflower or broccoli florets and diced lean crispy bacon (pancetta is even better) cooked with a sliced red chilli. Top with chopped parsley and a little grated Parmesan.
- Enjoy a quick **pasta and red bean salad**. Combine 1 cup of cooked pasta shapes with 1 cup of canned red kidney beans (drained), 3 finely chopped spring onions and a tablespoon of chopped fresh parsley. Toss with an oil and vinegar dressing made from 1 tablespoon of olive oil, 1 tablespoon of white wine vinegar, 1 teaspoon of Dijon mustard, a crushed clove of garlic and freshly ground black pepper. Serves 4.

GI 43

TORTELLINI

(mixed veal)
Tortellini are a small, crescent-shaped, filled pasta available in a range of fillings – including spinach and ricotta, chicken, veal, ham, mushrooms and cheese in a variety of combinations. The overall nutrient content will vary depending on the fillings. You can usually buy them fresh, frozen or vacuum packed and all you have to do is heat, whip up a sauce and serve with a salad.

- Toss cooked tortellini with fresh chopped herbs such as parsley and basil, a minced garlic clove and a little olive oil.
- Try this time-saving tortellini meal. Cook tortellini according to the packet instructions until al dente and serve with bought or homemade tomato sauce topped with a little grated Parmesan cheese. Serve with a big garden salad for a complete meal in minutes.

GI 48

FOOD	QUICK RECIPE IDEAS

GI 35

VERMICELLI

Rather like cappellini, vermicelli is a thin type of spaghetti that's available fresh and dried. Because it is so fine it cooks quickly, so watch the times. Serve with light sauces or add to soups and stir-fries.

Toss al dente vermicelli with:

- lightly steamed strips of zucchini, finely chopped parsley, a few walnut halves, a twist of black pepper and a little grated Parmesan cheese
- a bought or homemade tomato sauce with yellow and red marinated capsicum slices, anchovies, flaked canned tuna, olives, capers and basil.

If I eat twice as much, does the GI double?

The GI always remains the same, even if you double the amount of carbohydrate in your meal. This is because the GI is a relative ranking of foods containing the 'same amount' of carbohydrate. But if you double the amount of food you eat, you should expect to see a higher blood glucose response – i.e., your glucose levels will reach a higher peak and take longer to return to baseline compared with a normal serve.

LOW GI Rice

Carb-rich rice is one of the world's oldest and most cultivated grains – there are some 2000 varieties worldwide – and the staple food for over half the world's population. A soup, salad or stir-fry based around rice with a little fish, chicken, tofu or lean meat and plenty of vegetables will give you a healthy balance of carbs, fat and protein plus some fibre and essential vitamins and minerals.

Rice can have a very high GI value, or a low one, depending on the variety and its amylose content. Amylose is a kind of starch that resists gelatinisation. Although rice is a wholegrain food, when you cook it, the millions of microscopic cracks in the grains let water penetrate right to the middle of the grain, allowing the starch granules to swell and become fully 'gelatinised', thus very easy to digest.

So, if you are a big rice eater, opt for the low GI varieties with a higher amylose content such as Basmati or Doongara CleverRice. These high-amylose rices that stay firm and separate when cooked combine well with Indian, Thai and Vietnamese cuisines.

Brown rice is an extremely nutritious form of rice and contains several B vitamins, minerals, dietary fibre and protein. Chewier than regular white rice, it tends to take about twice as long to cook. The varieties available in Australia and New Zealand that have been tested to date generally have a high or moderate GI, so enjoy it occasionally, especially combined with low GI foods. Arborio risotto rice (GI 69) releases its starch during cooking and has a medium GI.

As with pasta and noodles, it's all too easy to overeat rice, so keep portions moderate. Even when you choose a low GI rice, eating too much can have a marked effect on your blood glucose. A cup of cooked rice combined with plenty of mixed vegetables can turn into three cups of a rice-based meal that suits any adult's daily diet.

FOOD	QUICK RECIPE IDEAS

GI 58

BASMATI RICE

Basmati is a long grain aromatic rice grown in the foothills of the Himalayas and is especially popular in India. When cooked the grains are dry and fluffy, so they make the perfect accompaniment for curries and sauces.

- Toss cooked rice in an oil and vinegar dressing with sultanas, chopped red and green capsicum, corn kernels and finely sliced red onion and celery to make a simple salad.
- To make a **spicy pilaf**, simmer a finely chopped onion in a little olive oil until soft, then add a cup of chopped button mushrooms and a crushed clove of garlic. Stir in ⅔ cup of Basmati rice, a teaspoon of garam masala and a cup of cooked chickpeas. Pour over 1½ cups of chicken stock, bring to the boil then reduce the heat to very low, cover and simmer gently for 10–12 minutes or until the rice is tender and all the liquid is absorbed.

GI 54–56

DOONGARA CLEVER RICE

This all-purpose white, long grain rice is a uniquely Australian developed and grown grain that was first commercially harvested about 20 years ago. Not only does it have a low GI value, but it is actually hard to overcook it. It's a rather forgiving grain, which means you get fluffy rice every time. It's also versatile and is a handy substitute for arborio rice in your favourite risotto recipe or in a paella.

- Rice on the run is great for lunch the next day, too. Pour a lightly beaten egg into an oiled frypan and cook over a medium heat until bubbly. Flip over to cook on the other side, turn onto a board and chop into slices. Sauté finely diced zucchini and red capsicum, a stick of thinly sliced celery and a grated carrot in a little oil in the pan. Add minced garlic, ginger and chopped shallots, stir till aromatic, then add a cup of cooked Basmati rice and stir until heated through. Sprinkle with soy sauce to serve.
- Make a delicious 'Doongara' rice pudding with low fat milk.

FOOD	QUICK RECIPE IDEAS

WILD RICE

Actually the seeds of a semi-aquatic grass and not a true grain, but it is right up there with brown rice in terms of nutrient-packed wholegrain benefits and a good source of minerals, fibre and B vitamins including niacin, B6 and folate. And it is gluten free. It has a chewy texture and nutty flavour and it takes longer to cook than white rice – 30–50 minutes.

- When you make a **rice salad**, combine wild rice with your favourite low (or lower) GI brown or white rice and toss with plenty of vegetables including green peas, corn kernels, chopped capsicum, chopped tomatoes and spring onions. Toss in a vinaigrette or tangy Asian style dressing and top with chopped herbs.
- Substitute wild rice in most recipes that call for white or brown rice but you will need to adjust the cooking time.

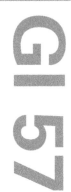

GI 57

Make a chicken pilaf

Heat 1 tablespoon canola oil in a large saucepan and cook 1 chopped onion over low–medium heat for 4–5 minutes or until it is starting to colour. Add 1 tablespoon grated fresh ginger, 500 g lean, skinless chicken thigh fillets chopped into chunks and 1 tablespoon mild curry powder and stir for about 3 minutes, until the chicken is golden all over. Add 1½ cups basmati rice, stirring to make sure the grains are well-coated. Then tip in 3 cups salt-reduced chicken stock and bring to the boil. Stir, cover, reduce the heat to low and simmer for 10 minutes. Place 200 g sliced green beans (and any other vegies you are using) on top of the rice, cover and simmer for another 5 minutes. Add 90 g spinach, remove from the heat and stand, covered, for 5 minutes. Stir the vegetables through the rice and serve with your chosen toppings.

LOW GI

Whole cereal grains

There are countless reasons to include more whole cereal grains in your diet, but it's hard to go past the fact that because you are eating the whole grain, you get all the benefits of its vitamins, minerals, protein, dietary fibre and protective anti-oxidants. Studies around the world show that eating plenty of wholegrain cereals reduces the risk of certain types of cancer, heart disease and type 2 diabetes.

A higher fibre intake, especially from whole cereal grains, is linked to a lower risk of cancer of the large bowel, breast, stomach and mouth. Eating these higher fibre foods can help you lose weight because they fill you up sooner and leave you feeling full for longer. They improve insulin sensitivity, too, and lower insulin levels. When this happens, your body makes more use of fat as a source of fuel – what could be better when you are trying to lose weight?

Are all 'wholegrain' foods low GI?

'Wholegrain' is one of the latest buzzwords in nutrition. You'll see it on everything from cornflake packets to rice crackers. Unfortunately, 'wholegrain' and 'low GI' have been used as though they are interchangeable terms. This is not the case.

Food labelling legislation requires that a food which is labelled 'wholegrain' contains all the components of whole cereal grains, present in their natural proportions. It doesn't mean that the grains are in their natural form and doesn't even hint at whether the food has a low GI. In fact, many processed wholegrain foods such as whole wheat bread and toasted bran flakes have a high GI. Why? It all comes down to the physical state of the fibre and the starch in the food.

The slow digestion and absorption of these foods will trickle fuel into your engine at a slower rate, keeping you satisfied for longer. We like to say that your body is doing the processing, not the manufacturer.

FOOD	QUICK RECIPE IDEAS
BARLEY, PEARL **One of the oldest cultivated cereals, nutritious and high in soluble fibre, helps to reduce the post-meal rise in blood glucose – it lowers the overall GI of a meal. Barley has one of the lowest GI values of any food. Use in place of rice as a side dish, in porridge or to add to soups, stews and pilafs. Substitute for rice to make risotto.**	• To make a satisfying **chunky lentil and barley soup**, cook a finely chopped onion gently in a little olive oil for about 10 minutes, or until soft and golden. Add 2 crushed cloves of garlic, ½ teaspoon of turmeric, 2 teaspoons of curry powder, ½ teaspoon of ground cumin and a teaspoon of minced chilli (or to taste) then add 4 cups of chicken stock or water. Stir in ½ cup of pearl barley, ½ cup of red lentils and a 400 gram can of tomatoes. Bring to the boil, cover and simmer for about 45 minutes or until the lentils and barley are tender. Season to taste and serve sprinkled with chopped fresh parsley or coriander. Serves 4
BUCKWHEAT GROATS **Gluten-free buckwheat is not a type of wheat or a true cereal at all – it's a herbaceous plant that produces triangular seeds used in exactly the same way as cereal grains. Buckwheat has a rather nutty flavour and is a good source of protein, B vitamins, magnesium, potassium and soluble fibre. Buckwheat flour is widely used for making pancakes, muffins, biscuits, and is an indispensable ingredient for Russia's blini and Japan's soba noodles.**	• To make **buckwheat and buttermilk pancakes**, combine 1 cup (100 g) of unprocessed oat bran with 2 cups of buttermilk in a bowl and let stand for 10 minutes. In a separate bowl, combine ½ cup (75 g) of chopped dried fruit medley, ½ cup of sifted buckwheat flour, 2 teaspoons of sugar, 1 teaspoon of bicarbonate of soda, 1 beaten egg and 2 teaspoons of melted margarine. Mix thoroughly then combine the two mixtures to make a batter and stand for 1 hour. Spray a large frypan with canola oil and heat to medium–hot, then spoon just enough batter into the pan to make a 10 cm pancake. Cook until bubbly on top and lightly browned underneath, then flip and cook on the other side for 2–3 minutes. Repeat for the rest of the batter. Serve with berries and low-fat yoghurt or maple syrup or floral honey.

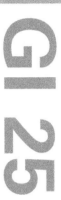

GI 25

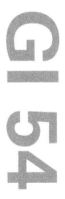

GI 54

FOOD	QUICK RECIPE IDEAS

GI 48

BULGUR

Also known as cracked wheat, bulgur is made from whole wheat grains that have been hulled and steamed before grinding to crack the grain. The wheat grain remains virtually intact – it is simply cracked – and the wheat germ and bran are retained, which preserves nutrients and lowers the GI. With its wheaty flavour you can use bulgur instead of rice or other grains in a range of recipes. Use it as a breakfast cereal, in tabbouli, or add it to pilafs, vegetable burgers, stuffing, stews, salads and soups.

- Try this super-nutritious, high fibre **mushroom and bulgur salad**. Make a marinade with 3 tablespoons of lemon juice, 3 tablespoons of olive oil, a crushed garlic clove and a tablespoon each of freshly chopped parsley and mint (or more if you like). Marinate 125 grams of sliced button mushrooms and 2 chopped spring onions in the mixture for about an hour. Place 1 cup of bulgur in a bowl, cover with hot water and let it stand for about 20–30 minutes until the water is absorbed and the bulgur softens. Drain well, squeezing out excess water. Toss the bulgur with the marinated mushrooms and spoon into a serving dish. Serves 4.

- To make **tabbouli**, cover ½ cup of bulgur with hot water and soak for 20–30 minutes to soften. Drain well and squeeze out the excess water. Add a cup of finely chopped flat leaf parsley, 3 or 4 chopped spring onions, 2 tablespoons of chopped mint and a chopped tomato. Stir in a dressing made with 2 tablespoons each of lemon juice and olive oil. Tabbouli is best made ahead of serving time to let the flavours develop. Serves 4.

- **Bulgar pilaf** has a far lower GI than rice pilaf. Serve it with casseroles or as a meal on its own with chopped vegetables. Sauté a thinly sliced brown onion in 1½ tablespoons of olive oil until it is translucent. Add a handful of crushed dry egg noodle vermicelli and stir until it is pale gold in colour. Add ½ cup of bulgur and 1 cup of hot chicken stock. Cover and simmer on low heat for about 7 minutes or until it looks dry. Cover and stand for 10 minutes before serving. Makes about 2 cups.

FOOD	QUICK RECIPE IDEAS
QUINOA Quinoa (pronounced keen-wah) is a small, round, quick-cooking grain somewhat similar in colour to sesame seeds. It's a nutritional powerpack – an excellent source of low GI carbs, fibre and protein, and rich in B vitamins and minerals including iron, phosphorus, magnesium and zinc. It cooks in about 10–15 minutes and has a light, chewy texture and slightly nutty flavour and can be used as a substitute for many other grains.	• Make the most of this super grain – substitute gluten-free quinoa for rice, couscous, cracked wheat or barley in soups, stuffed vegetables, salads, stews and even in 'rice' pudding. • To serve as a side dish, thoroughly rinse 1 cup of quinoa (if not pre-washed). Drain, place the grains in a medium-sized pot with 2 cups of water and bring to the boil. Reduce to a simmer, cover and leave to cook until all the water is absorbed. • Give your day a hearty start with **quinoa 'porridge'** by adding about ½ cup of finely sliced apples and a couple of tablespoons of sultanas to the pot while the quinoa is simmering. Add ½ teaspoon of cinnamon for extra flavour if you like. Serve with low-fat milk and sweeten with honey or sugar to taste.
SEMOLINA (cooked) Semolina is the coarsely milled inner part of the wheat grain called the endosperm. It is granular in appearance. The large particle size of semolina flour (compared with fine wheat flour) limits the swelling of its starch particles when cooked, which results in slower digestion, slower release of glucose into the blood stream and a lower GI.	• You can use it to make homemade pasta or gnocchi or simply cook it and eat it as a hot cereal or make it into a traditional milk pudding. Use semolina to thicken sauces and gravies instead of plain flour. Semolina is also used to make couscous (GI 65), a side dish that is quick and easy to prepare. • To make **semolina porridge**, mix about 1 tablespoon of semolina with 3 tablespoons of low-fat milk or water into a smooth paste. Slowly stir in ¾ cup of low-fat milk. Cook over a low heat, stirring continually for about 10 minutes to the desired consistency. Sweeten with a little honey or maple syrup, or serve with chopped fresh or canned fruit.

GI 51

GI 55

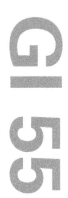

LOW GI

Legumes, including beans, peas & lentils

We have long known about the benefits of eating legumes. Not only do they keep in the cupboard for a year or more, they are an excellent source of protein, easy to prepare and cost very little. When you cook them, they more than double in weight – 1 cup of dry beans makes 2½ cups of cooked beans – and when you eat them, you'll feel satisfied for longer.

Also known as pulses, legumes are the edible dried seeds found inside the mature pods of leguminous plants. Legumes include various types of beans, peas, chickpeas and lentils. Green peas are legumes but we most often eat them fresh as a green vegetable, so we have included them in the vegetable section. Peanuts are legumes, too, but since they are usually thought of as nuts we have included them in that section.

Whether you buy them dried, or opt for canned convenience, you are choosing one of nature's lowest GI foods. They are high in fibre and packed with nutrients, providing protein, carbohydrate, B vitamins, folate and minerals. When you add legumes to meals and snacks, you reduce the overall GI of your diet because your body digests them slowly. This is primarily because their starch breaks down relatively slowly (or incompletely) during cooking and they contain tannins and enzyme inhibitors that also slow digestion.

Although they have an excellent shelf life, old beans take longer to cook than young, which is why it's a good idea to buy them from shops where you know turnover is brisk. Once home, store them in airtight containers in a cool, dry place – they will keep their colour better.

FOOD	QUICK RECIPE IDEAS

BAKED BEANS
(canned in tomato sauce)
Baked beans are a popular ready-to-eat form of legume, an easy way to introduce children to the world of beans, and available in convenient single-serve cans. Haricot (navy) beans are most commonly used for baked beans. If you make your own baked bean recipe, it will have a lower GI.

- Top half a jacket potato cooked in the microwave with a scoop or two of canned or homemade baked beans sprinkled with a little grated cheese.
- A scoop or two of baked beans is a healthy addition to any meal or a satisfying breakfast or light meal served on grainy toast.

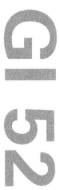

BLACK BEANS
(home-cooked)
The black bean or black kidney bean is the small, shiny bean with an earthy sweet flavour often used in South and Central American and Caribbean cooking, and Mexican dishes such as refried beans. Add them to chilli con carne or to bean soups and salads for extra flavour and texture. In Latin-American-style dishes, a spicy bean mix made with black or red kidney beans is often served over rice.

- Use leftover chicken and rice to make **tasty burritos**. Preheat the oven to 180°C. Wrap 6 large tortillas in foil and warm in the oven. Cook 1 chopped onion and 1 crushed clove of garlic in a tablespoon of vegetable oil, stirring occasionally until softened. Add 1 cup of chopped cooked chicken, 1 cup of cooked or canned black beans, 1 cup of cooked Basmati rice and 1 can of diced tomatoes. To serve, spoon about ¾ cup of the filling into the centre of the warmed tortilla. Sprinkle 1 tablespoon of grated low-fat cheese on top, fold in the ends, then roll the tortilla around the filling. Place in a large shallow baking dish. Sprinkle ½ cup of grated low-fat cheese on top of burritos, then cover with foil and heat in the oven for about 10 minutes, or until the cheese is melted and the filling is hot. Serve topped with chopped coriander. Makes 6.

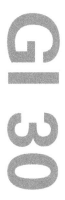

FOOD	QUICK RECIPE IDEAS

GI 42

BLACK-EYED BEANS
Also known as cowpeas, Southern peas and black-eyed peas, these beans are medium-sized, kidney-shaped and cream-coloured with a distinctive black 'eye' and a subtle flavour. They are a popular 'soul food' in the southern states of the US where they are traditionally served with pork. Add black-eyed beans to soups and stews or serve as a side dish.

- Cook chopped leeks, onions and carrots with crushed garlic in a little olive oil. Add cooked or canned black-eyed, kidney and borlotti beans, canned tomatoes plus fresh thyme and bay leaves and a chopped red chilli to make a **Mediterranean-style vegetable casserole**.
- For a **black-eyed bean salad**, soak a cup of black-eyed beans overnight then simmer in fresh water for about 30 minutes until tender. Drain and cool, then add chopped tomato and celery. Toss with a dressing of 2 tablespoons chopped parsley, 1 tablespoon seeded mustard, 1 crushed clove of garlic and 3 tablespoons each of olive oil and wine vinegar.

GI 41

BORLOTTI BEANS
(canned)
This medium-sized bean has a creamy texture, slightly nutty flavour and reddish-black to magenta streaks that fade to brown during cooking. It is widely used for soups, stews, casseroles and in salads and the delicious pasta and bean soup you will find served all over Italy (although they tend to use cannellini beans in the south).

- Combine a cup of cooked beans with ½ cup of semi-dried tomatoes and baby spinach leaves in a balsamic dressing.
- Add borlotti beans to a salad of tuna chunks, onion rings, tomato slices, olives and chopped fresh parsley.
- Mash cooked or canned borlotti beans with sweet potato or taro, ½ cup of heated low-fat milk and some freshly grated nutmeg. Leave some of the beans whole for texture.

FOOD	QUICK RECIPE IDEAS

BUTTER BEANS
(canned)
Sometimes called large lima beans, butter beans are a flat-shaped white bean with a smooth, creamy, slightly sweet flavour. Add to soups, stews and salads or simply heat and serve as a side dish topped with finely chopped fresh herbs.

- Add a cup of cooked butter beans and a crushed clove of garlic to steamed sweet potato (or taro or yam) and mash as usual. Season to taste with a little salt and freshly ground black pepper and add enough water or low-fat milk or soy milk for a creamy consistency.
- Dip pita crisps into a butter bean purée. Purée a drained can of butter beans (or any white bean) with a crushed clove of garlic in the food processor slowly, pouring in just enough oil and lemon juice to create the desired consistency.

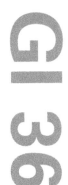
GI 36

CANNELLINI BEANS
(canned)
Also known as white kidney beans, cannellini beans are large, smooth-textured, mild-flavoured, kidney-shaped beans with a creamy white skin. They are used in soups, salads, stews, casseroles, bean pots such as the French cassoulet and in many Italian dishes.

- Add cannellini beans to puréed vegetable soups for a creamy texture. Simmer cauliflower florets until tender in chicken stock then blend with a cup of cooked beans and season to taste with salt and freshly ground black pepper. Top with freshly grated nutmeg and finely chopped parsley and serve.
- Make a salad of cannellini beans and finely sliced fennel tossed in a tangy lemon, oil and vinegar dressing and top with finely chopped flat leaf parsley.

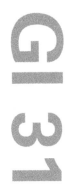
GI 31

FOOD	QUICK RECIPE IDEAS

GI 40

CHICKPEAS
(canned)
Also known as garbanzo beans or ceci, these versatile caramel-coloured legumes have a nutty flavour and firm texture. Popular in Middle Eastern, Mediterranean and Mexican cooking, they are the main ingredient in specialties such as hommous and felafel and the basis for many vegetarian dishes.

- Combine 2 oranges separated into segments, a drained and rinsed 400 gram can of chickpeas and a finely sliced fennel bulb (or two if small ones). Toss in a dressing made with olive oil, vinegar and orange juice for a tangy salad.
- Keep a can in the pantry or cooked chickpeas in the fridge and add them to soups, stews and salads or to a tomato-based sauce served with couscous or rice. After soaking, whole chickpeas can be roasted with salt and spices to make a crunchy low GI snack that's every bit as more-ish as potato chips!

GI 37

FOUR BEAN MIX
Canned bean mixes which include red kidney beans, chickpeas and lima and butter beans make it easy to add protein and boost flavour and fibre to meals including soups and stews. You can also add canned mixed beans to your salad wraps, sandwiches and rolls for a lunch that lasts.

- For a meal in minutes, combine drained and rinsed mixed beans with baby spinach leaves, chopped spring onions, cucumber, yellow capsicum, sliced radishes, finely sliced celery and halved or quartered cherry tomatoes and toss in a light lemony oil and vinegar dressing.
- Boost the flavour and fibre of a home-made tomato soup by adding a can of drained, rinsed four bean mix.

FOOD	QUICK RECIPE IDEAS

HARICOT BEANS
(home-cooked)
These small, white, oval-shaped beans, sometimes called navy beans, are the ones most often used in the manufacture of commercial baked beans. They have a mild flavour and combine well in soups and stews.

- Make your own **baked beans** to serve for breakfast on grainy toast or as a side dish. Combine a small chopped onion, 2 small diced capsicums (red or green) and 3 cups of cooked or canned haricot beans in a large casserole dish. Add $\frac{1}{3}$ cup of pure floral honey, 2 tablespoons of Dijon mustard, 1 tablespoon of white wine vinegar, $\frac{1}{2}$ cup of tomato sauce and a few twists of freshly ground black pepper. Mix well then cover and cook in a preheated oven (180°C) for about 45 minutes to an hour. Serves 6–8 as a side dish.

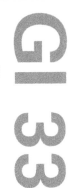

GI 33

HOMMOUS
(regular)
Hommous – puréed chickpeas, lemon juice, tahini, olive oil, garlic and sometimes ingredients such as roasted red peppers – is one of the most popular foods to emerge from the Middle East. It's widely available in the refrigerator section of supermarkets and fresh produce stores, in specialist delis, or as a takeaway from Lebanese or Turkish restaurants.

- Use hommous as a spread for sandwiches, as a topping on grilled fish, chicken, with baked potatoes, or in a wrap with kebabs and salad or a felafel roll.
- To make your own **hommous**, combine a 400 gram can of chickpeas (drained, reserving the liquid), ½ cup of tahini (sesame seed paste), a large clove of garlic, chopped, ⅓ cup of lemon juice, plus a little salt and freshly ground black pepper to taste. Process in a blender or food processor, adding enough of the reserved chickpea liquid to make a smooth consistency.
- It can be served as part of a mezze platter or used as a dip with pita bread, or raw or blanched vegetables such as carrot and celery sticks.

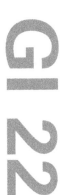

GI 22

FOOD	QUICK RECIPE IDEAS

GI 26–48

LENTILS

GI 26 (red, home-cooked)
GI 30 (green, home-cooked)
GI 48 (green, canned)
One of nature's superfoods – rich in protein, fibre and B vitamins and often used as substitutes for meat in vegetarian recipes – they have only a small effect on blood glucose levels. All colours and types of lentils have a similar low GI value, which is increased slightly if you opt to buy them canned and add them towards the end of cooking time. Lentils have a fairly bland, earthy flavour that combines well with onions, garlic and spices. They cook quickly to a soft consistency and are used to make Indian dhal, a spiced lentil purée.

- Make a meal of lentil soup and low GI bread – you will feel completely satisfied. Canned lentil soup (GI 44) is a convenient, quick meal when you don't have time to prepare your own.

- To make a **vegetarian lentil burger**, simmer a chopped onion in olive oil for a few minutes to soften. In a bowl thoroughly combine 2 cups of canned and drained lentils with the onion mix and 2 cups of mashed potato or sweet potato, season to taste with salt and freshly ground black pepper, adding a dash of Tabasco or chilli sauce for flavour. Form into patties and cook them on both sides until browned in the oven, on the barbecue or in a pan and combine with salad, tomato slices, chutney and grainy rolls.

- For **mashed lentils** an easy alternative to mashed potato, bring to the boil 250 ml of chicken or vegetable stock, ⅔ cup of split red lentils and 1 bay leaf, then simmer until the lentils are mushy and thick. Season with salt and freshly ground black pepper. You may also like to add a teaspoon of curry powder for extra flavour.

- Lentils thicken any kind of soup or extend meat casseroles.

FOOD	QUICK RECIPE IDEAS

MUNG BEANS

(home cooked)
Also known as green gram or golden gram, dried mung beans are small, olive-green beans that are used in many Asian cuisines. The starch from mung beans is used in making bean thread and cellophane noodles. A good source of fibre, iron and protein. You can buy sprouted mung beans in punnets – a useful source of vitamin C.

- Add mung bean sprouts as an extra vegetable to a stir-fry or fried rice at the end of cooking.
- For a **mung bean salad** combine 1 cup of mung bean sprouts, 1 cup of baby spinach, 1 cup of baby rocket, 1 sliced Lebanese cucumber, 1 punnet of baby tomatoes, halved, ½ an avocado, sliced, 1 small finely sliced red onion and ½ cup of pitted black olives in a large salad bowl with a dressing made from olive oil, balsamic vinegar and a dash of lemon juice. Serves 4.

GI 39

PEAS, SPLIT

(yellow or green split peas)
Like other legumes, dried peas are a nutritional storehouse and because they are slowly digested, a little goes a long way. Yellow or green split peas come from a variety of garden pea with the husk removed. They tend to disintegrate and are traditionally used for pea and ham soup and yellow split peas for making Indian dhal. Your local Indian takeaway will sell prepared dhals. Combined with flat bread and Basmati rice, dhal makes a delicious low GI light vegetarian meal.

- To make your own **dhal**, rinse and drain 1 cup of red lentils and place in a saucepan with ½ a teaspoon of turmeric and a pinch of chilli powder. Add 1½ cups of boiling water and cook for 15 minutes or until the lentils are very soft, but still retain their shape. Season to taste with salt. Heat 1 tablespoon of margarine or olive oil in a small frypan and gently cook a small finely chopped onion until soft and golden – about 10 minutes. Stir 1 teaspoon of garam masala into the onion mixture, stir briskly for 30 seconds, then add 1 teaspoon of coriander and combine with the lentils. Season to taste with salt and freshly ground black pepper. Add a squeeze of lime.

GI 25

FOOD	QUICK RECIPE IDEAS

GI 38

PINTO BEANS
(refried, canned)
This medium-sized mottled bean ('pinto' means painted) turns pinkish-brown when cooked. It's a staple in Latin-American cooking and used whole or made into refried beans as a filling for burritos or tacos.

- Make a colourful and **crunchy bean mix** for tacos. Combine 2 cups of cooked pinto beans with a finely diced green capsicum, a cup of juicy red chopped tomatoes, 2 sliced spring onions, 1 cup of sweetcorn kernels (straight off the cob is best), ½ teaspoon of ground cumin and salt and freshly ground black pepper to taste. Serve with tacos and bowls of guacamole, shredded lettuce and grated low-fat cheese. Serves 4.

GI 36

RED KIDNEY BEANS
(canned)
These tasty red beans are a popular addition to vegetarian and meat chilli dishes and nachos, tacos and burritos. Not only do red kidney beans play a leading role in Mexican and 'Tex-Mex' cuisines, a scoop is a sustaining side dish with main meals and adds substance to soups, stews and salads.

- Stir into a homemade or bought tangy tomato salsa to add a Mexican flavour.
- Create a **colourful bean salad** by combining a 400 gram can of kidney beans (drained) in a serving bowl with 1 cup each of cooked green beans and cooked yellow beans sliced on the diagonal. Finely slice half a red capsicum, half a green capsicum and 2 stalks of celery. Toss the beans and vegetables in a light dressing made with balsamic vinegar and olive oil. Coat the salad well – you will need about ½ a cup of dressing. Serves 4–6 as a side dish.

FOOD	QUICK RECIPE IDEAS
ROMANO BEANS (home-cooked) **Sometimes referred to as Italian flat beans, romano beans can be eaten as a snap bean when very young or as a dried bean during later stages of maturity. They are used in a wide variety of bean and chilli dishes, soups and salads.**	• To make a **spinach and bean stir-fry**, gently cook 2 chopped spring onions and a finely chopped clove of garlic in a little olive oil. Add a seeded and diced red capsicum and toss to heat through for 2–3 minutes. Stir in 2 cups of baby spinach leaves, 2 tablespoons of chopped fresh chives and 2 cups of cooked romano beans. When heated through, season to taste, and serve topped with freshly grated nutmeg alongside bulgur, quinoa or low GI rice. Serves 4. 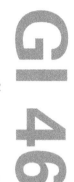
SOYBEANS (canned) **Soybeans and soy products are the nutritional powerhouse of the legume family. They have been a staple part of Asian diets for thousands of years and are an excellent source of protein. They're also rich in fibre, iron, zinc and vitamin B. They are lower in carbohydrate and higher in fat than other legumes, but the majority of the fat is polyunsaturated.**	• Use canned soybeans in place of other beans in any recipe. • Make a quick soybean and vegetable curry with chopped onions, garlic, carrots, tomatoes, cauliflower and broccoli using vegetable stock and your favourite curry paste. • Just one cup of soy milk constitutes a serving and can be used as a nutritionally balanced replacement for dairy milk, providing it is low-fat and calcium enriched. Try: – Soy milk on your breakfast cereal – A soy banana smoothie, or – A soy yoghurt for a snack. 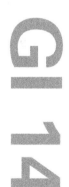

LOW GI

Nuts

Nuts are one of the richest sources of vitamin E, with a small handful of mixed nuts providing more than 20 per cent of the recommended daily intake. The vitamin E content may explain the findings from a recent study from Harvard University School of Public Health which found that increased nut consumption, including natural peanut butter, may improve the body's ability to balance glucose and insulin.

Peanut allergy

All processed peanuts are quality-controlled for the presence of fungus that produces a toxin called aflatoxin, one of the most carcinogenic substances known. Because peanuts in the shell are not screened, throw away any mouldy ones.

Peanut allergy is an increasingly common food allergy, especially in children. It occurs in approximately 1 in 50 children and 1 in 200 adults and is the allergy most likely to cause anaphylaxis (which involves swelling in the gut, respiratory tract and/or cardiovascular system) and death. Symptoms of allergy include itching, especially around the mouth, swelling tongue, flushed face, cramping, difficulty breathing, diarrhoea and vomiting. If peanut allergy is suspected urgent medical attention should be sought. One-third of all peanut-allergic people are also allergic to tree nuts such as brazil nuts, hazelnuts, walnuts, almonds, macadamia nuts, pistachios, pecans, pine nuts and cashews.

FOOD	QUICK RECIPE IDEAS

CASHEWS

Cashews, like all nuts, are cholesterol free and high in protein. Their carbohydrate content is quite low, but they do have a high fat content (almost half their total weight) but it is less than any other type of nut and three-quarters of it is heart-healthy polyunsaturated and monunsaturated fats. Cashews are also rich in several B vitamins and the minerals copper, magnesium and zinc.

- Cashews make a healthy addition to salads, rice dishes and desserts and are a popular ingredient in Asian stir-fries. Enjoy cashews several times a week if you wish, but keep the amounts you eat small and look for unsalted varieties.
- A delicious snack. Enjoy.
- Add a handful to Asian stir-fries.

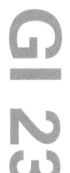

GI 22

PEANUTS, DRY ROASTED (UNSALTED)

A low carb but high fat, high protein food (50 per cent fat and 25 per cent protein), peanuts grow under the ground – they are also known as groundnuts. Technically a legume, they are an excellent source of vitamins B and E and so low in carbohydrate that their GI doesn't really count – although their fat content does! Because peanuts are such a tasty and convenient finger food they are easily overeaten, so give yourself a specific ration. And stick to it!

- Make up trail mixes with peanuts, sultanas, dried fruit and sunflower seeds for a no-fuss snack on the run.
- Sprinkle crushed nuts over salads for flavour and crunch or stir crushed nuts and chopped dried fruit through low-fat yoghurt.
- Add crushed peanuts to the mix when baking biscuits or slices.

GI 23

GI Fish & seafood

We can't measure a GI for fish because it doesn't contain any carbohydrate. However, it is an important part of a balanced diet and we now know that just one serve of fish or seafood a week may reduce the risk of a fatal heart attack by about 40 per cent. The likely protective components of fish are the very long chain omega–3 fatty acids. Our bodies only make small amounts of these fatty acids which is why we rely on dietary sources, especially fish and seafood.

Sustainable fish facts

Shopping for fish can be a bit of a minefield. Here's our guide to choosing sustainable fish when shopping.

Overfished* (*Identified by the Bureau of Rural Sciences as being overfished.)
Blue warehou (snotty trevalla, black trevally, sea bream) • Eastern gemfish (hake, king couta, silver kingfish) • Redfish (nannygai, red snapper) • Southern bluefin tuna (tuna) • Bigeye tuna (Indian Ocean tuna) • School shark (flake, snapper shark, tope) • Silver trevally (silver bream, white trevally) • Orange roughy (deep sea perch, sea perch)

Better choices
Blue grenadier (hoki) • Barramundi • Blue-eye trevalla (blue-eye cod, big eye, deep sea trevalla) • Bream • Yellowfin tuna • Flathead • King George whiting (spotted whiting, SA whiting) • Whiting (school, sand, trumpeter, yellowfin) • Mackerel • Mullet (bluetail, fantail, flicker, yellow eye) • Ling (pink ling, rock ling) • Snapper (red bream, cockney, squire) • Tailor (bluefish, skipjack) • Coral trout (various species)

GI

LOW

Lean meat, chicken, eggs & plant protein alternatives

As with fish and seafood, GI is not relevant to protein–rich meat, chicken and eggs. These foods are valuable inclusions in a healthy diet, however, not only for protein, but also for essential vitamins and minerals. Lean red meats are a good source of iron and zinc that will help to boost your energy levels by helping your blood to carry sufficient levels of oxygen throughout your body. Chicken and eggs contain less amounts of iron but are still a great source of nutrients, not to mention being a convenient food source to prepare and cook.

Plant sources of protein

The GI does not apply as these contain very little carbohydrates:

Tofu (soybean curd) is an easy way of using soy. It has a mild flavour itself but absorbs the flavours of other foods, making it delicious when it's been marinated in soy sauce, ginger and garlic and tossed into a stir-fry.

Mycoprotein (Quorn) is made from fermented fungus, and is low in saturated fat and a good source of protein, fibre, iron and zinc. It can be used in cooking or you will find it in ready-made meals such as casseroles, pies and curries.

Tempeh is made from fermented cooked soybeans and has a firm chewy texture and nutty mushroom-like flavour. An excellent source of protein, it also contains dietary fibre and phytochemicals from the soybeans. Try it sliced on sandwiches or in salads or use it in stir-fries and curries.

Seitan (pronounced say-*tahn*) is sometimes called 'wheat meat'. It comes from wheat gluten (the protein part of flour) and is an alternative to soy-based meat substitutes such as tofu. High in protein and low in fat, it's been a traditional food for Buddhists for centuries. It has a chewy texture, neutral taste and tends to absorb the flavour of the foods you cook it with. Sold chilled in tubs or frozen in blocks, chunks, strips or ground. Add it to cooked dishes at the last minute, heating just until it is warmed through.

LOW GI

Dairy foods

Dairy foods are recommended throughout childhood and beyond. In adults, they are linked to better weight control and higher insulin sensitivity. Not only are they an important source of calcium, but they also provide energy, protein, carbohydrate and vitamins A, B and D.

Low-fat varieties of milk, yoghurt, ice-cream and custard will give you high-quality protein energy and boost your calcium intake.

Cheese is a great source of micronutrients, but it is not a source of carbohydrate as its lactose is drawn off in the whey during production. This means that GI is not relevant to cheese. It is perfect for sandwich fillings, snacks and toppings for pasta and with gratin dishes. Cheese also contributes a fair number of kilojoules. Most cheese is around 30 per cent fat, much of it saturated. Ricotta and cottage cheese are good low-fat choices – usually less than 7 per cent fat.

Although there are a number of good reduced-fat cheeses available, others can lose out in the flavour stakes for a relatively small reduction in fat. If you are a real cheese lover and having a hard time finding a tasty low-fat one, try these tips for making the most of your higher fat cheese choices.

- Consider eating a little of a strong-flavoured cheese rather than a lot of something bland and tasteless.
- Shave a few strips of fresh Parmesan over pasta – a vegetable peeler does the job nicely. Grating and shaving helps a little cheese go a long way.
- Enjoy full-fat cheeses in small amounts occasionally. This includes regular types of cheddar, blue vein, Swiss, brie, camembert, Colby, gouda and havarti.
- Try some mozzarella cheese – whole milk or part skim – it may contain less fat than some reduced-fat cheeses. Grate and sprinkle over stuffed vegies such as capsicum or eggplant, baked potatoes and pizzas before cooking.

FOOD	QUICK RECIPE IDEAS
LOW-FAT DAIRY DESSERTS **From custard to Frûche (fromage frais) and ice-cream to mousse, or even rice 'pudding' yoghurt, supermarkets are filled with ready-to-eat, light, creamy, even aerated, dairy desserts. If you are watching your blood glucose levels, read the nutritional labels as some are much richer in carbs than others in a typical serving.**	• Top winter-warming desserts with a dollop of your favourite low fat dairy dessert or ice-cream. • Lightly grill fresh fruit such as peach or nectarine halves and top with a scoop of ice cream or fromage frais. • Enjoy a single serve low fat dairy dessert to refuel when you are on the run. • Enjoy a guilt-free after-dinner indulgence or a quick snack without adding too many kilojoules when you pick the reduced-fat or 'diet' versions.

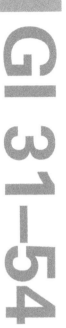

GI 31–54

What about lactose intolerance?

Lactose, the sugar in milk, is a disaccharide ('double sugar') that needs to be digested into its component sugars before our bodies can absorb it. The two sugars (glucose and galactose) compete with each other for absorption. Once absorbed, the galactose is mainly metabolised in the liver and produces very little effect on our blood glucose levels. The remaining sugar, glucose, is present in a small enough amount not to cause a spike in blood glucose.

Some people are lactose intolerant because the enzyme lactase is not active in their small intestine. Children who are lactose intolerant often outgrow this by five years of age. If you are lactose intolerant, you should still be able to enjoy cheese – which is virtually lactose free – and yoghurt. The micro-organisms in yoghurt are active in digesting lactose during passage through the small intestine. Alternatively, try lactose-reduced or lactose-free milk and milk products, or low GI, low-fat, calcium-enriched non-dairy alternatives such as soy milk. Note that rice milk has a high GI value (GI 92) and oat milk has a GI of 69.

FOOD	QUICK RECIPE IDEAS

GI 20–34

LOW-FAT MILK

Long valued for protein, the bone-building minerals calcium and phosphorus and valuable vitamins such as riboflavin (B$_2$). The low-fat flavoured milks are okay too, as they generally have relatively modest amounts of added sugar (about 4%) compared with soft drinks (11–12%). Some are also made with alternative sweeteners.

- Hot milk and honey makes a good nightcap. Research shows that people *do* sleep more soundly after a warm milk drink at night. Warming the milk activates an amino acid called tryptophan, which the body converts to serotonin, the hormone associated with calmness and wellbeing.

- When you are having a coffee break, choose a skim milk latte or cappuccino and get the low GI calcium boost.

- Add to your cereal or tea or coffee or simply drink as a snack or whip up in a fruit smoothie.

FOOD	QUICK RECIPE IDEAS

LOW-FAT OR NO FAT YOGHURT

Yoghurt has a naturally low GI and it's a great source of vitamins and minerals such as riboflavin, and calcium. The low GI values are thanks (mainly) to the combination of acidity and high protein and of course the fact that lactose, the sugar in milk, has a naturally low GI (46). How low does yoghurt go? Well, testing at the University of Sydney has found non-nutritive sweetened flavoured yoghurts have the lowest GI values (14–21) and contain fewer kilojoules, and around half the carbohydrate, than the nutritively sweetened versions (26–43). Here's a tip: Low fat yoghurt provides the most calcium for the least kilojoules (520 mg calcium in a 200 gram tub).

- Serve **chicken salad with a yoghurt dressing** made from a 200-gram tub of low fat plain yoghurt, 2 tablespoons of lemon juice, a couple of teaspoons of a tangy mango chutney and 2 tablespoons of finely chopped mint.

- Spice plain yoghurt with a little ground cumin and cardamom to make a sauce for topping burgers or falafel rolls. Add fresh mint for a finishing touch.

- Make a **spicy Indian 'lassi' drink** by blending 1 cup of low fat natural yoghurt with ½ teaspoon of ground cumin and a pinch of salt to taste. Chill. Just before serving, stir in ¼ teaspoon of finely minced onion and a few strips of finely sliced green chilli. Pour into a tall glass over ice blocks and serve – delicious as an appetiser before an Indian meal.

- Keep a tub of low fat plain yoghurt in the fridge, trying different brands until you find one you like. It's a great base for dips, salad dressings and sauces – sweet and savoury.

GI 24-40

LOW **GI**

Dairy alternatives

There are a number of alternatives to dairy products but as these are not as calcium-rich you need to look at ways of boosting your daily calcium intake. Soy products are not naturally high in calcium so it is best to choose calcium-fortified products if these are a key source of calcium in your diet.

Other non-dairy options that will boost your calcium intake are foods such as almonds, brazil nuts, sesame seeds, dried figs, dried apricots, soybeans, Asian greens such as bok choy, fish with edible bones such as salmon and sardines, calcium-enriched tofu and calcium-fortified breakfast cereals.

Soy milk – a healthy alternative

Soy milk is generally made by mixing soybeans – which are usually GM/GE free (always check the label) – with filtered water and flavourings to produce a milk-like product. You can buy reduced-fat, calcium-fortified soy milk, GI 16–44, fresh from the chilled dairy cabinet, in long-life packs and in powdered forms. You can also buy flavoured products. To ensure it is a suitable alternative to regular dairy milk, soy milk is often enriched with a range of vitamins and minerals including calcium and riboflavin (vitamin B12). Choose a low-fat, calcium-enriched milk and use it exactly as you would regular milk – on your breakfast cereal, with hot or cold drinks or in your cooking when making desserts and sauces.

FOOD	QUICK RECIPE IDEAS	
SOY MILK (REDUCED-FAT, CALCIUM-FORTIFIED) **Drinking this completely dairy- and lactose-free beverage is an easy way to include soy protein in your diet. Soy milk has become increasing popular, possibly because it tastes good and is recognised to be rich in phytoestrogens, nutrients that are known to have health benefits.**	• Mix it in with mashed sweet potato, pumpkin or potato; or in a combination of all three vegetables. • Try a soy latte or soy banana smoothie or use in other flavoured milk drinks. • Use it to make white sauce for lasagne or moussaka. • Make dairy desserts with soy milk.	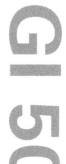GI 16–44
SOY YOGHURT **(fruit flavoured, sweetened with sugar)** **Soy yoghurt is usually made from soybeans or soy protein rather than soy milk. Look for calcium-enriched, low fat varieties.**	• Use in exactly the same way as you would dairy yoghurts as a snack or dessert, or added to smoothies and shakes. • It's a great base for dips, salad dressings and sauces – sweet and savoury.	GI 50

Part 5

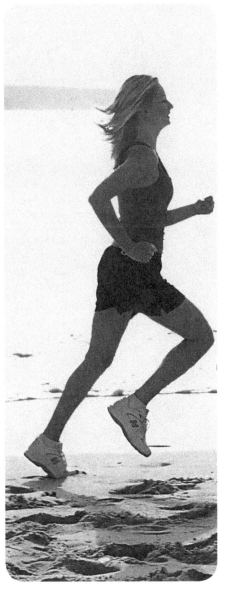

The Low GI shopper

- Low GI smart shopping
- The GI symbol
- The GI values

Chapter 17

Low GI smart shopping

Our shopping list will help you stock the pantry and fridge with the staples you require to turn out a meal in minutes. It includes everything you'll need for the low GI meal ideas in the food finder. To make your own shopping list, use the same headings. They will take you to the appropriate aisles of the supermarket or to the shops you usually favour.

We've included convenience foods such as canned beans, bagged salads, bottled sauces and pastes, canned fruits and chopped vegetables (fresh and frozen) in the list. There's no need to feel guilty about using these items. Remember, this book is about making eating a healthy, low GI diet as easy as possible and although some convenience items such as frozen vegetables or canned beans may be a little more expensive, the time savings and health benefits can outweigh the costs.

If you want to know more about some of the foods on the shopping list, check the Top 100 low GI food finder in Part 4. We have included lots of meal ideas and even some recipes in this section.

What to put in the shopping trolley

The perfect place to get started on healthy low GI eating is the supermarket, whether you are pushing a trolley up and down the aisles, or shopping online. This is where we make those hurried or impulsive decisions that have a big impact. Cadbury's milk chocolate is on sale, do you stock up or keep walking? One little decision – what a big impact.

Make a list

Spend a little time each day, or weekly if it suits, planning what to eat when. It makes life simpler. Meal planning is just writing down what you intend to eat for the main meals of the week, then checking your fridge and pantry for ingredients available and noting what you need to purchase. So study the GI tables, look at the meal ideas in this book and browse through some recipes with a notepad handy.

Nutritional Information

Servings per package: 3
Serving size: 150g

	Quantity per serving	Quantity per 100 g
Energy	608 kj	405 kj
Protein	4.2 g	2.8 g
Fat, total	7.4 g	4.9 g
– saturated	4.5 g	3.0 g
Carbohydrate, total	18.6 g	12.4 g
– sugars	18.6 g	12.4 g
Sodium	90 mg	60 mg
Calcium	300 mg (38%)*	200 mg

*Percentage of recommended dietary intake

Ingredients: Whole milk, concentrated skim milk sugar, strawberries (9%), gelatine, culture, thickener (1442).

The bakery

Fruit loaf	English-style muffins
Low GI bread	Pita bread
Wholegrain	
Sourdough	

The chilled foods section

Milk	Soy alternatives
Low fat	Low fat calcium-enriched soy milk
Skim	Soy yoghurt
Low fat flavoured	Dairy desserts
Margarine, canola	Fruche
Cheese	Custard
Reduced fat grated cheese	Fruit juice
Parmesan cheese	Apple juice
Reduced fat ricotta or cottage	Orange juice
cheese	Grapefruit juice
Reduced fat cheese slices	Cranberry juice
Yoghurt	Fresh noodles
Low fat plain/natural	Fresh pasta
Low-fat fruit or vanilla flavoured	Ravioli
Low fat drinking yoghurt	Tortellini
	Tofu
	Sushi
	Dips such as hommous

The freezer

Ice-cream	Beans
Reduced or low fat vanilla	Corn
or flavoured	Spinach
Frozen yoghurt	Mixed vegetables
Frozen fruit desserts or gelato	Stir-fry mix
Frozen vegetables	Broccoli
Peas	Cauliflower

Fresh fruit and vegetables

Basics

Sweet potato	Salad vegetables, depending on season
Taro	Lettuce (choose a variety)
Yam	Rocket
Sweetcorn	Tomato
Lemons or limes	Cucumber
Onions	Capsicum
Carrots	Spring onions
Garlic	Celery
Ginger	Bagged mixed salad greens
Chillies	Sprouts – mung bean, snowpea,

Leafy green and other seasonal
vegetables

	alfalfa etc.
Spinach or silverbeet	Avocado
Cabbage	Fresh herbs, depending on season
Broccoli	Parsley
Cauliflower	Basil
Asparagus	Mint
Asian greens such as bok choy	Chives
Leeks	Coriander
Fennel	Fresh fruit, depending on season
Snowpeas	Apples
Beans	Oranges
Zucchini or squash	Pears
Brussels sprouts	Grapes
Eggplant	Grapefruit
Mushrooms	Peaches
	Apricots
	Strawberries
	Mango

General groceries

Eggs

Beverages

  Tea

  Coffee

  Flavoured milk powders such as

  Milo

Herbs, spices, condiments and sauces

  Tube or jar of minced ginger,

  garlic, chilli

  Mustard

  Horseradish cream

  Tomato sauce

  Asian sauces

  Soy sauce

  Bottled pasta sauce

  Jar of curry paste

Deli items or pre-packed jars

  Sundried tomatoes

  Olives

Spreads

  Yellowbox honey

  Apricot jam

  Nutella

  Peanut butter

  Vegemite

Oils and vinegars

  Canola or olive oil cooking spray

  Olive oil

  Canola or vegetable oil

  Balsamic vinegar

  White wine vinegar

Breakfast cereals

  Traditional rolled oats

  Natural muesli

Low GI packaged breakfast cereal

Cereals and wholegrains

  Pasta

  Noodles, rice, buckwheat

  Rice – Basmati or Doongara

  Couscous

  Bulgur/cracked wheat

  Pearl barley

  Oat biscuits

Dried legumes

  Beans – keep a variety in the

  cupboard including cannellini,

  borlotti, lima, kidney, soy, pinto etc.

  Chickpeas

  Lentils

  Split peas

Canned foods

  Baked beans

  Mexi-beans

  Chickpeas

  Lentils

  Beans – keep a variety in the

  cupboard including cannellini,

  butter, borlotti, lima, kidney, soy,

  pinto etc

  Four bean mix

  Corn kernels

  Tomatoes, whole, crushed and

  tomato paste

  Tomato soup

  Tuna packed in spring water or oil

  Salmon packed in water

  Sardines

General groceries

Canned fruit and single serve tubs	Sultanas
Pears	Raisins
Peaches	Prunes
Mixed fruit salad	Apple rings
Dried fruit and nuts	Unsalted natural almonds, walnuts,
Apricots	cashews, etc.

Butcher/meat department

Lean ham	Lean minced beef
Lean beef for grills, barbecues and	Chicken
casseroles	Skinless chicken breast or drumsticks
Lean lamb fillets	Fish
Lean pork fillets	Any type of fresh fish

Making sense of food claims

Often the claims on the front of the package don't mean quite what you think. Here are some prime examples:

- Cholesterol free – be careful: the food may still be high in fat.
- Reduced fat – but is it low fat? Compare fat per 100 grams between products.
- Low in trans fat – but check the ingredient list for 'hydrogenated' or 'partially hydrogenated' oil. FDA regulations allow up to 0.5 grams of it to count as zero trans fat – the servings can add up.
- No added sugar – do you realize it could still raise your blood glucose?
- Lite or light – light in what? FDA regulations specify that these can mean that a nutritionally altered product contains one-third fewer calories or half the fat of the standard version—and if the food derives 50 per cent or more of its kilojoules from fat, the reduction must be 50 per cent of the fat. They could also mean simply light in color or texture – in which case qualifying information needs to be included, though exceptions are made for foods like light brown sugar that have a long history of use.

Making sense of nutritional labelling

To get the hard facts on the nutritional value of a food, look at the Nutrition Information table on the packaging. Here you'll find the details regarding the fat, calories/kilojoules, carbohydrate, fibre and sodium content of the food.

Reading the fine print – Remember, the GI alone doesn't identify a healthy food. If you like to keep some numbers in your head when you're shopping, then the following details are for you. Keep in mind that they are a general guide and shouldn't be used definitively to exclude or include foods in your diet.

Energy – This is a measure of how many kilojoules or calories we get from a food. For a healthy diet we need to eat more foods with a low energy density and combine them with smaller amounts of higher energy foods. To assess the energy density, look at the kJ per 100 grams. A low energy density is <500 kJ per 100 grams.

Fat – Seek low saturated fat content, ideally less than 20 per cent of the total fat. For example, if the total fat content is 10 grams, you want saturated fat less to be than 2 grams. Strictly speaking, a food can be labelled as low in saturated fat if it contains less than 1.5 grams saturated fat per 100 grams.

Total carbohydrate – This is the starch plus any naturally occurring and added sugars in the food. There's no need to look at the sugar figure separately since it's the total carbohydrate that affects your blood glucose level. You could use the total carbohydrate figure if you were monitoring your carbohydrate intake and to calculate the GL of the serving. The GL = grams of total carbohydrate × GI/100.

Fibre – Most of us don't eat enough fibre in our diet so seek out foods that are high in fibre. A high fibre food contains more than 3 grams of fibre per serving.

Sodium – This is a measure of the nasty part of salt in our food. Our bodies need some salt but most people consume far more than they need. Canned foods in particular tend to be high in sodium. Check the sodium content per 100 grams next time you buy – a low salt food contains less than 120 milligrams of sodium per 100 grams. Many packaged foods and convenience meals are well above this. Aim for less than 450 milligrams per 100 grams with convenience and ready-to-eat foods.

Can I believe what it says?

Consumers are increasingly interested in what is in the food they eat. That's where Food Standards Australia New Zealand (FSANZ) comes in. They are an independent organisation responsible for developing standards for food labelling to help us make informed choices about the food we buy and eat. Their principal role is to protect the health and safety of people in Australia and New Zealand through the maintenance of a safe food supply. For more information visit www.foodstandards.gov.au.

Chapter 18

The GI symbol

Look for the low GI symbol at the supermarket. It's an easy way to identify nutritious foods that have been GI tested. The GI symbol certification on a food label means that the food has been properly tested (according to the standardised method) and you can trust the GI value that's posted near the nutrition information panel. Unfortunately, some manufacturers make unverified and even false low GI claims.

Importantly, foods that carry the GI certification mark have been scientifically tested not just for their GI, but against a range of strict nutrient criteria. So you can be sure that the food is a healthier choice within its food group, no matter what the GI.

The GI symbol is your guarantee that the GI value stated near the nutrition information label is accurate, helping you select smart low GI carbohydrate foods with confidence to lower the overall GI of your diet.

www.glysymbol.com

The GI Symbol Program is run by the Glycemic Index Foundation, a not-for-profit organisation established by the University of Sydney, the Juvenile Diabetes Research Foundation and Diabetes Australia.

Things you should know about the GI symbol

- Foods that carry the certification mark are healthy in many respects. To be eligible, foods must meet other strict nutrient criteria relating to carbohydrate, total fat, salt, kilojoules and be a good source of fibre.
- Manufacturers pay a licence fee to use the certification mark on their products. The fee is paid to GI Limited, a non-profit partnership between the University of Sydney, Diabetes Australia and the Juvenile Diabetes Research Foundation. The fee helps to fund sensible, balanced communication about the GI, healthy eating and research.
- High GI foods can carry the symbol. Remember, you don't need to eat low GI all the time – an informed person can mix and match as he or she sees fit.
- If you have type 1 diabetes, you may need to consider the quantity of carbohydrate in each serving of food, in addition to the GI. Calculating the GL (grams of carbohydrate × GI/100) is one way of estimating the total glycemic effect.
- Beware of 'low glycemic' claims. 'Low glycemic' is a fuzzy term that can mean 'low carb', not 'slow carb'. Only slow carbs deliver the 'feel full' feeling and a host of other health benefits.
- A food may be reliably tested and not carry the certification mark. It's the manufacturer's choice, but as a consumer you may find it hard to distinguish between reliable and unreliable claims. Look for the GI symbol as your trusted signpost to healthier food choices.
- For more information about the certification mark, go to www.gisymbol. com.au
- To search a reliable GI database, go to www.glycemicindex.com

Subscribe to

GI News

for all the latest

ginews.blogspot.com

GI News is the free, monthly online newsletter from the University of Sydney's Human Nutrition Unit with almost 100 000 subscribers worldwide. It's easy to search for topics of interest and you can post your comments and queries on the site.

Each issues includes:

- The latest research on the glycemic index, carbohydrates, and diet and diabetes along with other hot nutrition topics

- GI Update from Prof Jennie Brand-Miller

- GI Symbol News from Dr Alan Barclay

- The latest GI values from SUGiRS in Australia and GI Labs in Canada

- Recipes from the GI News Kitchen, created by dietitian Johanna Burana, *Money Saving Meals* author Diane Temple, and from guest chefs and food writers including Damien Pignolet and Lyndey Milan

- The scoop on nutrition from dietitian Emma Stirling

- Busting food myths with dietitian and author Nicole Senior

Chapter 19

The GI values

These tables will help you put low GI food choices into your shopping trolley and on your plate.

Here we give you the best low GI food choices for each category. Each entry lists an individual food and its GI value. We also list the nominal serve size, the amount of carbohydrate, the carbohydrate exchange per serve, and the GL.

> **A low GI value is 55 and under**
> **A medium/moderate GI value is 56 to 69 inclusive**
> **A high GI value is 70 or more**

You can use the tables to:

❑ Find the GI of your favourite foods
❑ Compare carb-rich foods within a category (two types of bread or breakfast cereal for example)
❑ Identify the best carbohydrate choices
❑ Improve your diet by finding a low GI substitute for high GI foods
❑ Put together a low GI meal
❑ Find foods with a high GI but low GL.

Each individual food appears alphabetically within a food category, like 'Bread' or 'Fruit'. This makes it easy to compare the kinds of foods you eat every day and helps you see which high GI foods you could substitute with low GI versions. If you are unsure of the food category a food might fall under, we've also provided an index to individual foods that starts on page 385.

In this edition's tables, we have included the carbohydrate exchange value for each food. This value is most commonly used by people with diabetes in estimating their carbohydrate intake and is based on the amount of carbohydrate found in 1 slice of bread; 15 grams. Servings of food which contact 15 grams of carbohydrate can be 'exchanged' (or swapped) for 1 slice of bread, maintaining consistency in the amount of carbohydrate eaten. 1 carbohydrate exchange is an amount of food that contains 15 grams of carbohydrate.

We've also included a wider range of carbohydrate foods, even though their GI has not been measured. This is to make it clearer which foods have been tested and which haven't. These foods have been grouped under the Higher GI category. Unfortunately, we can't even make an assumption about the GI value of such foods unless they are very closely related to a food which has been tested. Only more testing will show us the GI value of more foods, so if you want to know the GI value of something you eat and you can't find it here, then contact the manufacturer and suggest they have their food tested.

Symbols in the tables

★ indicates that a food contains very little or no carbohydrate which means that the GI isn't relevant (or can't be tested). You will find this symbol beside foods like cheese, fish, chicken, meat and green leafy vegetables. We have included these foods because so many people ask us for their GI.

■ indicates that a food is high in saturated fat.

● indicates that a food does contain carbohydrate but has either not been GI tested or the results of the testing have not been published. To help you manage your blood glucose levels and reduce the overall GI of your diet you will find this symbol in these tables besides products like biscuits and cereals – carb-rich foods that we regularly buy. Although it's not possible to work out an accurate GI value for a product based on its ingredients, it is possible to make an educated guess as to whether it will be high or low GI, based on similar products that have been tested.

⊚ indicates that a food is part of the GI Symbol Program. Foods with the GI symbol have had their GI tested properly and are a healthy choice for their food category.

All foods have been tested using an internationally standardised method so you can make a fair comparison. Gram for gram of carbohydrates, the higher the GI, the higher the blood glucose levels after consumption. If you can't find the GI value for a food you regularly eat in these tables, check out our website (www. glycemicindex.com). We maintain an international database of published GI values that have been tested by a reliable laboratory. Alternatively, please write to the manufacturer and encourage them to have the food tested by an accredited laboratory such as the Sydney University Glycemic Index Research Service (SUGiRS). In the meantime, choose a similar food from the tables as a substitute.

Category Contents

Key to the tables

GISP: Identifies whether or not the food is part of the GI Symbol Program.

Food: Name of the food, grouped according to brand or type.

GI: GI value for the food or the range of values measured for the food or the varieties of food listed.

Serve: A nominal serving size of the food, based on common household measures of 250 ml cup, 20 ml tablespoon and 5 g teaspoon or popular, easily measured portions.

Carbohydrate: The carbohydrate content of the nominal serving, specified in grams.

Exchange: The carbohydrate exchange equivalent of the nominal serving, based on 15 g carbohydrate per exchange.

GL: The glycemic load for the nominal serving of the food – refer to p. 143 for explanation of the GL.

GISP	FOOD	GI	HOUSEHOLD MEASURE & WEIGHT	CARB (G) PER SERVE	CARB EXCHANGE PER SERVE	GL PER SERVE
	SWEET BISCUITS – LOW GI (LESS THAN OR EQUAL TO 55)					
	Arnott's					
	Snack Right Fruit Pillow, apple & blackberry, apple & sultana, wild berry	43–52	2 biscuits, 33g	24	1.5	12
	Snack Right Fruit Slice, mixed berry, sultana, apricot	48–52	2 biscuits, 20g	22	1.5	11
	Snack Right Fruit Slice, sultana choc	45	2 biscuits, 25g	17	1	8
	Generic					
	Chocolate chip cookies	43 ■	2 biscuits, 20g	16	1	7
	Coconut macaroons	32	2 biscuits, 20g	1	1	4
	100 Healthy Calories Fruit Cookies, Freedom Foods	47	2 biscuits, 25g	19	1	9
	Maltmeal Wafer, Griffins NZ	50	2 biscuits, 25g	17	1	9
	Oatmeal, Highland	55	2 biscuits, 20g	14	1	8
	Oatmeal	54	2 biscuits, 20g	14	1	8
	Rich tea	55	2 biscuits, 20g	13	1	7
	SWEET BISCUITS – HIGHER GI (MORE THAN 55 OR UNKNOWN) **(LESS THAN 10% TOTAL FAT, LESS THAN 1.5g SAT FAT/SERVE)**					
	Arnott's					
	Choc Ripple	•	2 biscuits, 18g	13	1	•
	Chocolate, Royals, dark chocolate	•	1 biscuit, 17g	11	1	•
	Chocolate, Royals, milk chocolate	•	1 biscuit, 17g	11	1	•
	Chocolate, Teddy Bear	•	1 biscuit, 17g	11	1	•
	Chocolate, Tee Vee Snacks	•	4 biscuits, 20g	13	1	•
	Full o' Fruit	•	2 biscuits, 20g	15	1	•
	Ginger Nut	•	1 biscuit, 13g	11	1	•
	Honey Jumbles	•	2 biscuits, 20g	16	1	•
	Hundreds & Thousands	•	2 biscuits, 17g	13	1	•
	Malt-O-Milk	•	3 biscuits, 21g	16	1	•
	Marie	•	2 biscuits, 16g	12	1	•
	Milk Arrowroot	69	2 biscuits, 16g	12	1	8
	Milk Coffee	•	2 biscuits, 17g	13	1	•
	Morning Coffee	79	3 biscuits, 17g	12	1	9
	Scalliwag	•	2 biscuits, 20g	15	1	•

★ little or no carbs ■ high in saturated fat ● untested/unknown Ⓖ GI Symbol partner

GISP	FOOD	GI	HOUSEHOLD MEASURE & WEIGHT	CARB (G) PER SERVE	CARB EXCHANGE PER SERVE	GL PER SERVE
	Shredded Wheatmeal	62	3 biscuits, 23g	15	1	9
	Spicy Fruit Roll	•	1 biscuit, 17g	12	1	•
	Teddy Bear	•	2 biscuits, 21g	15	1	•
	Tic Toc	•	2 biscuits, 18g	13	1	•
	Paradise					
	Vive Lites, caramel pecan	•	2 biscuits, 21g	16	1	•
	Vive Lites, choc chip mini cookies	•	1 mini pack, 30g	24	1	•
	Vive Wellbeing, date & ginger	•	2 biscuits, 18g	13	1	•
	Weight Watchers					
	Butternut	•	2 biscuits, 18g	14	1	•
	Fruit Slice	•	2 cookies, 23g	17	1	•
	Triple Choc	•	2 biscuits, 18g	11	1	•
	Generic					
	Golden Fruit, Griffins NZ	77	2 biscuits, 25g	17	1	13
	Shortbread, plain	64 ■	2 biscuits, 25g	16	1	10
	Vanilla wafer, cream-filled	77 ■	3 biscuits, 25g	18	1	14
	**SAVOURY BISCUITS — LOW GI (LESS THAN OR EQUAL TO 55)**					
	Arnott's					
	Jatz	55 ■	6 crackers, 25g	13	1	7
	Shapes, barbecue	48	10 crackers, 23g	15	1	7
	Ryvita varieties					
Ⓖ	Pumpkin Seeds & Oats crispbread	46	2 slices, 25g	14	1	6
Ⓖ	Sunflower Seeds & Oats crispbread	48	2 slices, 25g	14	1	7
	**SAVOURY BISCUITS — HIGHER GI (MORE THAN 55 OR UNKNOWN)**					
	Arnott's					
	Breton	67 ■	6 crackers, 26g	15	1	10
	Cruskits varieties					
	Corn	•	4 crackers, 19g	14	1	•
	Light	•	4 crackers, 23g	17	1	•
	Rye	•	4 crackers, 19g	12	1	•
	Jatz 97% fat free	•	5 crackers, 19g	15	1	•
	Salada varieties					
	Light original	•	1 cracker, 14g	11	1	•

★ little or no carbs ■ high in saturated fat ● untested/unknown Ⓖ GI Symbol partner

GISP	FOOD	GI	HOUSEHOLD MEASURE & WEIGHT	CARB (G) PER SERVE	CARB EXCHANGE PER SERVE	GL PER SERVE
	Light poppy & sesame	•	1 cracker, 14g	11	1	•
	Multigrain 97% fat free	•	1 cracker, 14g	11	1	•
	Original	•	1 cracker, 14g	10	1.5	•
	Wholemeal	•	1 cracker, 14g	9	1.5	•
	Generic					
	Sao	70 ■	3 crackers, 26g	16	1	11
	Thin Captain	•	3 crackers, 17g	12	1	•
	Vita-Weat varieties					
	9-Grain	•	2 sandwich, 23g	15	1	•
	9-Grain	•	4 regular, 25g	14	1	•
	Cracked Pepper	•	4 regular, 23g	16	1	•
	Grain Snacks, all varieties	•	1 packet, 20g	13	1	•
	Grain Sticks	•	1 packet, 20g	13	1	•
	Original	•	4 regular, 25g	16	1	•
	Sesame	•	4 regular, 23g	13	1	•
	Soy & Linseed	•	4 regular, 23g	13	1	•
	Water cracker	78	6 crackers, 18g	14	1	11
	Paradise					
	Vive Lites Wholemeal crispbread	•	4 biscuits, 28g	20	1.5	•
	Vive Wellbeing 7 Grains crispbread	•	4 biscuits, 32g	20	1.5	•
	Generic					
	Corn Thins, puffed corn, Real Foods	87	4 slices, 23g	16	1	14
	Norwegian crispbread, Kavli	71	4 thin, 20g	13	1	9
	Rice cake, puffed	82	2 slices, 20g	15	1	12
	Rice cracker	91	12 crackers, 20g	16	1	15

★ little or no carbs   ■ high in saturated fat   ● untested/unknown   Ⓖ GI Symbol partner

GISP	FOOD	GI	HOUSEHOLD MEASURE & WEIGHT	CARB (G) PER SERVE	CARB EXCHANGE PER SERVE	GL PER SERVE
	BREAD & BAKERY PRODUCTS – LOW GI (LESS THAN OR EQUAL TO 55)					
	Bakers Delight					
	Cape Seed					
	loaf	48	1 toast slice, 45g	13	1	6
	roll	48	89g	27	2	13
	Cape Fruit & Nut roll	55	89g	33	2	18
	Hi-Fibre Lo-GI, white					
	block loaf	52	1 toast slice, 40g	17	1	9
	dinner roll	52	30g	15	2	8
	roll	52	65g	30	1	16
	Wholemeal Country Grain					
	block loaf	53	1 toast slice, 40g	15	1	8
	dinner roll	53	34g	13	1	7
	long roll	53	65g	27	2	14
	round roll	53	65g	27	2	14
	Bill's Bakery					
	Sourdough Multigrain	•	1 slice, 35g	15	1	•
	Bürgen varieties					
ⓖ	Fruit & Muesli	53	1 slice, 42g	19	1	10
ⓖ	Grains with Barley	50	1 slice, 49g	13	1	7
ⓖ	Pumpkin Seeds	51	1 slice, 42g	11	1	6
ⓖ	Rye	53	1 slice, 42g	14	1	7
ⓖ	Soy & Linseed	52	1 slice, 42g	13	1	7
ⓖ	Wholemeal with Seeds	39	1 slice, 42g	9	0.5	4
	Buttercup					
	Fruit & Spice loaf	54	1 thick slice, 30g	15	1	8
	Country Life varieties					
	Country Grain & Organic Rye	53	1 slice, 32g	10	0.5	5
	Low GI Gluten free, white	53	1 slice, 32g	19	1	10
	Golden Hearth (Gold Coast Bakeries)					
	Heavy Wholegrain Organic	53	1 large slice, 50g	21	1.5	11
	Tip-Top varieties					
ⓖ	9-Grain Original	53	1 slice, 37g	13	1	7

★ little or no carbs   ■ high in saturated fat   ● untested/unknown   ⓖ GI Symbol partner

GISP	FOOD	GI	HOUSEHOLD MEASURE & WEIGHT	CARB (G) PER SERVE	CARB EXCHANGE PER SERVE	GL PER SERVE
☺	9-Grain Pumpkin Seed	52	1 slice, 37g	13	1	7
☺	9-Grain Wholemeal	53	1 slice, 38g	12	1	6
	Spicy Fruit loaf	54	1 slice, 36g	19	1.5	10
	Woolworth's Select					
	Traditional white corn tortilla	53	1 regular, 56g	27	2	14
	Reduced carb tortilla	51	1 regular, 43g	16	1	8
	Diego's					
☺	White corn tortillas	53	1 regular, 56g	27	2	14
☺	Reduced carb wraps	51	1 regular, 43g	11	1	6
	Specialty Breads					
	Continental fruit loaf	47	1 thick slice, 45g	24	1.5	11
	Pumpernickel	50	1 slice, 47g	21	1.5	11
	Sourdough, wheat	54	1 large slice, 64g	33	2	18
	Sourdough, rye	48	1 large slice, 64g	28	2	13
	Spelt multigrain	54	1 slice, 34g	15	1	8

BREAD & BAKERY PRODUCTS – HIGHER GI (MORE THAN 55 OR UNKNOWN)

	Bakers Delight					
	Apricot Delight					
	log	56	1 slice, 43g	24	1.5	13
	roll	56	80g	48	3	27
	scroll	56	105g	60	4	34
	Authentic sourdough					
	loaf	58	1 toast slice, 33g	16	1	9
	roll	58	115g	59	4	34
	Block loaf, wholemeal	71	1 toast slice, 38g	14	1	10
	Chia, white	63	1 toast slice, 40g	17	1	11
	Tiger loaf, white	71	1 toast slice, 37g	17	1	12
	Toasty Fruit loaf	61	1 toast slice, 37g	25	1.5	15
	Bürgen					
	Oatbran & Honey	63	1 slice, 42g	12	1.5	8
	Buttercup					
	Wonder White Lower GI	59	1 slice, 35g	13	1	8

★ little or no carbs   ■ high in saturated fat   ● untested/unknown   ☺ GI Symbol partner

GISP	FOOD	GI	HOUSEHOLD MEASURE & WEIGHT	CARB (G) PER SERVE	CARB EXCHANGE PER SERVE	GL PER SERVE
	Country Life					
	Gluten free, multigrain	79	1 slice, 30g	13	1	10
	Naturis					
	Gluten free, buckwheat	72	1 slice, 48g	17	1	12
	Tip-Top					
	EnerGI, white sandwich	58	1 slice, 37g	17	1	10
	Raisin toast, Retreats	63	1 slice, 33g	19	1	12
	Sunblest, white	71	1 slice, 30g	14	1	10
	Sunblest, wholemeal	71	1 slice, 30g	12	1	9
	Specialty Breads & Baked Foods					
	Bagel	72	1 large, 85g	43	3	31
	Baguette, traditional French	77	¼ loaf, 62g	33	2	25
	Breadcrumbs, white		¼ loaf, 30g	20	1.5	●
		●	100g	66	4.5	●
	Chapatti	59	1 small, 35g	14	1	8
		●	100g	39	2.5	●
	Croissant	67	1 large, 70g	24	1.5	16
	Crumpet, white	69	100g	42	3	29
	mini-finger	69	30g	13	1	9
	round	69	50g	16	1	11
	square	69	70g	23	1.5	16
	Doughnut, commercial, cinnamon	75	1 regular, 50g	25	1.5	30
	English muffin	77	1 regular, 64g	23	1.5	18
	Foccacia	●	1 piece, 50g	21	1.5	●
	Fruit	●	1 slice, 31g	16	1	●
	Fruit bun, iced	●	1 regular, 85g	39	2.5	●
	Gluten free, commercial	●	1 medium slice, 30g	16	1	●
	Hamburger bun	61	1 regular, 90g	45	3	27
	Hotdog bun, white	68	1 regular, 62g	33	2	22
	Hot cross bun, fruit	●	1 regular, 85g	49	3	●
	Hot cross bun, choc chip	●	1 regular, 65g	41	2.5	●
	Italian bread	73	1 slice, 40g	18	1	13
	Italian breadsticks, grissini	●	3 sticks, 25g	18	1	●
	Lavash, white	●	1 piece, 67g	36	2.5	●
	Lavash, wholemeal	●	1 piece, 67g	33	2	●
	Kaiser roll, white	73	1 regular, 108g	60	4	44

★ little or no carbs   ■ high in saturated fat   ● untested/unknown   ⓒ GI Symbol partner

GISP	FOOD	GI	HOUSEHOLD MEASURE & WEIGHT	CARB (G) PER SERVE	CARB EXCHANGE PER SERVE	GL PER SERVE
	Lebanese bread, wholemeal	•	1 large, 100g	48	3	•
	Lebanese bread, white, Seda Bakery	75	1 large, 100g	53	3.5	40
	Matzo, Jewish bread	•	1 piece, 30g	24	1.5	•
	Melba toast, plain	70	30g	23	1.5	16
	Multigrain	65	1 slice, 34g	15	1	10
	Naan	•	1 piece, 15cm diam.	46	3.5	•
	Wrap, Mountain	•	1 piece 25g	14	1	•
	Pancakes, buckwheat, gluten free, packet mix, Orgran	102	1/10 pkt, 37.5g	29	2	30
	Pancakes, gluten-free, packet mix, Freedom Foods	61	1 serve, 80g	53	3.5	32
	Pancakes, homemade	•	1 regular, 56g	16	1	•
	Pancakes, shaker mix, Green's	67	1 regular, 50g	23	1.5	15
	Pappadum, microwaved	•	4 regular, 24g	11	1	•
	Pikelets, homemade	•	4 regular, 100g	48	3	•
	Pikelets, commercial, Golden	85	1 regular, 25g	9	0.5	8
	Pikelets, shake mix	•	1 regular, 35g	16	1	•
	Pita bread, white	57	1 regular, 60g	33	2	19
	Roll, white	71	1 regular, 65g	34	2	24
	Roll, white, dinner	71	1 small, 30g	16	1	11
	Roll, wholemeal	70	1 regular, 65g	26	2	18
	Roll, cheese & bacon	•	1 regular, 75g	27	2	•
	Rye bread, light	68	1 slice, 30g	14	1	10
	Rye bread, dark	76	1 slice, 30g	13	1	10
	Rye bread, wholemeal	58	1 slice, 30g	13	1	8
	Scone, plain, homemade	•	1 regular, 40g	16	1	•
	Scone, plain, packet mix, Defiance	92	1 regular, 40g	16	1	15
	Scone, fruit	•	1 regular, 40g	22	1.5	•
	Sliced bread, white	71	1 slice, 32g	14	1	10
	Sliced bread, wholemeal	71	1 slice, 32g	12	1	9
	Stuffing, bread	74	100g	22	1.5	16
	Taco shell, corn	68	1 large, 20g	11	1	7
	Turkish pide	87	1 small roll, 85g	40	2.5	35
	Waffles, plain	76	1 regular, 33g	19	1	14

★ little or no carbs ■ high in saturated fat ● untested/unknown Ⓖ GI Symbol partner

GISP	FOOD	GI	HOUSEHOLD MEASURE & WEIGHT	CARB (G) PER SERVE	CARB EXCHANGE PER SERVE	GL PER SERVE
	BREAKFAST CEREALS – LOW GI (LESS THAN OR EQUAL TO 55)					
	Generic					
	Oat Bran, raw, unprocessed	55	⅓ cup, 30g	15	1	8
	Natural muesli	40	½ cup, 45g	27	2	11
	Porridge, steel-cut oats with water	52	¾ cup, 170g	17	1	9
	Rice Bran, extruded	19	⅓ cup, 30g	14	1	3
	Semolina, cooked	55	1 cup, 245g	17	1	9
	Kellogg's					
	All-Bran	44	¾ cup, 45g	20	1.5	9
	Frosties	55	¾ cup, 30g	27	2	15
	Guardian	37	⅔ cup, 30g	19	1	7
	Komplete	48	½ cup, 45g	31	2	15
	Sustain	55	¾ cup, 45g	33	2	18
	Freedom Foods					
	Gluten-free muesli	39	40g	13	1	5
	Hi-Lite	54	100g	68	4.5	37
	Quick Oats porridge	●	100g	62	4	●
	Yeast-free muesli	44	40g	13	1	6
	Goodness Superfoods					
	Digestive 1st	39	45g	21	1.5	8
	Heart 1st	46	45g	20	1.5	9
	Protein 1st	36	45g	17	1	6
	Monster Muesli					
	Multi-Grain porridge	55	60g	35	2.5	19
	Morning Sun					
◉	Apricot & Almond muesli	49	⅔ cup, 60g	34	2	17
◉	Peach & Pecan muesli	49	⅔ cup, 60g	38	2.5	19
	Vogel's					
	Grain Clusters, classic	54	45g	29	2	15
	Muesli Cluster Spice	51	45g	27	2	14
	Muesli Fruit & Nut	48	45g	24	1.5	12
	Ultra-Bran	45	45g	22	1.5	10

★ little or no carbs   ■ high in saturated fat   ● untested/unknown   ◉ GI Symbol partner

GISP	FOOD	GI	HOUSEHOLD MEASURE & WEIGHT	CARB (G) PER SERVE	CARB EXCHANGE PER SERVE	GL PER SERVE
	Woolworth's Select					
	Natural Swiss Bircher muesli	52	½ cup, 50g	30	2	16
	Naytura Fruit & Nut muesli	48	30g	14	1	7
	BREAKFAST CEREALS – HIGHER GI (MORE THAN 55 OR UNKNOWN)					
	Generic					
	Buckwheat, puffed	65	14g	12	1	8
	Porridge, regular, oats with water	58	1 cup, 260g	21	1.5	12
	Rice porridge	88	100g	9	0.5	8
	Shredded wheat	75	1 biscuit, 24g	16	1	12
	Traditional rolled oats	57	30g	18	1	10
	Wheat flake	69	1 biscuit, 15g	10	0.5	7
	Lowan					
	Fusion muesli, all varieties	•	45g	26–28	2	•
	Grizzlies	•	35g	26	2	•
	Honey O's	•	35g	29	2	•
	Muesli, all varieties	•	45g	26–28	2	•
	Quick Oats	•	30g	18	1	•
	Rice Flakes	•	55g	41	2.5	•
	Rice Porridge	•	50g	34	2	•
	Rolled Oats	59	½ cup, 50g	31	2	18
	Kellogg's					
	All-Bran varieties					
	Dual	•	¾ cup, 40g	26	2	•
	Tropical	•	½ cup, 45g	25	1.5	•
	Wheat Flakes	•	⅔ cup, 30g	21	1.5	•
	Wheat Flakes, honey almond	•	½ cup, 40g	24	1.5	•
	Corn Flakes	77	30g	25	1.5	19
	Crispix	87	1 cup, 30g	26	2	23
	Crunchy Nut varieties					
	Corn Flakes	72	⅔ cup, 30g	25		18
	Clusters	•	⅔ cup, 30g	23	1.5	•
	Nutty	•	⅔ cup, 30g	22	1.5	•
	Froot Loops	69	¾ cup, 30g	26	2	18

★ little or no carbs   ■ high in saturated fat   ● untested/unknown   Ⓖ GI Symbol partner

GISP	FOOD	GI	HOUSEHOLD MEASURE & WEIGHT	CARB (G) PER SERVE	CARB EXCHANGE PER SERVE	GL PER SERVE
	Just Right varieties					
	Antioxidant	•	¾ cup, 45g	33	2	•
	Original	60	¾ cup, 45g	32	2	19
	Tropical	•	¾ cup, 45g	33	2	•
	Mini-Wheats varieties					
	Blackcurrant	72	⅔ cup, 40g	28	2	20
	5 Grains, no fruit filling	58	¾ cup, 40g	27	2	16
	Nutri-Grain	66	1 cup, 30g	21	1.5	14
	Rice Bubbles	87	1 cup, 30g	26	2	23
	Special K varieties					
	Advantage	•	1 cup, 40g	26	2	•
	Chocolatey Flakes	•	⅔ cup, 35g	24	1.5	•
	Forest Berries	•	¾ cup, 30g	21	1.5	•
	Honey Almond	•	⅔ cup, 30g	22	1.5	•
	Original	56	¾ cup, 30g	21	1.5	12
	Sultana Bran varieties					
	Crunch	•	⅔ cup, 45g	32	2	•
	Original	64	¾ cup, 45g	29	2	18
Sanitarium						
	Fibre Life varieties					
	Bran Flakes	•	35g	23	•	•
	Bran & Oats with Berry	•	45g	29	•	•
	Granola Clusters, all varieties	•	50g	35	2.5	•
	Honey Weets	•	30g	24	•	•
	Light 'n' Tasty, all varieties	68	40g	27–29	2	19
	Muesli, all varieties	•	50g	29–34	2	•
	Puffed Wheat	80	30g	21	•	17
	Skippy corn flakes	93	30g	24	•	22
	Weet-Bix varieties					
	Bites, all varieties	•	45g	30–34	2	•
	Hi-Bran	61	2 biscuits, 40g	22	1.5	13
	Kids	•	1 biscuit, 15g	10	0.5	•
	Lite	•	1 biscuit, 30g	20	1.5	•

★ little or no carbs   ■ high in saturated fat   ● untested/unknown   Ⓖ GI Symbol partner

GISP	FOOD	GI	HOUSEHOLD MEASURE & WEIGHT	CARB (G) PER SERVE	CARB EXCHANGE PER SERVE	GL PER SERVE
	Multigrain	•	1 biscuit, 24g	17	1	•
	Organic	•	2 biscuits, 30g	20	1.5	•
	Original	69	2 biscuits, 33g	22	1.5	15
	Uncle Tobys					
	Bran Plus	•	45g	12	1	•
	Cheerios	•	30g	22	1.5	•
	Healthwise varieties					
	Digestive Wellbeing	66	45g	31	2	20
	Heart Wellbeing	•	45g	29	2	•
	Muesli, Original Swiss Style	62	30g	18	1	11
	Plus varieties					
	Fibre Lift	•	45g	29	2	•
	Protein Lift	•	45g	33	•	•
	Sports Lift	•	45g	32	•	•
	Quick Oats	82	30g	17	1	14
	Oatbrits	•	42g	26	2	•
	Vita Brits varieties					
	Original	68	33g	23	1.5	16
	Weeties	•	30g	20	1.5	•

★ little or no carbs   ■ high in saturated fat   ● untested/unknown   Ⓖ GI Symbol partner

GISP	FOOD	GI	HOUSEHOLD MEASURE & WEIGHT	CARB (G) PER SERVE	CARB EXCHANGE PER SERVE	GL PER SERVE
			DAIRY PRODUCTS			
	Milk					
	Regular, whole, 4% fat	27–31	1 cup, 250ml	12	1	4
	Dairy Farmers	31	250ml	12	1	4
	Fat-reduced, 1–2% fat	20–30	1 cup, 250ml	15	1	4
	Farmer's Best with Omega-3, Dairy Farmers	27	250ml	19	1	5
	HiLo, Pura	20	250ml	14	1	3
	Lite Start, Pura	30	250ml	15	1	5
⊙	Lite White, Dairy Farmers	30	250ml	14	1	4
	Skim, <1% fat	20–34	1 cup, 250ml	12	1	3
⊙	Dairy Farmers	32	250ml	12	1	4
	Shape, calcium-enriched	34	250ml	17	1	6
	Skimmer, Pura	20	250ml	14	1	3
	Tone, Pura	30	250ml	16	1	5
	Buttermilk	•	½ cup, 125ml	6	<0.5	•
	Other milk products					
	Cheese	★	40g	0	•	•
	Condensed milk, canned, whole	61	½ cup, 125ml	69	4.5	42
	Condensed milk, canned, skim	•	½ cup, 125ml	75	5	•
	Evaporated milk, canned, whole	•	½ cup, 125ml	13	1	•
	Evaporated milk, canned, reduced fat or skim	•	½ cup, 125ml	14	1	•
	Powdered milk, whole, dry powder	•	4 tbsp, 30g	11	11	•
	Powdered milk, skim, dry powder	•	2 tbsp, heaped, 25g	13	1	•
	Fermented milk drink, Yakult	46	1 bottle, 65ml	12	1	6
	Fermented milk drink, Yakult Light	36	1 bottle, 65ml	9	0.5	3
	Flavoured milk					
	Big M, chocolate or strawberry	37	1 carton, 600ml	56–60	4	22
	Commercial, full-fat milk	34	300ml	28	2	•
	Commercial, low-fat, artificially sweetened	24	300ml	18	1	4

★ little or no carbs   ■ high in saturated fat   ● untested/unknown   ⊙ GI Symbol partner

GISP	FOOD	GI	HOUSEHOLD MEASURE & WEIGHT	CARB (G) PER SERVE	CARB EXCHANGE PER SERVE	GL PER SERVE
	Commercial, low-fat, sugar sweetened	34	300ml	22	1.5	7
	Malted milk powder, Nestle, 20 g in full-fat milk	45	200ml	24	1.5	11
	Malt Milo powder, Nestle, 20 g in full-fat milk	37	¾ cup, 200ml	24	1.5	9
☺	20g in reduced-fat milk	40	200ml	25	1.5	10
☺	20 g in skim milk	46	200ml	24	1.5	11
	Masters varieties					
	Mocha milk	32	1 carton, 600ml	62	4	20
	Light, 99% fat free, chocolate or mocha flavour	27	1 carton, 600ml	49–55	3.5	14
	Reduced-fat, chocolate or strawberry flavour	35	1 carton, 600ml	49–59	4.5	19
	Milo powder, Nestle					
	20 g in full-fat milk	33	¾ cup, 200ml	24	1.5	8
☺	20 g in reduced-fat milk	36	200ml	24	1.5	9
☺	20 g in skim milk	39	200ml	24	1.5	9
	Nesquik powder, 12g in reduced-fat milk					
	chocolate flavour	41	¾ cup, 200ml	21	1.5	9
	strawberry flavour	35	¾ cup, 200ml	22	1.5	8
	Rush, low-fat, heavenly vanilla malt, ultimate chocolate, wicked latte flavours, Paul's	26–31	1 bottle, 500ml	27–30	2	9
	Smoothie varieties					
	banana	30	1 cup, 250ml	26	2	8
	fruit	35	1 cup, 250ml	30	2	11
	mango	32	1 cup, 250ml	27	2	9
	Sustagen varieties					
	Dutch Chocolate	31	1 carton, 250ml	41	3	13
	sport drink	43	2 scoops in water, 40g	26	2	11
	Up & Go, drink, Sanitarium	43–46	350ml	39	2.5	18
	Milk alternatives					
	Oat milk, Vitasoy	69	1 cup, 250ml	23	1.5	16

★ little or no carbs ■ high in saturated fat ● untested/unknown ☺ GI Symbol partner

GISP	FOOD	GI	HOUSEHOLD MEASURE & WEIGHT	CARB (G) PER SERVE	CARB EXCHANGE PER SERVE	GL PER SERVE
	Rice milk					
	Australia's Own, low-fat	92	1 cup, 250ml	34	2	31
	Vitasoy	79	1 cup, 250ml	24	1.5	19 ·
	Soy milk					
	So Natural Calciforte, calcium-enriched	40	1 cup, 250ml	8	0.5	3
	So Natural, Original	44	1 cup, 250ml	12	1	5
	Soy milk, low fat	•	1 cup, 250ml	15	1	•
	So Natural Light, calcium-enriched	44	1 cup, 250ml	8	0.5	4
	Vitasoy, Calci Plus	24	1 cup, 250ml	15	1	4
	Vitasoy, high fibre, 98.5% fat-free	16	1 cup, 250ml	14	1	2
	Yoghurt					
☉	Brownes Diet No Fat, various flavours	24–40	1 tub, 200g	15	1	4–6
	Jalna varieties					
	Bio Dynamic, bush honey flavour	26	½ cup, 125g	16	1	4
	Fat Free, natural	19	½ cup, 125g	9	0.5	2
	Greek style	12	½ cup, 125g	8	0.5	1
	Leben European style	11	½ cup, 125g	9	0.5	1
	Premium Blend, creamy vanilla	18	1 tub, 200g	30	2	5
☉	Nestle Diet, various flavours	19–21	1 tub, 175g	11	1	2
	Vaalia, low-fat varieties					
	apricot, mango & peach flavour	26	1 tub, 150g	22	1.5	6
	French vanilla	26	1 tub, 175g	29	2	8
	lemon crème	43	1 tub, 150g	27	2	12
	luscious berries	28	¾ cup, 200g	31	2	9
	passionfruit	32	1 tub, 175g	29	2	9
	tempting strawberry	28	1 tub,175g	28	2	8
	Yoplait varieties					
	Lite, all flavours	25–37	1 tub, 175g	23–29	1.5–2	8
	Forme, various flavours	16–20	1 tub, 175g	11	1	2
	Generic Yoghurt					
	Natural, plain, unflavoured, low fat	14	½ cup, 125g	8	0.5	1
	Flavoured	41	1 tub, 200g	24	1.5	10

★ little or no carbs   ■ high in saturated fat   ● untested/unknown   ☉ GI Symbol partner

GISP	FOOD	GI	HOUSEHOLD MEASURE & WEIGHT	CARB (G) PER SERVE	CARB EXCHANGE PER SERVE	GL PER SERVE
	Flavoured, low fat, artificially sweetened	20	½ cup, 125g	7	1	1
	Custard					
	Homemade, from custard powder, with milk and sugar	43	½ cup, 125ml	14	1	6
	Reduced fat, commercial	•	½ cup, 125ml	19	1	•
	Paul's Trim, vanilla, reduced fat	37	½ cup, 125ml	19	1	7
	Ice-cream, regular, full fat					
	Paddlepop varieties					
	banana, chocolate, rainbow	50–52	1 serve, 68ml	11	1	6
	Moo, chocolate	48	1 serve, 68ml	13	1	6
	Moo, strawberry	51	1 serve, 68ml	14	1	7
	Sara Lee, French vanilla, ultra chocolate flavour	38	2 scoops, 100g	18	1	7
	Vanilla	47	2 scoops, 100g	21	1.5	10
	Ice-cream, reduced-fat					
◎	Chocollo, low-fat, Wendy's	24	1 junior scoop, 80g	11	1	3
◎	Chocollo, low-fat Wendy's,	24	1 junior scoop in waffle cone	55	1.5	22
	Light 98% fat free, Vanilla, Bulla	36	2 scoops, 100g	23	1.5	8
	Low carbohydate, chocolate	32	2 scoops, 100g	4	<0.5	1
	Low fat, low sugar, Peter's No Sugar Added	•	2 scoops, 100g	8	0.5	•
	Vanilla	•	2 scoops, 100	28	2	•
	Frozen Yoghurt					
	Vanilla	46	½ cup, 125ml	21	1.5	10
	Dairy Desserts					
	Aero Mousse	37	1 tub, 62g	10	0.5	4
	Fromage frais	35	1 tub, 125g	15	1	5
	Instant pudding, packet mix made with whole milk, chocolate or vanilla	47	100g	16	1	8
	Nestle Diet varieties					
	chocolate mousse	31	1 tub, 62g	10	0.5	3
	crème caramel	33	1 tub, 125g	12	1	4

★ little or no carbs   ■ high in saturated fat   ● untested/unknown   ◎ GI Symbol partner

GISP	FOOD	GI	HOUSEHOLD MEASURE & WEIGHT	CARB (G) PER SERVE	CARB EXCHANGE PER SERVE	GL PER SERVE
	Fruche					
	Apricot Danish	•	1 tub, 150g	21	1.5	•
	Berry Crumble	•	1 tub, 150g	22	1.5	•
	Citrus Cheesecake	•	1 tub, 150g	21	1.5	•
	Fromage frais					
	Strawberry fields	•	1 tub, 150g	23	1.5	•
	Tropical mango	•	1 tub, 150g	23	1.5	•
	Vanilla crème	49	1 tub, 150g	25	1.5	12
	Layers					
	Vanilla on apple & cranberry	44	1 tub, 150g	25	1.5	11
	Vanilla on mixed berries	49	1 tub, 150g	26	2	13
	Vanilla on strawberry & pomegranate	50	1 tub, 150g	25	1.5	13
	Yoplait Le Rice					
	apple cinnamon	52	1 tub, 150g	28	2	15
	chocolate	•	1 tub, 150g	27	2	•
	classic vanilla	45	1 tub, 150g	27	2	12
	smooth caramel	41	1 tub, 150g	29	2	12
	forest berries	45	1 tub, 150g	29	2	13
	raspberry & white chocolate	51	1 tub, 150g	28	2	14
	tropical mango	54	1 tub, 150g	28	2	15

★ little or no carbs　■ high in saturated fat　● untested/unknown　© GI Symbol partner

GISP	FOOD	GI	HOUSEHOLD MEASURE & WEIGHT	CARB (G) PER SERVE	CARB EXCHANGE PER SERVE	GL PER SERVE
	FRUIT – LOW GI (LESS THAN OR EQUAL TO 55)					
	Fresh fruit					
☉	Apple, unpeeled	38	1 medium, 166g 100g	18 12	1	7
	Apricot, raw	34	2 regular, 112g 100g	8 7	0.5	3
	Banana	52	1 medium, 120g 100g	24 14	1.5	12
	Blueberries	53	½ cup, 80g 100g	9 11	0.5	5
	Custard apple	54	1 regular, 327g 100g	52 16	3.5	28
	Grapefruit	25	1 medium, 207g 100g	7 3	0.5	2
☉	Grapes	53	⅔ cup, 112g 100g	17 15	1	9
	Kiwifruit	53	1 regular, 95g 100g	9 10	0.5	5
	Mango, unpeeled	51	1 regular, 207g 100g	26 8	2	13
	Nectarine	43	1 small, 87g 100g	7 8	0.5	3
	Orange	42	1 large, 193g 100g	15 6	1	16
	Peach	42	1 medium, 145g 100g	9 6	0.5	4
☉	Pear, unpeeled	38	1 medium, 166g 100g	22 14	1.5	8
	Plum	39	2 regular, 132g 100g	10 7	1	4
	Strawberries	40	1 punnet, 250g 100g	8 3	0.5	3
	Dried Fruit					
	Apple	29	4 rings, 25g 100g	16 67	1	5

★ little or no carbs   ■ high in saturated fat   ● untested/unknown   ☉ GI Symbol partner

GISP	FOOD	GI	HOUSEHOLD MEASURE & WEIGHT	CARB (G) PER SERVE	CARB EXCHANGE PER SERVE	GL PER SERVE
	Apricot	31	10 halves, 35g 100g	16 44	1	5
	Dates	39–45	5 regular, 25g 100g	17 67	4	7
	Fruit & nut mix	15	¼ cup, 50g 100g	24 48	1.5	4
	Peach	35	3 halves, 40g 100g	16 40	1	6
	Pear	43	1 half, 18g 100g	11 60	1	5
	Prunes	40	4 regular, 32g 100g	14 33	1	6
	Sultanas	56	1½ tbsp, 21g 100g	15 75	1	8
	Tropical fruit & nut mix	49	¼ cup, 50g 100g	14 28	1	7
	Canned fruit					
	Apple, canned, Woolworth's Select	42	½ cup, 125g 100g	10 8	0.5	4
	Apricot, canned in natural juice	51	4 halves, 72g 100g	8 10	0.5	4
	Cherries, sour, pitted	41	¼ cup, 130g 100g	12 9	1	5
	Fruit salad, canned in juice	54	1 cup, 263g 100g	26 8	2	14
	Grapefruit, ruby red segments canned in juice, Woolworth's Select	47	½ cup, 120g 100g	21 17	1.5	10
	Mandarin, segments, canned in fruit juice	47	½ cup,130g 100g	18 14	1	8
	Orange & grapefruit segments, canned in fruit juice, Woolworth's Select	53	½ cup, 120g 100g	19 15	1	10
	Peach, canned in natural juice	45	½ cup, 132g 100g	12 9	1	5
	Peaches & grapes, canned in fruit juice, Woolworth's Select	46	½ cup, 120g 100g	12 10	1	6

★ little or no carbs   ■ high in saturated fat   ● untested/unknown   ⓒ GI Symbol partner

GISP	FOOD	GI	HOUSEHOLD MEASURE & WEIGHT	CARB (G) PER SERVE	CARB EXCHANGE PER SERVE	GL PER SERVE
	Peaches & pineapple, canned in fruit juice, Woolworth's Select	45	½ cup, 120g 100g	13 10	1	6
	Pear, canned in fruit juice	43	½ cup, 120g 100g	13 10	1	6
	Pear, halves, canned in reduced sugar syrup, SPC Lite	25	½ cup, 120g 100g	14 11	1	4
	Pineapple, canned in juice, drained, Woolworth's Select	43	1 cup chunks, 200g 100g	20 10	1	9
	Pineapple pieces, canned in fruit juice	49	½ cup, 128g 100g	13 10	1	6
	Pineapple & papaya pieces, canned in fruit juice, Woolworth's Select	53	½ cup, 120g 100g	17 14	1	9
Juices						
	Apple juice, no added sugar	40	1 cup, 250ml	28	2	11
☺	Apple, filtered, pure, Wild About Fruit	44	1 cup, 250ml	30	2	13
	Apple, Granny Smith, pure, Ducat's	44	1 cup, 250ml	30	2	13
☺	Apple, with fibre, Wild About Fruit	37	1 cup, 250ml	28	2	10
	Apple blackcurrant, no added sugar, Berri	45	1 cup, 250ml	26	2	12
☺	Apple & cherry, pure, Wild About Fruit	43	1 cup, 250ml	33	2	14
☺	Apple & mango, pure, Wild About Fruit	47	1 cup, 250ml	34	2	16
☺	Apple, pineapple & passionfruit, Wild About Fruit	48	1 cup, 250ml	33	2	16
	Carrot juice, freshly made	43	1 cup, 250ml	14	1	6
	Cranberry Juice Cocktail, Ocean Spray	52	1 cup, 250ml	31	2	16
	Grapefruit juice, unsweetened	48	1 cup, 250ml	20	1.5	10
	Orange juice, fresh, unsweetened	50	1 cup, 250ml	18	1	9
	Orange juice, unsweetened, from concentrate, Quelch	53	1 cup, 250ml	18	1	10
	Pineapple juice, unsweetened	46	1 cup, 250ml	34	2	16
	Prune juice, Golden Circle Healthy Life Natural	43	1 cup, 250ml	38	1.5	16
	Tomato juice, no added sugar, Berri	38	1 cup, 250ml	9	0.5	3
	Vegetable juice	43	1 cup, 250ml	9	0.5	4

★ little or no carbs ■ high in saturated fat ● untested/unknown ☺ GI Symbol partner

GISP	FOOD	GI	HOUSEHOLD MEASURE & WEIGHT	CARB (G) PER SERVE	CARB EXCHANGE PER SERVE	GL PER SERVE
	FRUIT – HIGHER GI (MORE THAN 55 OR UNKNOWN)					
	Fresh fruit					
	Avocado	★	120g	<1	0	0
	Blackberries	●	10 regular, 50g	4	<0.5	●
			100g	8		
	Breadfruit	62	¼ cup, 55g	15	1	9
			100g	27		
	Cherries	63	1 cup, 124g	15	1	9
			100g	11		
	Fig, raw, fresh, unpeeled	●	1 large, 64g	5	<0.5	●
			100g	8		
	Fruit salad, fresh, with melon	●	1 cup, 206	19	1	●
			100g	8		
	Guava	●	1 regular, 90g	3	<0.5	●
			100g	4		
	Honeydew melon, peeled	●	1 cup, 180g	12	1	●
			100g	7		
	Lemon	★	1 whole, 80g	1.5	0	●
	Lime	★	1 whole, 60g	1.5	0	●
	Loquat (5 large)	●	5 large, 100g	5	<0.5	●
	Lychees, B3 variety	57	7 regular, 90g	15	1	9
			100g	16		
	Mandarin	●	1 medium, 86g	7	0.5	●
			100g	7		
	Mulberries	●	1 cup, 148g	6	<0.5	●
			100g	4		
	Nashi pear	●	1 medium, 187g	21	1.5	●
			100g	11		
	Paw paw	56	1 cup cubed, 148g	10	0.5	6
			100g	7		
	Persimmon	●	1 medium, 168g	27	2	●
			100g	16		
	Pineapple	59	1 cup, diced 164g	13	1	8
			100g	10		

★ little or no carbs ■ high in saturated fat ● untested/unknown © GI Symbol partner

GISP	FOOD	GI	HOUSEHOLD MEASURE & WEIGHT	CARB (G) PER SERVE	CARB EXCHANGE PER SERVE	GL PER SERVE
	Pomegranate, peeled	•	100g	14	1	•
	Prickly pear, peeled	•	100g	9	0.5	•
	Quince, peeled	•	1 medium, 393g 100g	43 11	3	•
	Rambutan	•	100g	16	1	•
	Rockmelon/cantaloupe, without skin	88	1 cup diced, 189g 100g	8 6	0.5	7
	Rockmelon/cantaloupe, with skin	★	100g	4	68	3
	Raspberries	★	100g	7	0.5	•
	Rhubarb, stewed, unsweetened	★	125g	2	<0.5	•
	Tamarillo, peeled	•	100g	3	<0.5	•
	Tangelo, peeled	•	100g	8	0.5	•
	Watermelon, with skin (without skin)	78	100g 100g	3 6	<0.5	2
Canned fruit						
	Apricot, canned in light syrup	64	4 halves, 90g 100g	12 13	1	8
	Lychees, canned in syrup, drained	79	7 regular, 90g 100g	16 17	1	13
	Peach, canned in light syrup	57	½ cup, 132g 100g	17 13	1	10
Dried Fruit						
	Cranberries, sweetened	64	2 tbsp, 25g 100g	16 65	1	10
	Currants	•	2 tbsp, 24g 100g	16 65	1	•
	Fig	61	2 regular, 20g 100g	21 55	1.5	13
	Mixed fruit	•	100g	65	4	•
	Raisins	61	1½ tbsp, 20g 100g	16 79	1	10
	Sultanas	56	1½ tbsp, 20g 100g	15 79	1	8

★ little or no carbs   ■ high in saturated fat   ● untested/unknown   Ⓖ GI Symbol partner

GISP	FOOD	GI	HOUSEHOLD MEASURE & WEIGHT	CARB (G) PER SERVE	CARB EXCHANGE PER SERVE	GL PER SERVE
	LEGUMES					
	Baked beans					
	Canned In Tomato Sauce	52	½ cup, 150g	18	1	9
	Heinz varieties, canned					
	Barbecue sauce	47	1 sml can, 220g	34	2	16
	Cheesy tomato sauce	44	1 sml can, 220g	28	2	12
	Ham sauce	53	1 sml can, 220g	31	2	16
	Mild curry sauce	49	1 sml can, 220g	34	2	17
	Sweet chilli sauce	46	1 sml can, 220g	33	2	15
	Tomato sauce	49	1 sml can, 220g	30	2	15
	Black-eye beans					
	Dried, uncooked	•	100g	60	4	•
	soaked, boiled	42	½ cup, 75g	17	1	7
	Borlotti beans					
	Dried, uncooked	•	100g	35	3	•
	Canned, drained, Edgell	41	½ cup, 75g	12	1	5
	Butter beans					
	Soaked, boiled	26	½ cup, 75g	8	1	2
	Canned, drained, Edgell	36	½ cup, 80g	11	1	4
	Cannellini beans					
	Cooked from dried beans	•	½ cup, 86g	12	1	•
	Canned, drained, Edgell	31	½ cup, 128g	15	1	5
	Chickpeas					
	Canned, drained	40	½ cup, 80g	11	1	4
	Canned, drained, Edgell	38	1 can, 75g	13	1	5
	Hommus, Chris' Traditional	22	2 tbsp, 40g	3	<0.5	1
	Four bean mix					
	Canned, drained, Edgell	37	1 can, 75g	12	1	4
	Haricot/Navy bean					
	Dried, uncooked	•	100g	35	3	•
	Boiled	33	½ cup, 88g	12	1	4

★ little or no carbs　■ high in saturated fat　● untested/unknown　Ⓖ GI Symbol partner

GISP	FOOD	GI	HOUSEHOLD MEASURE & WEIGHT	CARB (G) PER SERVE	CARB EXCHANGE PER SERVE	GL PER SERVE
	Lentils					
	Average of green, red, brown, dried	•	100g	35	2	•
	Average of green, red, brown, boiled	•	100g	10	0.5	•
	Brown, canned	42	½ cup, 80g	13	1	5
	Green, dried, boiled	30	⅔ cup, 125g	17	1	5
	Green, canned	48	⅔ cup, 135g	17	1	8
	Red, dried, boiled	26	⅔ cup, 125g	18	1	5
	Red, dried, split, boiled 25 min	21	125g	15	1	3
	Dhal	•	1 cup, 195g	29	2	•
	Mung beans					
	Boiled	39	⅔ cup, 127g	15	1	4
	Red kidney beans					
	Dried, uncooked	•	100g	36	2.5	•
	Dried, boiled	51	100g	9	1	5
	Canned, drained, Edgell	36	1 can, 75g	11	1	4
	Pinto beans					
	Refried, canned, Casa Fiesta	38	½ cup, 113g	20	2	8
	Steamed	33	½ cup, 150g	23	2	8
	Snake beans					
	Snake beans	★	70g	0	•	•
	Soup Mix					
	Dry, standard	•	100g	50	3.5	•
	Dry, Italian	•	100g	40	2.5	•
	Soy beans					
	Dried, uncooked	•	100g	13	1	•
	Dried, boiled	18	1 cup, 170g	4	<0.5	1
	Canned, drained, Edgell	14	½ cup, 100g	3	<0.5	0
	Split peas					
	Dried, uncooked, yellow/green	•	¼ cup, 53g	25	1.5	•
	Dried, boiled, yellow/green	25	1 cup, 180g	13	1	3

★ little or no carbs   ■ high in saturated fat   ● untested/unknown   Ⓒ GI Symbol partner

GISP	FOOD	GI	HOUSEHOLD MEASURE & WEIGHT	CARB (G) PER SERVE	CARB EXCHANGE PER SERVE	GL PER SERVE
	MEAT, SEAFOOD & PROTEIN					
	Bacon	★ ■	50g	0	•	•
	Beef, lean	★	120g	0	•	•
	Brawn	★ ■	75g	0	•	•
	Calamari rings, squid, not battered or crumbed	★	70g	0	•	•
	Chicken, no skin	★	110g	0	•	•
	Duck	★ ■	140g	0	•	•
	Eggs	★ ■	120g	0	•	•
	Fish	★	120g	0	•	•
	Ham, lean	★	24g	0	•	•
	Lamb	★	120g	0	•	•
	Liver Sausage	★ ■	30g	0	•	•
	Liverwurst	★ ■	30g	0	•	•
	Oysters, natural, plain	★	85g	0	•	•
	Pork, lean	★	120g	0	•	•
	Prawns	★	150g	0	•	•
	Salami	★ ■	120g	0	•	•
	Salmon, fresh or canned in water or brine	★	150g	0	•	•
	Sardines	★	60g	0	•	•
	Sausages, fried	28 ■	100g	3	<0.5	1
	Scallops, natural, plain	★	160g	0	•	•
	Shellfish	★	120g	0	•	•
	Steak, lean	★	120g	0	•	•
	Tofu, bean curd, plain, unsweetened	★	100g	0	•	•
	Trout, fresh or frozen	★	63g	0	•	•
	Tuna, fresh or canned in water or brine	★	120g	0	•	•
	Turkey, lean	★	140g	0	•	•
	Veal	★	120g	0	•	•

★ little or no carbs   ■ high in saturated fat   ● untested/unknown   © GI Symbol partner

GISP	FOOD	GI	HOUSEHOLD MEASURE & WEIGHT	CARB (G) PER SERVE	CARB EXCHANGE PER SERVE	GL PER SERVE
	RICE, PASTA, NOODLES & GRAINS – LOW GI (LESS THAN OR EQUAL TO 55)					
	Barley					
	Pearl, raw	•	2 tbsp, 32g	15	1	•
	Pearl, boiled	25	1 cup, 190g	40	3.5	10
	Bulgur (burghul)					
	Raw	•	2 tbsp, 25g	15	1	•
	Boiled	•	1 cup, 265g	46	3	•
	Soaked in water	48	100g	28	2	13
	Buckwheat					
	Groats, raw	•	2 tbsp, 29g	21	1.5	•
	Groats, boiled	54	1 cup, 180g	34	2	18
	Couscous					
☺	Gourmet pearl couscous, cooked, boiled, Blu	52	½ cup	19	1	10
	Rice					
	Doongara rice, CleverRice, SunRice	54–56	1 cup, 170g	44	3	24
	Long-grain rice, white, boiled 15 min, Mahatma	50	1 cup, 170g	46	3	23
	Noodles					
	Instant '2-minute' noodles, Woolworth's Select	52	1 pkt, 360g	42	3	22
	Mung bean noodles, Lungkow bean thread, dried, boiled	39	1 cup, 180g	45	3	18
	Rice noodles, fresh, boiled	40	1 cup, 180g	39	2.5	16
	Soba noodles, instant, served in soup	46	1 cup, 180g	49	3	23
	Quinoa					
	Dry	•	¼ cup, 43g	27	2	•
	Boiled, Nature First Organic	53	⅓ cup, 62g	13	1	7
	Semolina					
	Raw	•	2 tbsp, 26g	17	1	•
		•	100g	66	4.5	•
	Cooked	55	1 cup, 245g	17	1	10

★ little or no carbs   ■ high in saturated fat   ● untested/unknown   ☺ GI Symbol partner

GISP	FOOD	GI	HOUSEHOLD MEASURE & WEIGHT	CARB (G) PER SERVE	CARB EXCHANGE PER SERVE	GL PER SERVE
	Pasta					
	Capellini	45	1 cup, 150g	45	3	20
	Fettuccine, egg	40	1 cup, 180g	46	3	18
	Fusilli twists, tricolour	51	1 cup, 150g	42	3	21
	Lasagne, beef, commercial	47	200g	30	2	14
	Latina Fresh Pasta					
	Agnolotti, ricotta & spinach	47	½ pkt, 280g	83	5.5	39
	Fettuccine, egg	54	½ pkt, 360g	92	6	50
	Lasagne sheets	49	1 regular, 47g	23	1.5	11
	Ravioli, beef	43	½ pkt, 315g	70	4.5	30
	Ravioli, chicken & garlic	44	½ pkt, 279g	76	5	33
	Ravioli, Kids beef & vegetable	47	½ pkt, 155g	49	3.5	23
	Ravioli, Kids, cheese & vegetable	51	½ pkt, 155g	51	3.5	26
	Ravioli, wholegrain, ricotta & spinach	39	½ pkt, 220g	58	4	23
	Tortellini, mixed veal	48	½ pkt, 305g	80	5	38
	Vetta varieties					
☉	Lasagne sheets	53	1 regular, 19g	13	1	7
☉	Macaroni, boiled 8–10 min	49	1 cup, 150g	40	2.5	20
☉	Spaghetti, boiled 8–10 min	49	1 cup, 180g	48	3	24
	Macaroni	47	1 cup, 150g	40	2.5	19
	Spaghetti	44	1 cup, 180g	48	3	21
	Spaghetti, protein-enriched	27	1 cup, 180g	14	1	4
	Spaghetti, wholemeal	42	1 cup, 180g	42	3	18
	Spirali, white, durum wheat	43	1 cup, 150g	44	3	19
	Star Pastina, white, boiled 5 min	38	1 cup, 150g	48	3	18
	Vermicelli	35	1 cup, 180g	48	3	17
	White, boiled	•	1 cup, 140g	35	2.5	•
	White, dry	•	⅓ cup, 45g	30	2	•
	Instant pasta					
	Pasta & sauce, prepared, Continental	33–43	½ pkt, 140g	19–22	1.5	33–43
	Pasta & sauce, prepared, Woolworth's Select	48–57	¼ pkt, 110g	20–23	1.5	48–57

★ little or no carbs   ■ high in saturated fat   ● untested/unknown   ☉ GI Symbol partner

GISP	FOOD	GI	HOUSEHOLD MEASURE & WEIGHT	CARB (G) PER SERVE	CARB EXCHANGE PER SERVE	GL PER SERVE
	Gluten-free pasta					
	Rice pasta, Freedom Foods	51	1 cup, 180g	47	3	24
	**RICE, PASTA, NOODLES & GRAINS – HIGHER GI (MORE THAN 55 OR UNKNOWN)**
	Cornmeal/Polenta					
	Raw	•	2 tbsp, 20g	14	1	•
	Boiled	68	1 cup, 250g	22	4	15
	Couscous					
	Raw	•	¼ cup, 40g	30	2	•
	Cooked, soaked	65	1 cup, 160g	15	2.5	10
	Flours					
	Wheat, white	•	1 tbsp, 13g	8	0.5	•
	Wheat, wholemeal	•	1 tbsp, 13g	8	0.5	•
	Millet, raw	•	100g	63	•	•
	Millet, boiled	71	100g	23	1.5	16
	Noodles					
	Buckwheat noodles	59	180g	42	3	25
	Instant Noodles: 2-Minute Noodles, Maggi, 99% fat free	67	1 pkt, 320g	61	4	41
	Rice vermicelli, dried, boiled	58	¼ pkt, 250g	50	3.5	29
	Rice pasta, brown, boiled	92	1 cup, 180g	38	2.5	35
	Asian, shelf stable noodles, e.g. Hokkein, Singapore	•	½ pkt, 110g	35	2.5	•
	Udon, plain	62	½ pkt, 200g	50	3.5	31
	Pasta					
	Gnocchi, cooked	68	100g	29	2	20
	Macaroni & cheese, prepared, Kraft	64	302g	76	5	49
	Gluten-free pasta					
	Corn pasta, Orgran	78	1 cup, 180g	42	3	33
	Rice and maize pasta, Ris'O'Mais, Orgran	76	1 cup, 180g	49	3.5	37
	Spaghetti, canned in tomato sauce, Orgran	68	1 can, 220g	27	2	18

★ little or no carbs   ■ high in saturated fat   ● untested/unknown   Ⓖ GI Symbol partner

GISP	FOOD	GI	HOUSEHOLD MEASURE & WEIGHT	CARB (G) PER SERVE	CARB EXCHANGE PER SERVE	GL PER SERVE
Rice						
	raw	•	¼ cup, 50g	40	2.5	•
	boiled	•	1 cup, 170g	45	3	•
	Arborio/risotto rice, boiled, SunRice	69	1 cup, 170g	49	3	34
	Basmati rice, white, boiled	58	1 cup, 170g	47	3	27
	Broken Rice, Thai, white, cooked in rice cooker	86	1 cup, 170g	49	3	42
	Brown rice, boiled/pelde	86	1 cup, 170g	43	3	37
	Calrose rice, brown, medium-grain, boiled	76	1 cup, 170g	45	3	34
	Calrose rice, white, medium-grain, boiled	87	1 cup, 170g	48	3	42
	Glutinous rice, white, cooked in rice cooker	98	½ cup, 170g	36	2.5	35
	Instant rice, white, cooked 6 min with water	87	1 cup, 170g	48	3	42
	Japanese-style sushi rice, SunRice	73	1 cup, 170g	46	3	34
	Jasmine fragrant rice, SunRice	89	1 cup, 170g	45	3	40
	Medium-Grain, Brown SunRice	59	1 cup, 170g	49	3	29
	Parboiled rice, Pelde, Sungold	87	1 cup, 170g	49	3	43
	Sri Lankan Red Rice, boiled	59	1 cup, 170g	45	3	27
	Sunbrown Quick rice, Ricegrowers, boiled	80	1 cup, 170g	43	3	34
	White long-grain rice, Premium, SunRice	59	1 cup, 170g	45	3	27
	Wild rice, boiled	57	½ cup, 75g	15	1	9
Spelt						
	Dry	•	100g	59	4	•
	Cooked	•	100g	23	1.5	•
Wheat						
	Wheat bran, unprocessed	•	100g	16	1	•
	Wheatgerm	•	100g	30	2	•

★ little or no carbs   ■ high in saturated fat   ● untested/unknown   Ⓒ GI Symbol partner

GISP	FOOD	GI	HOUSEHOLD MEASURE & WEIGHT	CARB (G) PER SERVE	CARB EXCHANGE PER SERVE	GL PER SERVE
	SNACKFOODS & TREATS – LOW GI (LESS THAN OR EQUAL TO 55)					
	Cakes & Pastries					
	Banana cake, homemade	51	1 slice, 80g	38	2.5	19
	Bavarian, chocolate honeycomb, Sara Lee Lite	31	¼ cake, 93g	25	1.5	8
	Carrot cake, commercially made	38	1 sml slice, 50g	19	1	7
	Chocolate brownies	42	1 serve, 56g	30	2	13
	Chocolate cake, pkt mix, with frosting, Betty Crocker	38	1 slice, 110g	52	3.5	20
	Chocolate mud cake	43	1 slice, 100g	54	3.5	29
	Chocolate crackles	43	1 serve, 12g	1	1	●
	Crumble, apple berry, commercially made	41	1 slice, 165g	34	2	14
	Danish, apple & peach, Sara Lee Lite	50	⅛ pkt, 67g	29	2	15
	Fruit cake, commercial, Big Sister	53	1 slice, 50g	28	2	15
	Pavlova, prepared with fresh cream, strawberries, banana and passionfruit	49	1 slice, 120g	33	2	16
	Pound cake	54	1 sml slice, 50g	23	1.5	12
	Sponge cake, plain, unfilled	46	1 slice, 25g	14	1	6
	Vanilla cake, from pkt mix with frosting, Betty Crocker	42	1 slice, 65g	31	2	13
	Savoury Snacks					
	Chickpea chips, Freedom Foods	44	⅕ pkt, 50g	25	1.5	11
	Corn chips	42	1 pkt, 50g	26	2	11
	Grain Waves Wholegrain chips, original, Smith's	51	1 pkt, 40g	25	1.5	13
	Confectionery					
	Chocolate	42–49	4 sml squares, 24g	15	1	7
	Chocolate coated almonds	21	5–6 almonds, 30g	8	0.5	2
	Chocolate, dark, Dove	23	4 sml squares, 24g	13	1	3
	Chocolate, fructose sweetened	20	4 sml squares, 24g	15	1	3
	Chocolate, white, Milky Bar, Nestle	44	1 fun size, 15g	8	0.5	4
	Jelly, diet, made from crystalswith water	★	½ cup, 120g	0	●	●

★ little or no carbs   ■ high in saturated fat   ● untested/unknown   Ⓖ GI Symbol partner

GISP	FOOD	GI	HOUSEHOLD MEASURE & WEIGHT	CARB (G) PER SERVE	CARB EXCHANGE PER SERVE	GL PER SERVE
	Jelly, made from commercial jelly crystals	53	½ cup, 120g	19	1	10
	M&M's, peanut, Mars Confectionery	33	1 fun size, 14g	8	0.5	3
	Milo bar, Nestle	40	1 serve, 21g	15	1	6
	Rum balls, Woolworth's	50	1 serve, 25g	14	1	7
	Snickers bar, Mars Confectionery	41	1 fun size, 22g	13	1	5
	Twix bar, Mars Confectionery	44	1 fun size, 16g	10	4	4
	Yummiees jelly lollies, Allseps	43	4 lollies, 15g	5	<0.5	2
Muffins						
	Apple, homemade	46	1 regular, 60g	29	2	13
	Apple blueberry, Sara Lee	49	1 regular, 60g	25	1.5	12
	Apple, oat, sultana	54	1 regular, 50g	26	2	14
	Blueberry, Sara Lee	50	1 regular, 60g	31	2	16
	Chocolate	53	1 regular, 60g	30	2	16
	Choc-butterscotch	53	1 regular, 50g	28	2	15
	Choc-chip, Sara Lee	52	1 regular, 60g	32	2	17
	Double chocolate	46	1 regular, 60g	34	2	16
Nuts						
	Almonds	•	½ cup, 75g	3	<0.5	•
	Cashews	22	½ cup, 100g	26	2	6
	Chestnut, roasted	•	5 kernels, 100g	34	2	•
	Dried fruit & nut mix, commercial	32	¼ cup, 50g	22	1.5	7
	Macadamia	•	½ cup, 75g	3	<0.5	•
	Mixed nuts, roasted, salted	24	½ cup, 100g	25	1	6
	Peanut, dry roasted	23	½ cup, 100g	9	0.5	2
	Pecan	10	½ cup, 100g	5	<0.5	1
	Pine nut	•	½ cup, 100g	5	<0.5	•
	Sesame seeds	★	11g	0	<0.5	•
	Walnut	•	½ cup, 53g	<0.5	•	•
Snack Bars						
Bakers Delight, Fit2Go Bars						
	Cranberry & Nuts bar	51	1 bar, 77g	25	1.5	13
	Fruit & Cinnamon bar	53	1 bar, 77g	28	2	15

★ little or no carbs   ■ high in saturated fat   ● untested/unknown   ☺ GI Symbol partner

GISP	FOOD	GI	HOUSEHOLD MEASURE & WEIGHT	CARB (G) PER SERVE	CARB EXCHANGE PER SERVE	GL PER SERVE
	Freedom Foods					
	Hi-Lite breakfast bar	53	1 bar, 35g	21	1.5	11
	Omega Bar, gluten-free, seed & nut	21	1 bar, 40g	17	1	4
	Superberry breakfast bar	54	1 bar, 35g	20	1.5	11
	Healtheries Simple Snack Bar					
	apricot & yoghurt	40	1 bar, 45g	23	1.5	9
	berry & yoghurt	51	1 bar, 45g	24	1.5	12
	chocolate	35	1 bar, 45g	25	1.5	9
	Ironman PR bar, chocolate	39	1 bar, 65g	26	2	10
	Mother Earth Baked Fruit Stick, apricot-filled	50	1 bar, 19g	13	1	7
	Sunripe School Straps,					
ⓒ	blackberry sour buzz	35	1 bar, 15g	10	0.5	4
ⓒ	strawberry & wildberry	40	1 bar, 15g	10	0.5	4
	Trim Low-GI protein snack bar, Aussie Bodies					
	Berryliscious	46	1 bar, 50g	15	1	7
	Chocorama	31	1 bar, 50g	14	1	4
	Uncle Tobys, muesli bar varieties					
ⓒ	Chewy, forest fruit	48	1 bar, 31g	20	1.5	10
ⓒ	Chewy, white choc chip	54	1 bar, 31g	20	1.5	11
ⓒ	Chewy, choc chip	54	1 bar, 31g	20	1.5	11
ⓒ	Crunchy, apricot	54	1 bar, 31g	20	1.5	11
ⓒ	Crunchy, forest fruit	48	1 bar, 31g	20	1.5	10
ⓒ	Crunchy, choc chip	54	1 bar, 31g	20	1.5	11
	Drinks					
	Coca-Cola	53	1 can, 375ml	40	2.5	21
	Coffee, black, no milk or sugar	★	1 cup, 250ml	0	0	•
	Lemonade	54	1 can, 375ml	42	3	23
	Ribena blackcurrant fruitsyrup, reconstituted	52	250ml	32	2	17
	Soft drink, diet	★	250ml	0	0	•

★ little or no carbs   ■ high in saturated fat   ● untested/unknown   ⓒ GI Symbol partner

GISP	FOOD	GI	HOUSEHOLD MEASURE & WEIGHT	CARB (G) PER SERVE	CARB EXCHANGE PER SERVE	GL PER SERVE
	SNACKFOODS & TREATS – HIGHER GI (MORE THAN 55 OR UNKNOWN)					
	Cakes & Pastries					
	Angel food cake	67	1 sml piece, 57g	31	2	21
	Cupcake, strawberry iced	73	1 serve, 38g	26	2	19
	Fruit mince pies, Mr Kipling	58	1 serve, 59g	35	2	20
	Lamington	87	1 serve, 50g	29	2	25
	Puff pastry	56	100g	40	2.5	22
	Savoury Snacks					
	Burger Rings	90	1 pkt, 50g	29	2	26
	Chips, potato	57	1 mini pkt, 25g	12	1	7
	Poppin Microwave Popcorn varieties, Green's Foods					
	Butter	62	1 pkt, 100g	50	3.5	31
	Lite	67	1 pkt, 85g	48	3	32
	plain	72	1 cup, 9g	5	<0.5	4
	Prawn cracker	•	1 pkt, 50g	33	<0.5	•
	Pretzels	•	1 cup, 42g	27	2	•
	Pretzels, oven-baked, traditional wheat flavour, Parkers	84	10 pretzels, 19g	15	1	13
	Rice crackers	91	11 crackers, 19g	15	1	14
	Twisties, Smith's	74	1 pkt, 30g	19	1	14
	Confectionery					
	Gummi confectionery	94	6 pieces, 24g	15	•	14
	Jelly beans	78	10–15 lollies, 30g	28	2	22
	Licorice, soft	78	1 stick, 12g	9	0.5	7
	Life Savers, peppermint candy, Nestle	70	1 pkt, 22g	21	1.5	15
	Mars Bar, Mars Confectionery	62	1 fun size, 22g	16	1	10
	Marshmallows, plain, pink & white	62	4 small, 20g	16	1	10
	Milky Way bar, Mars Confectionery	62	1 fun size, 14g	10	0.5	6
	Skittles, fruit candies, Mars Confectionery	70	1 fun size, 25g	23	1.5	16
	Muffins					
	Apricot, coconut & honey	60	1 regular, 50g	26	2	16
	Banana, oat & honey	65	1 regular, 50g	26	2	17

★ little or no carbs   ■ high in saturated fat   ● untested/unknown   Ⓒ GI Symbol partner

GISP	FOOD	GI	HOUSEHOLD MEASURE & WEIGHT	CARB (G) PER SERVE	CARB EXCHANGE PER SERVE	GL PER SERVE
	Blueberry, commercially made	59	1 regular, 57g	29	2	17
	Bran, commercially made	60	1 regular, 57g	24	1.5	14
	Carrot, commercially made	62	1 regular, 57g	32	2	20
	Oatmeal, from pkt mix	69	1 regular, 50g	35	2	24
	Snack Bars					
	Roll-Ups, processed fruit snack, Uncle Tobys	99	1 serve, 15g	11	1	11
	Soft Drinks					
	Cordial, orange, reconstituted	66	1 cup, 250ml	20	1.5	13
	Fanta	68	1 can, 375ml	51	2	35
	Solo, lemon squash	58	1 can, 375ml	44	3	26

★ little or no carbs   ■ high in saturated fat   ● untested/unknown   Ⓖ GI Symbol partner

GISP	FOOD	GI	HOUSEHOLD MEASURE & WEIGHT	CARB (G) PER SERVE	CARB EXCHANGE PER SERVE	GL PER SERVE
	SPREADS & SWEETENERS – LOW GI (LESS THAN OR EQUAL TO 55)					
	Agave Nectar, premium, Sweet Cactus Farms	19	1 tsp, 5g	3	<0.5	1
	Divine Date spread, Buderim Ginger	29	1 tbsp, 25g	16	1	5
☺	Fruisana Fructose, pure	19	1 sachet, 10g	10	0.5	2
	Ginger, sucrose free, Buderim Ginger	10	4 pieces, 20g	15	1	2
	Honey					
	ironbark	48	2 tsp, 14g	12	1	6
	red gum	53	2 tsp, 14g	12	1	6
	stringybark	44	2 tsp, 14g	12	1	5
	yapunya	52	2 tsp, 14g	12	1	6
	yellowbox	35	2 tsp, 14g	12	1	4
☺	LoGiCane, low GI cane sugar	50	1 tsp, 4g	4	<0.5	2
	Maple syrup, pure	54	1 tbsp, 27g	18	1	10
	Marmalade, ginger, Buderim Ginger	50	1 tbsp, 18g	13	1	7
	Marmalade, orange	55	2 tbsp, 25g	16	1	9
	Nutella, hazelnut spread, Ferrero	25	2 tsp, 10g	5	<0.5	1
	Strawberry jam, regular	51	1 tbsp, 25g	17	1	9
☺	Sweetaddin	19	2 tsp, 10g	10	1	2
	SPREADS & SWEETENERS – HIGHER GI (MORE THAN 55 OR UNKNOWN)					
	Golden syrup	63	2 tsp, 14g	10	0.5	6
	Honey	•	2 tsp, 14g	12	1	•
	Blended	64	2 tsp, 14g	12	1	8
	Salvation Jane	64	2 tsp, 14g	12	1	8
	Maple-flavoured syrup, Cottees	68	1 tbsp, 20g	11	1	7
	Sugar	68	1 tsp, 5g	5	<0.5	3
	Treacle	68	3 tsp, 20g	13	1	9
	Vinegar	★	1 tsp, 5ml	0	0	•

★ little or no carbs   ■ high in saturated fat   ● untested/unknown   ☺ GI Symbol partner

GISP	FOOD	GI	HOUSEHOLD MEASURE & WEIGHT	CARB (G) PER SERVE	CARB EXCHANGE PER SERVE	GL PER SERVE
	TAKEAWAY, PRE-PREPARED & CONVENIENCE FOODS **— LOW GI (LESS THAN OR EQUAL TO 55)**					
	Burrito, corn tortilla, refried beans & tomato salsa	39	1 serve, 100g	23	1.5	9
	Cannelloni, spinach & ricotta, prepared convenience meal	15	1 serve, 300g	54	3.5	8
	Chicken nuggets, frozen, reheated in microwave 5 min	46	6 nuggets, 100g	16	1	7
	Dosai, served with chutney	55	1 serve, 150g	39	2.5	21
	Fajitas, chicken	42	1 serve, 300g	42	3	18
	Fish fingers	38	4 fingers, 100g	18	1	7
	Lasagne, beef, commercially made	47	1 serve, 300g	35	2.5	16
	Meat pie	45	1 regular, 175g	41	2.5	18
	Party pies, beef, commercial	45	1 regular, 38g	10	0.5	5
	Moussaka, lamb, prepared convenience meal	35	1 serve, 300g	27	2	9
	Pizza Hut varieties					
	Supreme, thin & crispy,	30	1 slice, 71g	17	1	5
	Super Supreme, pan	36	1 slice, 94	23	1.5	8
	Veggie Supreme, thin & crispy	49	1 slice, 63g	16	1	8
	Generic					
	Pork Puff, Asian, BBQ pork, commercial	55	1 portion, 54g	17	1	9
	Spaghetti Bolognaise	52	1 serve, 360g	48	3	25
	Sushi, salmon	48	2 med pieces, 100g	14	1	7
	Vine leaves, stuffed with rice & lamb, served with tomato sauce	30	1 serve, 100g	15	1	5
	Pasta sauce Latina Fresh varieties					
	Bolognese sauce	24	½ tub, 212g	15	1	4
	Creamy Sun dried tomato	19	½ tub, 212g	18	1	3
	Italian tomato & garlic	40	½ tub, 212g	14	1	6
	Mediterranean sauce	40	½ tub, 212g	10	1.5	4
	Soups					
	Barley & vegetable	41	1 cup, 250ml	28	2	11

★ little or no carbs   ■ high in saturated fat   ● untested/unknown   Ⓖ GI Symbol partner

GISP	FOOD	GI	HOUSEHOLD MEASURE & WEIGHT	CARB (G) PER SERVE	CARB EXCHANGE PER SERVE	GL PER SERVE
	Campbell's Country Ladle Chicken & vegetable with wholegrain pasta	43	½ can, 250ml	9	0.5	4
	Minestone, traditional	39	1 can, 290ml	18	1	7
	Carrot, canned	35	1 cup, 250ml	13	1	5
	Lentil, canned	44	1 cup, 250ml	21	1.5	9
	Tomato, canned	45	1 cup, 250ml	17	1	8
TAKEAWAY, PRE-PREPARED & CONVENIENCE FOODS — HIGHER GI (MORE THAN 55 OR UNKNOWN)						
	Baked potato with baked beans	62	1 serve, 140g	37	2.5	23
	Battered fish, commercial	•	1 serve, 100g	14	1	•
	Chiko roll	•	1 serve, 100g	26	2	•
	Chips, takeaway	•	1 serve, 100g	26	2	•
	Crumbed calamari	•	1 serve, 100g	16	1	•
	Dim sim, commercial, deep fried	•	1 serve, 100g	27	2	•
	French fries, frozen, reheated in microwave	75	1 serve, 150g	29	2	22
	Fried chicken, e.g. KFC	•	1 serve, 100g	6	<0.5	•
	Pork Bun, Asian, commercial	69	1 bun, 60g	25	1.5	17
	Potato scallop	•	1 serve, 100g	27	2	•
	Sausages and mash, prepared, convenience meal	61	1 serve, 500g	67	4.5	41
	Shepherds pie	66	1 serve, 500g	74	5	49
	Steak, mashed potato & mixed vegetables, homemade	66	1 serve, 360g	53	3.5	35
	Taco shells, cornmeal-based, baked	68	2 regular, 26g	14	1	10
Soups						
	Chicken & mushroom	58	1 cup, 250ml	18	1	10
	Clear consommé, chicken or vegetable	★	1 cup, 205ml	0	0	•
	Green pea, canned	66	1 cup, 250ml	41	2.5	27
	Pumpkin, creamy, Heinz Very Special	76	1 cup, 290ml	29	2	22
	Spicy Thai instant soup, low fat	56	1 cup, 250ml	31	2	17
	Split pea, canned	60	1 cup, 250ml	27	2	16
	Vegetable	60	1 cup, 250ml	18	1	11

★ little or no carbs   ■ high in saturated fat   ● untested/unknown   Ⓖ GI Symbol partner

GISP	FOOD	GI	HOUSEHOLD MEASURE & WEIGHT	CARB (G) PER SERVE	CARB EXCHANGE PER SERVE	GL PER SERVE
	**STARCHY VEGETABLES – LOW GI (LESS THAN OR EQUAL TO 55)**					
	Carrot	39	1 medium, 61g	3	<0.5	1
	Carrot juice	43	1 cup, 250ml	14	1	6
	Cassava, peeled, diced, boiled	46	1 cup, 140g	42	3	19
	Corn on cob	48	1 medium, 77g	16	1	8
	Corn, loose kernels	48	½ cup, 87g	17	1	8
	Corn, canned	46	½ cup, 88g	16	1	7
	Corn, creamed, canned	•	⅓ can, 86g	14	1	•
	Parsnip, boiled	52	1 cup, 100g	10	1	5
	Parsnip, baked	•	100g	12	1	•
	Peas, green, fresh or frozen, boiled	51	½ cup, 80g	6	0.5	3
	Peas, canned	•	100g	9	0.5	•
Ⓖ	Potato, Carisma, unpeeled, boiled	55	1 medium, 125g	16	1	9
	Pumpkin, raw	•	1 cup, 100g	6	0.5	•
	Pumpkin, baked	•	1 cup, 100g	8	0.5	•
	Pumpkin, butternut, boiled, mashed	51	2 scoops, 100g	8	0.5	4
	Taro	54	½ cup, 100g	25	1	14
	Tomato juice	38	1 cup, 250ml	14	0.5	6
	Vegetable juice	43	1 cup, 250g	9	0.5	4
	Yam, peeled, boiled	54	1 cup, 100g	25	2.5	14
	**STARCHY VEGETABLES – HIGHER GI (MORE THAN 55 OR UNKNOWN)**					
	Beetroot, fresh, boiled	•	1 whole, 82g	7	0.5	•
	Beetroot, canned	64	4 slices, 32g	3	0	2
	Mixed vegetables, frozen e.g., peas, carrot, swede, beans, sweetcorn	•	½ cup	11	1	•
	Potato, baked, peeled, without oil	•	2 med chunks, 100g	20	2	•
	Potato, baked, jacket, in foil, without oil	•	1 large, 200g	28	2	•
	Potato chips, frozen, oven heat	•	15–20 chips, 100g	45	13	•
	Potato, Desiree, peeled, boiled 35 min	101	1 medium, 150g	17	1	17
	Potato Gems	•	12 gems	31	2	•
	Potato, Hash Browns	•	1 patty	12	1	•
	Potato, mashed, instant, Edgell	86	¼ pkt, 150g	20	1.5	17

★ little or no carbs   ■ high in saturated fat   ● untested/unknown   Ⓖ GI Symbol partner

GISP	FOOD	GI	HOUSEHOLD MEASURE & WEIGHT	CARB (G) PER SERVE	CARB EXCHANGE PER SERVE	GL PER SERVE
	Potato, mashed potato, with butter and milk	•	½ cup, 100g	11	1	•
	Potato, Nardine, peeled, boiled	70	1 medium, 150g	25	1.5	18
	Potato, new	78	2 small, 140g	18	1	14
	Potato, new, canned, microwaved	65	3–4 small, 120g	17	1	11
	Potato, Nicola, unpeeled, boiled whole 15 min	58	3 small, 150g	16	1	9
	Potato, Pontiac, peeled, boiled 15 min, mashed	91	½ cup, 150g	20	1.5	18
	Potato Pontiac, peeled, boiled whole 30–35 min	72	1 medium, 150g	18	1	13
	Potato Pontiac, peeled, microwaved 7 min	79	1 medium, 150g	18	1	14
	Potato, Sebago, peeled, boiled 35 min	87	1 medium, 150g	17	1	15
	Potato, wedges, with skin, frozen, oven heat	•	2 large, 50g	44	3	•
	Pumpkin, boiled	66	1 cup, 100g	7	0.5	5
	Swede, diced	72	1 cup, 170g	7	0.5	5
	Sweet potato, orange, peeled, cut into pieces, boiled 8 min	61	100g	15	1	9
	Sweet potato, purple skin, white flesh raw, diced	•	100g	14	1	•
	Sweet potato, purple skin white flesh, peeled, cut into pieces, boiled 8 min	75	1 cup, 150g	21	1	16
	Tapioca, boiled	93	1 cup, 250g	18	1	17
	Tapioca, raw, dry	•	2 tbsp	25	1.5	•
	Tapioca, pudding, creamed, homemade	81	1 cup	35	2.5	28

★ little or no carbs   ■ high in saturated fat   ● untested/unknown   Ⓖ GI Symbol partner

GISP	FOOD	GI	HOUSEHOLD MEASURE & WEIGHT	CARB (G) PER SERVE	CARB EXCHANGE PER SERVE	GL PER SERVE
	GREEN/SALAD VEGETABLES – LOW GI (LESS THAN OR EQUAL TO 55)					
	Alfalfa sprouts	★	6g	0	0	•
	Artichokes, globe, fresh or canned in brine	★	80g	1	0	•
	Artichoke, Jerusalem	•	3 medium, 145g	13	1	•
	Asparagus	★	100g	1	0	•
	Bean sprouts, raw	★	14g	0	0	•
	Bok choy	★	100g	1	0	•
	Broad beans, fresh, raw	•	½ cup, 55g	1	0	•
	Broccoli	★	60g	0	0	•
	Brussels sprouts	★	100g	2	0	•
	Cabbage	★	70g	1	0	•
	Capsicum	★	80g	2	0	•
	Cauliflower	★	60g	1	0	•
	Celery	★	40g	0	0	•
	Chillies, fresh or dried	★	20g	0	0	•
	Chives, fresh	★	4g	0	0	•
	Cucumber	★	45g	0	0	•
	Eggplant	★	100g	2.5	0	•
	Endive	★	30g	0	0	•
	Fennel	★	90g	0	0	•
	Garlic	★	5g	0	0	•
	Ginger	★	10g	0	0	•
	Herbs, fresh or dried	★	2g	0	0	•
	Leeks	★	80g	3	0	•
	Lettuce	★	50g	0	0	•
	Mushrooms	★	35g	0.5	0	•
	Okra	★	80g	1	0	•
	Onions, raw, peeled	★	30g	2	0	•
	Onions, stir-fried without extra oil	★	100g	8	0.5	•
	Radishes	★	15g	0	0	•
	Rocket	★	30g	0	0	•
	Shallots	★	10g	0	0	•

★ little or no carbs ■ high in saturated fat ● untested/unknown Ⓖ GI Symbol partner

GISP	FOOD	GI	HOUSEHOLD MEASURE & WEIGHT	CARB (G) PER SERVE	CARB EXCHANGE PER SERVE	GL PER SERVE
	Silverbeet	★	35g	0	0	•
	Snowpea sprouts	★	15g	0	0	•
	Spinach	★	75g	0	0	•
	Spring onions	★	15g	0	0	•
	Squash, yellow	★	70g	2	0	•
	Tomato	★	150g	3	0	•
	Turnip	★	120g	4	0	•
	Watercress	★	8g	0	0	•
	Zucchini	★	100g	1.5	0	•
GREEN/SALAD VEGETABLES – HIGHER GI (MORE THAN 55 OR UNKNOWN)						
	Broad beans, frozen, reheated	63	½ cup, 75g	2	<0.5	1

★ little or no carbs   ■ high in saturated fat   ● untested/unknown   ⓒ GI Symbol partner

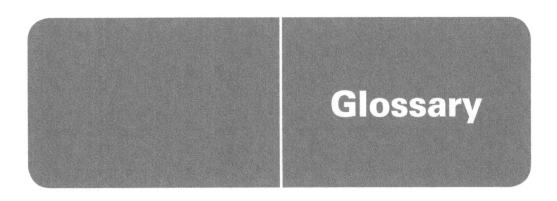

Glossary

An A to Z of key terms used throughout this book

A1c See **HbA1c**.

Alternative sweeteners include nutritive sweeteners (which add kilojoules to the diet) and non-nutritive sweeteners, which are kilojoule free.

Nutritive sweeteners, including sugars, sugar-alcohols and oligosaccharides (medium-sized chains of glucose), are simply different types of carbohydrate with varying levels of sweetness. The sugar alcohols sorbitol, mannitol and maltitol are generally not as sweet as table sugar, provide fewer kilojoules, and have less of an impact on blood glucose levels.

Non-nutritive sweeteners (such as Equal, Splenda, Stevia, NutraSweet, or saccharin, for example) are all much sweeter than table sugar and have essentially no effect on your blood glucose levels because most are used in such small quantities and are not absorbed into or metabolised by the body. Because they are used in only minute amounts, the number of kilojoules they provide is insignificant. Non-nutritive sweeteners made of protein molecules often break down when heated for long periods and lose their sweetness.

Area under the curve refers, in the context of the GI testing of food, to the mathematical space under blood glucose response to any food. It is calculated using a computer program.

Atherosclerosis, or hardening of the arteries, is a slow, progressive disease that produces problems such as angina, heart attack or stroke. Most heart disease is caused by atherosclerosis–clogging on the inside wall of the coronary arteries through the slow build-up of fatty deposits (called plaque) that narrow the arteries and reduce the blood flow. If the plaque ruptures, clots form, causing a more acute, total blockage. If the blood vessel is providing blood to the heart, the result is a heart attack. Atherosclerosis can affect the arteries to the heart and in the brain, kidneys and the arms and legs.

Autoimmune disease is a disorder in which the body's immune system mistakenly attacks and destroys body tissue or organs that it believes to be foreign; type 1 diabetes (see below) is an autoimmune condition.

Beta cells produce the hormone insulin. They are found grouped together in 'islands' (the Islets of Langerhans) in the pancreas.

Blood glucose (blood sugar or **glucose**) is the most common kind of sugar found in the blood and is a major source of energy for most of the body's organs and tissues and the only source of fuel for the brain. When the body's digestive organs process carbohydrates, they end up mostly as glucose, which passes through the walls of the intestine into the bloodstream to the liver and eventually into general circulation. From here glucose enters individual cells or tissues throughout the body to be used for fuel and energy.

Blood glucose level (BGL) is the amount of glucose in the bloodstream. If you haven't eaten in the past few hours (and you don't have diabetes), your blood glucose level will normally fall within the range of 4–6 mmol/L. If you eat, this will rise, but rarely above 10 mmol/L, unless you have diabetes. The extent of the increase will vary depending on your glucose tolerance (your own physiological response) and the type of food you have just eaten.

Blood pressure is the pressure of the blood on the inside walls of your blood vessels caused by the beating of the heart. It is expressed as a ratio such as '120/80.' The first number is the *systolic* pressure, or the pressure when the heart pushes the blood out into the arteries. The second number is the *diastolic* pressure, or the pressure when the heart rests between beats. High blood pressure (or hypertension), above 140/90, is the most common cardiovascular risk factor. High blood pressure is more prevalent in people with diabetes and increases the risk of stroke, heart attack and diseases of the kidney and eye. Your blood pressure should be measured when you visit your doctor for checkups or at least twice a year, with a goal of 130/80 mm Hg or lower.

Blood sugar. See **blood glucose**.

BMI (Body Mass Index) is a measure that evaluates body relative to height to find out if an individual is underweight, in the healthy weight range, overweight, or obese. It has limitations: it can overestimate body fat in athletes and others who have a muscular build, such as body builders, and in pregnant women, and it can underestimate body fat in older people or people with a disability who have lost muscle mass. It's not appropriate for children and young people under eighteen. For an easy online calculator, go to www.nhlbisupport.com/bmi/

BMI categories:

Less than 18.5	Underweight
18.5–24.9	Healthy weight range
25–29.9	Overweight
Over 30	Obese

For Maori and Pacific Island people: BMI is 20–26 for the healthy weight range, 27–31 for overweight, and over 32 for obese.

Calorie (or kilocalorie, to be technically correct) is the old unit that measures the energy you get from the food you eat (your energy intake). The term is used in the United States, while Australians use kilojoules, the metric equivalent. You can convert calories to kilojoules by multiplying by 4.2; you can convert kilojoules to calories by dividing by 4.2.

Carbohydrate is one of the three main macronutrients in food; protein and fat are the other two. Carbohydrate is the starchy part of foods like rice, bread, legumes, potatoes and pasta and the sugars in foods like fruit, milk and honey and most types of fibre. Some foods contain a large amount of carbohydrate (cereals, potatoes, sweet potatoes, yams, taro and legumes), while other foods, such as carrots, broccoli and salad vegetables, are very dilute sources. *See also* **fibre**, **starches** and **sugars**.

Carbohydrate counting is a method of meal planning for people with diabetes based on counting the grams of carbohydrate in food. It ignores the type of carbohydrate and its GI.

Carbohydrate exchange is an amount of food typically containing an average of 15 grams of carbohydrate. It is one of several approaches to meal planning for people with diabetes. Lists set out the serving sizes of different carb foods. A dietitian assigns a certain number of exchanges to each meal over the course of the day. The system is intended to promote consistency in the amount of carbohydrate eaten from day to day. It was developed long before research on the glycemic index was published, and thus the emphasis is on carbohydrate quantity rather than carbohydrate quality.

Cardiovascular disease, or CVD, refers to the diseases that involve the heart and/or blood vessels (arteries and veins), particularly those related to atherosclerosis in the heart, brain and lower limbs.

Cardiovascular system is the heart and blood vessels. It is the means by which blood is pumped from the heart and circulated through the body. As the blood circulates, it carries nourishment and oxygen to all the body's tissues. It also removes waste products.

Coeliac disease is a condition in which the lining of the small intestine is damaged due to an immune reaction from the body to gluten, a small protein. Gluten is found in certain grain foods, such as wheat, rye, triticale (a hybrid of wheat and rye) and barley, and in much smaller amounts in oats (as a contaminant). The only treatment for coeliac disease at present is a gluten-free diet.

Central obesity, or a high waist measurement, is often a better predictor of your health risks than BMI. Abdominal fat increases your risk of heart disease, high blood pressure and diabetes. The cutoff waist measurements are:

For people of Caucasian (European) origin:

Men	94 cm
Women	80 cm

For people from South Asia, China and Japan:

Men	90 cm
Women	80 cm

Until more specific data are available:

Ethnic South and Central Americans should use South Asian data. Sub-Saharan Africans should use European data. Eastern Mediterranean and Middle East (Arab) populations should use European data.

Cholesterol is a soft waxy substance found in the blood and in all the body's cells. It is an important part of a healthy body because it is part of the membrane around all the body's cells and is a major component of many of the hormones the body produces. Most of the cholesterol the body needs can be manufactured by the liver. It is found in animal foods (eggs, milk, cheese, liver, meat and poultry), but not plants. High levels of cholesterol in the blood are related to excessive intake of saturated fat, rather than dietary cholesterol. A high level can lead to blocked arteries, heart attack and stroke. Cholesterol and other fats can't dissolve in the blood. They have to be transported to and from the cells by special carriers called *lipoproteins*. The most common ones are low-density lipoprotein (LDL) cholesterol and high-density lipoprotein (HDL) cholesterol.

HDL cholesterol is known as 'good' cholesterol because higher levels of HDL protect against heart attack and stroke. HDL tends to sweep excess cholesterol from the blood back to the liver, where it is eliminated from the body.

LDL cholesterol is the main form of cholesterol in the blood and does most of the damage to blood vessels; it's a red flag for cardiovascular disease. If there is too much LDL cholesterol in the blood, it can slowly build up in the walls of the blood vessels that feed the heart, brain and other important organs, causing a heart attack or stroke.

Recommended ranges for people with diabetes:

Total cholesterol	<5.1 mmol/L
Triglycerides	<1.7 mmol/L
HDL cholesterol	
men:	>1.0 mmol/L
women:	>1.3 mmol/L
LDL cholesterol	<2.5 mmol/L

Total cholesterol/HDL ratio men: <5.0; women: <4.0

Complications are the harmful effects of diabetes, including damage to the blood vessels, heart, nervous system, eyes, feet, kidneys, teeth and gums. Studies show that keeping blood glucose, blood pressure and cholesterol levels within the recommended ranges can help to prevent or delay these problems.

Diabetes *Type 1 diabetes* is characterised by high blood glucose levels due to the body's complete inability to produce insulin. It occurs when the body's immune system attacks the insulin-producing beta cells in the pancreas and destroys them. The pancreas then produces very little or no insulin. Type 1 diabetes occurs most often in young people but can develop in adults.

Type 2 diabetes is characterised by high blood glucose levels caused by an insufficiency of insulin and the body's inability to use insulin efficiently. It occurs when the body becomes excessively **insulin resistant.** The pancreas compensates initially by producing more insulin, then eventually becomes 'exhausted' and fails to produce enough insulin. Type 2 diabetes occurs most often in middle-aged and older people but is being seen increasingly in younger people at the time of puberty. See also **gestational diabetes**.

Energy The foods we eat provide energy (fuel for the body), which is measured in kilojoules or calories. Just how much energy a food provides depends on the amount of carbohydrate, protein and fat it contains. The technical term for this used to be 'calorie', but 'kilojoule' tends now to be accepted internationally. The terms *kilojoule* and *calorie* allow us to talk about how much energy a food contains and how much energy is burned up during exercise.

Energy density The number of kilojoules in a food, per gram or per serving size.

Fasting blood glucose is a blood test in which a sample of your blood is drawn after an overnight fast (8–12 hours) to measure the amount of glucose in your blood. The test is used to diagnose diabetes and pre-diabetes and to monitor people who already have type 2 diabetes.

Fat is one of the three main nutrients in food and provides 37 kilojoules per gram. Today's health message is to focus on the good fats (mono- and omega 3-polyunsaturated fats) and avoid the bad fats (saturated fats and trans fats). All fats are actually mixtures of saturated and unsaturated fats.

Saturated fats are solid or semisolid at room temperature. They are found in both plant and animal foods. Saturated fats raise blood cholesterol levels by increasing the amount of cholesterol produced by the liver, causing it to build up in the bloodstream and become part of the plaque that forms on the walls of the blood vessels.

Monounsaturated fat is a type of unsaturated fat that can be found in both animal and plant foods. It's considered to be healthy fat; in fact, studies show that it can boost levels of good HDL cholesterol and that a diet rich in monounsaturated fats may reduce the risk of heart disease. Rich sources include olive oil, canola oil and nuts.

Polyunsaturated fat is a type of unsaturated fat that also comes from both animal and plant foods. It's healthier than saturated fat, but some forms lower levels of both bad LDL cholesterol *and* good HDL cholesterol. Sources include safflower, sunflower, soybean, corn and cottonseed oils. Salmon, tuna and other fish contain large amounts of omega–3 polyunsaturated fats, which are the healthiest of all.

Transfatty acids or *trans fats* occur naturally in small amounts in the fat of dairy products and meat. They are also formed by hydrogenation – a chemical process that changes a liquid oil into a solid fat. In the United States, fried fast foods, some margarines, crackers, biscuits and snack foods are high in trans fat but Australian products are usually not. Trans fats can raise cholesterol levels and are linked with an increased risk of cardiovascular disease.

Fatty liver disease is the buildup of excessive amounts of triglycerides and other fats inside liver cells; also known as non-alcoholic fatty liver (NAFL) or *steatohepatitis* or *NASH* (non-alcoholic steatohepatitis).

Fibre Dietary fibres are mainly carbohydrate molecules made up of many different sorts of *monosaccharides*. They are different from starches and sugars in that they are not broken down by human digestive enzymes, and they reach the large intestine largely unchanged. Once there, bacteria begin to ferment and break down the fibres. Dietary fibre comes mainly from the outer bran layers of grains (corn, oats, wheat and rice and in foods containing these grains), fruits and vegetables, and nuts and legumes (dried beans, peas and lentils). There are three main types of fibre-soluble, insoluble and resistant starch.

Soluble fibres can be dissolved in water – the gel, gum and often jellylike components of apples, oats and legumes. Some soluble fibres are very viscous when in solution. By slowing down the time it takes for food to pass through the stomach and small intestine, soluble fibre can lower the glycemic response to a food. Good sources include porridge, oat bran, nuts and seeds, legumes (beans, peas and lentils), apples, pears, strawberries and blueberries.

Insoluble fibres such as cellulose, are insoluble, meaning they are not soluble in water and don't reduce blood glucose directly. Indirectly, they improve insulin sensitivity and glucose tolerance. They are dry and bran-like and are commonly called *roughage*. All cereal grains and products that retain the outer coat of the grain they are made from are sources of insoluble fibre, e.g. whole-wheat bread and All-Bran®, but not all foods containing insoluble fibre are low GI. Insoluble fibres will only lower the GI of a food when they exist in their original, intact form; for example, in whole grains of wheat. Here they act as a physical barrier, delaying access of digestive enzymes and water to the starch within the cereal grain. Good sources include whole grains, wholemeal breads, barley, couscous, brown rice, bulghur, wheat bran, seeds and most vegetables.

Resistant starch. See page 374.

Fructose. See **sugars**.

Fuel hierarchy The body runs on fuel the way a car runs on gasoline. The fuels the body burns are derived from a mixture of the protein, fat, carbohydrate and alcohol you consume. The fuel hierarchy describes the priority for burning the fuels in food. Alcohol is burned first, because the body has no place to store unused alcohol and it is potentially toxic to many of the body's organs and tissues. Excess protein comes second, followed by carbohydrate, while fat is last in line. In practice, the fuel mix is usually a combination of carbohydrate and fat in varying proportions – after meals the mix is mainly carbohydrate; before meals it is mainly fat.

Gestational diabetes can develop during pregnancy but usually goes away following the birth of the baby. Type 2 diabetes often develops later in life. Hormones released by the placenta during pregnancy reduce the effectiveness of the mother's insulin. This insulin resistance of pregnancy is normal, but in some women it is more than the beta-cells can deal with. It is usually managed successfully with healthy eating and regular physical activity. Some women may require insulin as well.

Glucose is a simple form of sugar (a *monosaccharide*) that is created when the body's digestive processes break down the carbohydrate foods you eat such as bread, cereals and fruit. It is this glucose that is absorbed from the intestine and becomes the fuel that circulates in the bloodstream.

Glucose tolerance test (**GTT**) a test used in the diagnosis of diabetes and pre-diabetes. Glucose in the blood is measured at regular intervals for a couple of hours before and after a person has drunk 75 g of pure glucose, after an overnight fast.

Glycemia is the concentration of glucose in the blood. Hence the adjective **glycemic**.

Glycemic index (**GI**) Ranks carbohydrate foods according to their glycemic potency. Some carbs break down quickly during digestion and release glucose rapidly into the bloodstream; others break down gradually and slowly trickle glucose into the blood stream. The glycemic index, or GI, is a numerical ranking on a scale of 0 to 100 that describes this difference. It is a measure of carbohydrate quality. After testing hundreds of carbohydrate foods around the world, scientists have found that foods with a low GI will have less effect on your blood glucose than foods with a high GI. High-GI foods tend to cause spikes in your glucose levels, whereas low GI foods tend to cause gentle increases. All foods are compared with a reference food and tested using an internationally standardised method.

Glycemic Index Symbol Program is a program that helps consumers make nutritious carbohydrate choices, whatever the GI. Manufacturers must have their carbohydrate foods GI tested at an accredited laboratory and show the value on the food's packaging. Foods that are part of the GISP must meet strict nutrition criteria to ensure that they are healthy foods. They are easily identified by the program's distinct symbol 🌀. More details can be found at

the program's web site,
www.gisymbol.com.au

Glycemic load (**GL**) is a number that depends on both the quality of the carbohydrate (its GI) and the quantity of carbohydrate in the meal. You can think of the GL as the *amount* of carbohydrate adjusted for its glycemic impact. It is calculated by multiplying the GI of a food by the available carbohydrate content (carbohydrate minus fibre) in the serving (expressed in grams), divided by 100 (GL = GI ÷ 100 × available carbs per serving).

Glycemic response or **glycemic impact** describes the actual change or pattern of change in blood glucose after you have consumed a food or a meal. Glucose response can be fast or slow, short or prolonged. It varies from person to person, from day to day, and with the amount of carbohydrate and the kind of carbohydrate in the meal.

Glycosylated haemoglobin . See **A1c**.

Gram is a unit of weight in the metric system. One typical slice of bread is 15 grams.

Glycogen is the name given to the glucose stores in the body. It can be readily broken down into glucose to maintain normal blood glucose levels. Approximately 60 per cent of the body's glycogen is found in the muscles and 40 per cent in the liver. The total stores of glycogen in the body are relatively small, however, and will be exhausted in about twenty-four hours during fasting or starvation.

HbA1c (also called **A1c**), **haemoglobin A1c**, or **glycosylated or glycolated haemoglobin**) a blood test that measures your average blood glucose level over the previous 2–3 months. It indicates the percentage of haemoglobin (the part of the red blood cell that carries oxygen) that ahs become 'glycated'. *Glycated* means it has a glucose molecule riding on its back. This is always proportional to the amount of glucose in the blood. The higher the level of HbA1c, the greater the risk of developing diabetic complications. If you have diabetes, it should be measured 2–4 times a year, depending on your type, and you should aim to keep it under 7 per cent.

HDL cholesterol. See **cholesterol**.

High blood glucose. See **hyperglycaemia**.

Hormones are 'chemical messengers' made in one part of the body and released into the bloodstream to trigger or regulate particular functions of another part of the body. For example, insulin is a hormone made in the pancreas that plays a master role in growth and metabolism.

Hyperglycaemia is a condition that occurs when there are excessively high levels of glucose in the blood. The symptoms usually occur when blood glucose levels go above 270 mg/dL (15 mmol/L), and include extreme thirst, frequent urination and large volumes of urine, weakness and weight loss. If left untreated it can lead to the *ketoacidosis* and eventually unconsciousness, coma and death.

Hyperinsulinemia is a condition when the level of insulin in the blood is higher than normal. It is caused by excessive secretion of insulin by the pancreas and is related to **insulin resistance**.

Hypertension. See **blood pressure**.

Hypoglycaemia (also called an insulin reaction) occurs when a person's blood glucose falls below normal levels – usually less than 3.5 mmol/L. It is treated by consuming a carb-rich food, such as a glucose tablet or juice. It may also be treated with an injection of *glucagon* if the person is unconscious or unable to swallow. See also **reactive hypoglycaemia**.

Immune system is the body's defence system, which protects itself from viruses, bacteria and any 'foreign' substances.

Impaired fasting glucose is a condition in which the fasting blood glucose level is elevated >6.1 mmol/L) after an overnight fast but is not high enough to be classified as diabetes. It is sometimes called **pre-diabetes**.

Impaired glucose tolerance is a condition in which the blood glucose level is elevated (>7.8mmol/L) after a two-hour oral glucose tolerance test but is not high enough to be classified as diabetes. It is now called **pre-diabetes**. People with impaired glucose tolerance are at increased risk of developing diabetes, heart disease and stroke.

Insulin is a hormone produced by the pancreas that facilitates the passage of glucose into muscle cells, where it is used to create energy for the body. The pancreas should automatically produce the right amount of insulin to move glucose into the cells. When the body cannot make enough insulin, it has to be taken by injection or through use of an insulin pump. It can't be taken by mouth, because it will be broken down by the body's digestive juices. Insulin is not only involved in regulating blood glucose levels, but it also plays a key part in determining whether we burn fat or carbohydrate to meet our energy needs – it switches muscle cells from fat burning to carb burning. For this reason, lowering insulin levels is one of the secrets to weight control.

Insulinemia simply means the presence of insulin in the blood; hyperinsulinemia is excessive amounts of insulin in the blood.

Insulin resistance means that your muscle and liver cells are resisting glucose uptake. Chances are you'll have very high insulin levels even long after a meal, as the body tries to metabolise the carbohydrate in the meal. When insulin levels in the body are chronically raised, the cells that usually respond to insulin become resistant to its signals. The body then responds by secreting more and more insulin, a never-ending vicious cycle that spells trouble on many fronts. Insulin resistance is at the root of pre-diabetes and type 2 diabetes, many forms of heart disease and polycystic ovarian syndrome (PCOS).

Insulin resistance syndrome. See **metabolic syndrome**.

Insulin sensitivity If you are insulin sensitive, your muscle and liver cells take up glucose rapidly without the need for a lot of insulin. Exercise keeps you insulin sensitive; so does a moderately high carbohydrate intake.

Ketones are the breakdown products of fat, which can be used as a source of fuel if required. They occur in higher concentrations when the body is unable to use glucose as a fuel source. Ketones are strong acids, and when they are produced in large quantities they can upset the body's delicate acid-base balance. They are normally released into the urine, but if levels are very high or if the person is dehydrated, they may begin to build up in the blood. High blood levels of ketones may cause bad breath, loss of appetite, nausea or vomiting, fast, deep breathing (to blow off the acid in the form of carbon dioxide), and excessive urination (to eliminate the extra acid). In severe cases, it may lead to coma and death. In a pregnant woman, even a moderate amount of ketones in the blood may harm the baby and impair brain development. The excessive formation of ketones in the blood is called *ketosis*. Large amounts of ketones in the urine may signal *diabetic ketoacidosis*, a dangerous condition that is caused by very high blood glucose levels.

Ketosis is the metabolic state in which the body is burning only fat for fuel. Normally, carbohydrates are the main source of fuel for your brain and nervous system, kidneys, and many other organs.

Kilojoule (kJ) is the metric system for measuring the amount of energy produced when food is completely metabolised in the body. You can convert kilojoules to calories by dividing by 4.2; you can convert calories to kilojoules by multiplying by 4.2.

LDL cholesterol. See **cholesterol**.

Lipid profile is a blood test that measures total cholesterol, triglycerides and HDL cholesterol. LDL cholesterol is then usually calculated from the results, though it can sometimes be measured separately. Your lipid profile is one measure of your risk of cardiovascular disease.

Lipids is a term for fat in the body and in food. The most common lipids are cholesterol and triglycerides (sometimes called triacylglycerols).

Macronutrients are the three main components in foods: **carbohydrate**, **protein** and **fat**.

Metabolic syndrome is a cluster of risk factors for heart disease and diabetes. A person with metabolic syndrome will have central or abdominal obesity plus two of the following risk factors: high triglycerides, low HDL cholesterol, raised blood pressure, raised blood glucose. Tests on patients with the metabolic syndrome show that insulin resistance is very common.

Metabolism is the term used to describe how the cells of the body chemically change the food you consume and make the protein, fats and carbohydrates into forms of energy or use them for growth and repair.

mg/dL stands for milligrams per decilitre – a unit of measure that shows the concentration of a substance in a specific amount of fluid. In the United States, blood glucose test results are reported as mg/dL. Medical journals and other countries, including Canada, use millimoles per liter (mmol/L). To convert blood glucose levels to mg/dL from mmol/L, multiply mmol/L by 18. Example: 10 mmol/L × 18 = 180 mg/dL.

mmol/L stands for millimoles per litre – a unit of measure that shows the concentration of a substance in a specific amount of fluid. In most of the world, including Canada, blood glucose test results are reported as mmol/L. In the United States, milligrams per deciliter (mg/dL) is used. To convert blood glucose results to mmol/L from mg/dL, divide mg/dL × 18. Example: 180 mg/dL ÷ 18 = 10 mmol/L.

Monounsaturated fat. See **fats**.

Nurses' Health Study Established in 1976 by Dr Frank Speiser at Harvard's Channing Laboratory, one of the largest ongoing studies of the risk factors in women for developing major chronic diseases. The study follows registered nurses, because due to their medical background, they can easily and accurately answer specific, health-related questions. Every two years, more than 100,000 nurses provide personal information about diseases and health, including diet and nutrition, smoking, hormones, and general quality of life. The study is now conducted under the aegis of the Harvard School of Public Health.

Obesity is defined as when a person's BMI is >30 kg/m2. The risk of developing pre-diabetes, type 2 diabetes, heart disease, stroke and arthritis is very high when a person is obese.

Overweight is defined as when a person's BMI is between 25 and 29.9 kg/m2. The healthy weight range is 18.5–24.9 kg/m2. The risk of developing pre-diabetes, type 2 diabetes, heart disease and stroke starts to increase when a person is overweight.

Pancreas is a vital organ near the stomach that secretes the digestive juices that help break down food during digestion and produces the hormones insulin and glucagon.

PCOS (polycystic ovarian syndrome) can have a number of different causes. Elements of PCOS are thought to affect one in four women in developed countries. At the root of PCOS is insulin resistance. The signs of PCOS range from subtle symptoms such as faint facial hair to a 'full house' syndrome-lack of periods, infertility, heavy body-hair growth, acne or skin pigmentation, obstinate body fat, diabetes and cardiovascular disease.

Postprandial glucose The increase in blood glucose that occurs immediately after a meal that contains appreciable (>10 grams per serving) amounts of carbohydrate.

Pre-diabetes is a condition in which blood glucose levels are higher than normal but not high enough for a diagnosis of diabetes. People with pre-diabetes may have impaired fasting glucose or impaired glucose tolerance. Some people have both. Studies show that most people with pre-diabetes will develop type 2 diabetes within ten years if they don't make lifestyle changes such as losing weight, eating a healthy diet and exercising more. They are also at increased risk of having a heart attack or stroke.

Protein is one of the three main macronutrients from food along with fat and carbohydrate. The body uses protein to build and repair body tissue-muscles, bones, skin, hair and virtually every other body part are made of protein. The best sources are meat, egg, fish, seafood, poultry and dairy foods. Other sources are plant proteins-legumes (beans, chickpeas and lentils), tofu, cereal grains (especially whole grains) and nuts and seeds. Because our bodies can't stockpile amino acids (the building blocks of protein) from one day to the next as it does fat or carbs, we need a daily supply. Women on average need about 45 grams of protein a day (more if they are pregnant or breast-feeding) and men about 55 grams. Active people may need more, as do growing children and teenagers. In practice, we eat much more protein than we actually need and break the excess down as a source of energy.

Polyunsaturated fat. See **fats**.

Reactive hypoglycaemia is a lay term to describe blood glucose levels rising too quickly after you have eaten, causing the release of too much insulin. This then draws too much glucose out of the blood, your blood glucose levels fall below normal, and you suffer a variety of unpleasant symptoms, including sweating, tremor, anxiety, palpitations, weakness, restlessness, irritability, poor concentration, lethargy and drowsiness. Most doctors believe it is in people's imaginations – but it's not.

Resistant starch is the starch that completely resists digestion in the small intestine. It cannot contribute to glycemia because it is not absorbed but passes through to the large intestine, where it acts just like dietary fibre to improve bowel health. Sources of resistant starch are foods such as unprocessed cereals and whole grains, firm (unripe) bananas, legumes and especially starchy foods that have been cooked and then cooled (such as cold potatoes). Resistant starch is also added to some refined cereal products, including breads and breakfast cereals, to increase their fibre content.

Retinopathy is damage to the retina of the eye caused by high blood glucose and blood pressure. It is a major cause of blindness in people with diabetes. Modern laser therapy may be used to treat people with this condition.

Risk factor is anything that increases your chances of developing a disease.

Satiety is the feeling of fullness and satisfaction we experience after eating. Carbohydrate-rich foods and protein provide the best satiety.

Saturated fats. See **fats**.

Starches are long chains of sugar molecules. They are called *polysaccharides* (poly meaning many). They are not sweet-tasting. There are two sorts – amylose and amylopectin. *Amylose* is a straight-chain molecule, like a string of beads. These tend to line up in rows and form tight, compact clumps that are harder to gelatinise and therefore digest. *Amylopectin* is a string of glucose molecules with lots of branching points, such as you see in some types of seaweed. Amylopectin molecules are larger and more open and the starch is easier to gelatinise and digest. See also **resistant starch**.

Starch gelatinisation occurs when starch granules have swollen and burst during cooking – the starch is said to be fully gelatinised. The starch in raw food is stored in hard, compact granules that make it difficult to digest. Most starchy foods need to be cooked for this reason. During cooking, water and heat expand the starch granules to different degrees; some granules actually burst and free the individual starch molecules. The swollen granules and free starch molecules are very easy to digest, because the starch-digesting enzymes in the small intestine have a greater surface area to attack. A food containing starch that is fully gelatinised will therefore have a high GI value.

Sugars are a type of carbohydrate. The simplest is a single-sugar molecule called a *monosaccharide* (mono meaning one, saccharide meaning sweet). Glucose is a monosaccharide that occurs in food (as glucose itself and as the building block of starch). If two monosaccharides are joined together, the result is a *disaccharide* (di meaning two). *Sucrose*, or common table sugar, is a disaccharide, as is *lactose*, the sugar in milk. As the number of monosaccharides in the chain increases, the carbohydrate becomes less sweet. Maltodextrins are *oligosaccharides* (oligo meaning a few) that are 5 or 6 glucose residues long and commonly used as a food ingredient. They taste only faintly sweet.

Syndrome X. See **metabolic syndrome**.

Trans fats. See **fats**. **Triglycerides**, also known as **triacylglycerols** or **blood fats**, are another type of fat linked to increased risk of heart disease. Having too much triglyceride often goes hand in hand with having too little HDL cholesterol. Having high levels of triglycerides can be inherited, but it's most often associated with being overweight or obese. People with diabetes should aim to keep their triglyceride levels under 1.7 mmol/L, as they are at greater risk of cardiovascular disease.

Type 1 diabetes. See **diabetes**.

Type 2 diabetes. See **diabetes**.

Unsaturated fat. See **fats**.

Vasodilation is the normal increase in the diameter of blood vessels that occurs after a meal.

Further reading

Sources and references

Amano, Kawakubo and Lee, 'Correlation between dietary glycemic index and cardiovascular disease risk factors among Japanese women', *European Journal of Clinical Nutrition*, 58(11), 1472–8, 2004.

Bahadori, Yazdani-Biuki, Krippl et al, 'Low-fat, high-carbohydrate (low-glycaemic index) diet induces weight loss and preserves lean body mass in obese healthy subjects: results of a 24-week study', *Diabetes, Obesity and Metabolism*, 7(3), 290–3, 2005.

Barclay, Flood, Rochtchina et al, 'Glycemic Index, dietary fibre and risk of type 2 diabetes in a cohort of older Australians', *Diabetes Care*, 30, 2811–2813, 2007.

Benton and Nabb, 'Carbohydrate, memory, and mood', *Nutrition Reviews*, 61(5), S61–7, 2003.

Benton, 'Carbohydrate ingestion, blood glucose and mood', *Neuroscience and Biobehavioral Reviews*, 26(3), 293–308, 2002.

Benton, Ruffin, Lassel et al, 'The delivery rate of dietary carbohydrates affects cognitive performance in both rats and humans', *Psychopharmacology*, 166(1), 86–90, 2003.

Beulens, de Bruijne, Stolk et al, 'High dietary glycemic load and glycemic index increase risk of cardiovascular disease among middle-aged women: a population-based follow-up study', *Journal of the American College of Cardiology*, 50(1), 14–21, 2007.

Brand-Miller, Hayne, Petocz et al, 'Low-glycemic index diets in the management of diabetes: a meta-analysis of randomized controlled trials', *Diabetes Care*, 26(8), 2261–7, 2003.

Chiu, Hubbard, Armstrong et al, 'Dietary glycemic index and carbohydrate in relation to early age-related macular degeneration', *American Journal of Clinical Nutrition*, 83(4), 880–6, 2006.

Davis, Miller, Mitchell et al, 'More favorable dietary patterns are associated with lower glycemic load in older adults', *Journal of the American Dietetic Association*, 104(12), 1828–35, 2004.

DeMarco, Sucher, Cisar et al, 'Pre-exercise carbohydrate meals: application of glycemic index', *Medicine and Science in Sports and Exercise*, 31(1), 164–70, 1999.

Ebbeling, Leidig, Sinclair et al, 'A reduced-glycemic load diet in the treatment of adolescent obesity', *Archives of Pediatric and Adolescent Medicine*, 157(8), 773–9, 2003.

FAO/WHO, Expert consultation, Carbohydrates in human nutrition, FAO Food and Nutrition Paper, 66, 1997.

Foster-Powell, Holt, Brand-Miller et al, 'International table of glycemic index and glycemic load values: 2002', *American Journal of Clinical Nutrition*, 76(1), 5–56, 2002.

Frost, Wilding and Beecham, 'Dietary advice based on the glycaemic index improves dietary profile and metabolic control in type 2 diabetic patients', *Diabetic Medicine*, 11(4), 397–401, 1994.

Galgani, Aguirre, Díaz et al, 'Acute effect of meal glycemic index and glycemic load on blood glucose and insulin responses in humans', *Nutrition Journal*, 5(5), 22, 2006.

Gilbertson, Brand-Miller, Thorburn et al, 'The effect of flexible low glycemic index dietary advice versus measured carbohydrate exchange diets on glycemic control in children with type 1 diabetes', *Diabetes Care*, 24(7), 1137–43, 2001.

Halton, Willett, Liu et al, 'Low-carbohydrate-diet score and the risk of coronary heart disease in women', *New England Journal of Medicine*, 355(19), 1991–2002, 2006.

Higginbotham, Zhang, Cook et al, 'Dietary glycemic load and risk of colorectal cancer in the Women's Health Study', *Journal of the National Cancer Institute*, 96(3), 229–233, 2004.

Hodge, English, O'Dea et al, 'Glycemic index and dietary fiber and the risk of type 2 diabetes', *Diabetes Care*, 27(11), 2701–6, 2004.

Holmes, Liu, Hankinson et al, 'Dietary carbohydrates, fiber, and breast cancer risk', *American Journal of Epidemiology*, 159(8), 732–739, 2004.

Järvi, Karlström, Granfeldt et al, 'Improved glycemic control and lipid profile and normalized fibrinolytic activity on a low-glycemic index diet in type 2 diabetic patients', *Diabetes Care*, 22(1), 10–18, 1999.

Jenkins, Woleve and Kalmusky, 'Low glycemic index carbohydrate foods in the management of hyperlipidemia', *American Journal of Clinical Nutrition*, 42(4), 604–17, 1985.

Jenkins, Wolever, Taylor et al, 'Glycemic index of foods: a physiological basis for carbohydrate exchange', *American Journal of Clinical Nutrition*, 34(3), 362–6, 1981.

Kirwan, O'Gorman, Evans et al, 'A moderate glycemic meal before endurance exercise can enhance performance', *Journal of Applied Physiology*, 84(1), 53–9, 1998.

Larsson, Friberg, Wolk et al, 'Carbohydrate intake, glycemic index and glycemic load in relation to risk of endometrial cancer: A prospective study of Swedish women', *International Journal of Cancer*, 120(5), 1103–7, 2007.

Liu, Willett, Stampfer et al, 'A prospective study of dietary glycemic load, carbohydrate intake, and risk of coronary heart disease in US women', *American Journal of Clinical Nutrition*, 71, 1455–61, 2000.

McMillan-Price, Petocz and Atkinson, 'Comparison of 4 diets of varying glycemic load on weight loss and cardiovascular risk reduction in overweight and obese young adults: a randomized controlled trial', *Archives of Internal Medicine*, 166(14), 1466–75, 2006.

Michaud, Fuchs, Liu et al, 'Dietary glycemic load, carbohydrate, sugar, and colorectal cancer risk in men and women', *Cancer Epidemiology, Biomarkers & Prevention*, 14(1), 138–43, 2005.

Moses, Luebcke, Davis et al, 'Effect of a low-glycemic-index diet during pregnancy on obstetric outcomes', *American Journal of Clinical Nutrition*, 84(4), 807–12, 2006.

Murakami, Sasaki and Takahashi, 'Dietary glycemic index and load in relation to metabolic risk factors in Japanese female farmers with traditional dietary habits', *American Journal of Clinical Nutrition*, 83(5), 1161–9, 2006.

Nabb and Benton, 'The effect of the interaction between glucose tolerance and breakfasts varying in carbohydrate and fibre on mood and cognition', *Nutritional Neuroscience*, 9(3), 161–8, 2006.

Oh, Willett, Manson et al, 'Carbohydrate intake, glycemic index, glycemic load, and dietary fiber in relation to risk of stroke in women', *American Journal of Epidemiology*, 161(2), 161–169, 2005.

Opperman, Venter, Oosthuizen et al, 'Meta-analysis of the health effects of using the glycaemic index in meal-planning', *British Journal of Nutrition*, 92(3), 367–81, 2004.

Papanikolaou, Palmer, Binns et al, 'Better cognitive performance following a low-glycaemic-index compared with a high-glycaemic-index carbohydrate meal in adults with type 2 diabetes', *Diabetologia*, 49(5), 855–62, 2006.

Patel, McCullough, Pavluck et al, 'Glycemic load, glycemic index, and carbohydrate intake in relation to pancreatic cancer risk in a large US cohort', *Cancer Causes Control*, 18(3), 287–94, 2007.

Rizkalla, Taghrid, Laromiguiere et al, 'Improved plasma glucose control, whole-body glucose utilization, and lipid profile on a low-glycemic index diet in type 2 diabetic men: a randomized controlled trial', *Diabetes Care*, 27(8), 1866–72, 2004.

Salmeron, Ascherio, Rimm et al, 'Dietary fiber, glycemic load, and risk of NIDDM in men', *Diabetes Care*, 20, 545–550, 1997.

Salmeron, Manson, Stampfer et al, 'Dietary fiber, glycemic load, and risk of non-insulin dependant diabetes mellitus in women', *Journal of the American Medical Association*, 277, 472–477, 1997.

Schaumberg, Liu, Seddon et al, 'Dietary glycemic load and risk of age-related cataract', *American Journal of Clinical Nutrition*, 80(2), 489–95, 2004.

Schulze, Liu, Rimm et al, 'Glycemic index, glycemic load, and dietary fiber intake and incidence of type 2 diabetes in younger and middle-aged women', *American Journal of Clinical Nutrition*, 80(2), 348–56, 2004.

Slyper, Jurva, Pleuss et al, 'Influence of glycemic load on HDL cholesterol in youth', *American Journal of Clinical Nutrition*, 81(2), 376–9, 2005.

Spieth, Harnish, Lenders et al, 'A low-glycemic index diet in the treatment of pediatric obesity', *Archives of Pediatric and Adolescent Medicine*, 154(9), 947–51, 2000.

Standards Australia, 'Glycemic Index of foods', Australian Standard 4694, 2007.

Stevenson, Williams, McComb et al, 'Improved recovery from prolonged exercise following the consumption of low glycemic index carbohydrate meals', *International Journal of Sport Nutrition and Exercise Metabolism*, 15(4), 333–49, 2005.

Thomas, Brotherhood, Brand et al, 'Carbohydrate feeding before exercise: effect of glycemic index', *International Journal of Sports Medicine*, 12(2), 180–6, 1991.

Thomas, Elliott, Baur et al, 'Low glycaemic index or low glycaemic load diets for overweight and obesity', *Cochrane Database of Systematic Reviews*, 18(3), 5105, 2007.

Tsai, Leitzmann, Willett et al, 'Dietary carbohydrates and glycaemic load and the incidence of symptomatic gall stone disease in men', *Gut*, 54(6), 823–8, 2005.

Tsai, Leitzmann, Willett et al, 'Glycemic load, glycemic index, and carbohydrate intake in relation to risk of cholecystectomy in women', *Gastroenterology*, 129(1), 105–12, 2005.

Wolever and Bolognesi, 'Prediction of glucose and insulin responses of normal subjects after consuming mixed meals varying in energy, protein, fat, carbohydrate and glycemic index', *Journal of Nutrition*, 126(11), 2807–12, 1996.

Wolever and Jenkins, 'The use of the glycemic index in predicting the blood glucose response to mixed meals', *American Journal of Clinical Nutrition*, 43(1), 167–72, 1986.

Wolever, Hamad, Chiasson et al, 'Day-to-day consistency in amount and source of carbohydrate associated with improved blood glucose control in type 1 diabetes', *Journal of the American College of Nutrition'*, 18(3), 242–7, 1999.

Wolever, Vorster, Björck et al, 'Determination of the glycaemic index of foods: interlaboratory study', *European Journal of Clinical Nutrition*, 57(3), 475–82, 2003.

Wolever, Yang, Zeng et al, 'Food glycemic index, as given in glycemic index tables, is a significant determinant of glycemic responses elicited by composite breakfast meals', *American Journal of Clinical Nutrition*, 83(6), 1306–12, 2006.

Zhang, Liu, Solomon et al, 'Dietary fiber intake, dietary glycemic load, and the risk for gestational diabetes mellitus', *Diabetes Care*, 29, 2223–2230, 2006.

Thank you

Many people, all experts in their fields, have contributed to the life of this book across many editions. Thank you one and all!

First, we would like to acknowledge those who have contributed to particular chapters in this edition: Alan Barclay; Joanna McMillan (Chapter 4); Anthony Leeds (Chapter 9); Professor Nadir R Farid (Chapter 10); Kate Marsh (Chapter 10); Heather Gilbertson (Chapter 11) and Emma Stevenson (Chapter 12). We are especially indebted to our publishers in Sydney and the United States for their passion, commitment and attention to every detail. We thank Hachette and their committed team.

Our thanks go to Catherine Saxelby, whose wise advice got us off to a flying start back in 1996. We remain eternally grateful to Philippa Sandall, our literary agent, who has contributed to the success of all the books in the series. Thanks to all those who have supported the GI approach and recommended our books, including dietitians and doctors, and especially the Australian Diabetes Council and the Juvenile Diabetes Research Foundation.

Many readers (lay and professional) have given us feedback and played a role in the success of the series, some of whom deserve special mention: Shirley Crossman, Martina Chippendall, Helen O'Connor, Rudi Bartl, Toni Irwin, Michelle Norman, David Jenkins, David Ludwig, Simin Liu, Ted Arnold, Warren Kidson, Bob Moses, Ian Caterson, Stewart Truswell, Gareth Denyer, Fiona Atkinson, Scott Dickinson, Johanna Burani and David Mendosa.

Lastly, we thank our wonderful, long-suffering partners and families, in particular John Miller and Ruth Colagiuri, for all those nights and weekends when we were otherwise occupied.

About the authors

Professor Jennie Brand-Miller is Professor of Human Nutrition in the Human Nutrition Unit at the University of Sydney and a past president of the National Nutrition Society of Australia.

Kaye Foster-Powell is an accredited practising dietitian with more than 20 years' experience in diabetes management. A graduate of the University of Sydney (BSc Master of Nutrition & Dietetics) she has conducted research into the glycemic index of foods and its practical applications. She is a Diabetes Specialist Dietitian with Sydney West Diabetes Service and co-author of the Low GI Diet series.

Stephen Colagiuri is now Professor of Medicine in the new Institute of Obesity, Nutrition and Exercise at the University of Sydney. A Fellow of the Royal Australasian College of Physicians, he has more than one hundred scientific papers to his name, many concerned with the importance of postprandial glycemia and carbohydrates in the diet of people with diabetes. He is a practising endocrinologist and a leading researcher and policy maker who is recognised nationally and internationally.

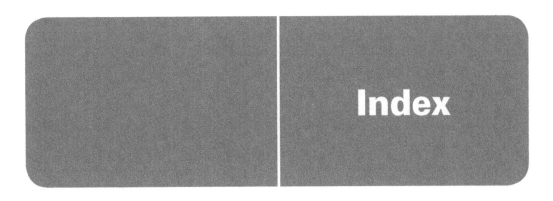

Index

PROFESSOR JENNIE BRAND-MILLER'S
LOW**GI**DIET
Cookbooks

Delicious and healthy GI-friendly recipes from the low-GI eating pioneers.

The Low GI Vegetarian Cookbook

A collection of over eighty delicious and tempting recipes, illustrated with mouth-watering photography including recipes for breakfasts, light lunches and snacks, main courses and desserts and sweet treats including Asian, Indian and Mediterranean style dishes.

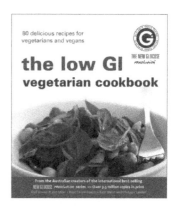

The Low GI Family Cookbook

Whether you have a toddler or a teenager, this cookbook shows you how easy it is to combine the essentials of healthy eating with the proven benefits of low GI carbs and make a real difference to your whole family's long-term health and wellbeing – with over 100 healthy recipes the whole family will love.

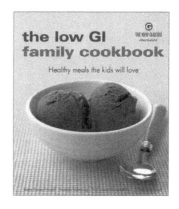

The Low GI Diet Cookbook

Science has proven that low GI, slowly digested carbohydrates are key to healthy and sustained weight loss. *The Low GI Diet Cookbook* brings you over seventy tempting recipes based on these established principles. Packed with beautiful photographs, handy tips, and with a complete breakdown of fat, protein and carb content, calorie values and GI values for every recipe, covering everything from sustaining breakfasts and brunches, substantial but healthy dinner dishes, to quick salads and sweet treats.

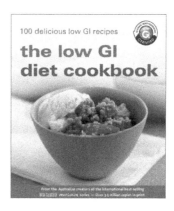

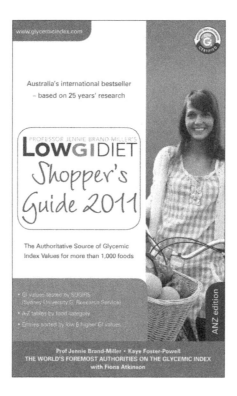

Find all the latest GI values with Australia's #1 low GI shopper's guide.

GI values are the key to lowering the GI of your diet. This guide will help you compare your favourite foods and preferred brands so you can make the substitutions that really matter. In this easy-to-use book we give you:

- **The GI values of over 1,000 foods**
- **A–Z tables by food category**
- **A low or high GI rating for each food**
- **Handy household measures (new for this edition!) and expanded nutrient data for each food – carbohydrate content and glycemic load per serving**
- **A shopping list of low GI essentials**
- **A guide to eating out**
- **Healthy takeaway food options**
- **Ideas for gluten-free eating and living**
- **Sugars and sweeteners section**